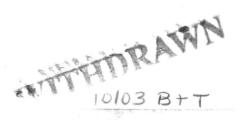

Women Are Not
Small Men

Women Are Not Small Men

Life-Saving Strategies for Preventing and Healing Heart Disease in Women

Nieca Goldberg, M.D.

BALLANTINE BOOKS | NEW YORK

A Ballantine Book
Published by The Ballantine Publishing Group
Copyright © 2002 by Nieca Goldberg, M.D.
Illustrations copyright © 2002 by Colleen A. Daley

All rights reserved under International and Pan-American Copyright Conventions.
Published in the United States by The Ballantine Publishing Group, a division of
Random House, Inc., New York, and simultaneously in Canada by Random House
of Canada Limited, Toronto.

Ballantine is a registered trademark and the Ballantine colophon is a trademark
of Random House, Inc.

www.ballantinebooks.com

Library of Congress Cataloging-in-Publication Data
Goldberg, Nieca.
Women are not small men : life-saving strategies for preventing and healing heart
disease in women / Nieca Goldberg.— 1st ed.
p.   cm.
1. Heart diseases in women—Popular works. I. Title.
RC672 .G59 2002
616.1'2'0082—dc21   2001049943

ISBN 0-345-44098-6

Manufactured in the United States of America

First Edition: February 2002

10 9 8 7 6 5 4 3 2 1

I dedicate this book
to my husband, Robert,
the heart of my life
and the life of my heart.

Contents

Part II: Examining Your Heart   123

Part III: The Women's Healthy Heart Program 199

Part IV: Medical Treatments for Cardiovascular Disease

Acknowledgments

The task of raising awareness and improving the treatment of heart disease in women is a team effort, and I would like to acknowledge the support and encouragement of my family, friends, colleagues, and patients for this book.

I want to thank Nicholas DePasquale, M.D., Gladys George, and the Lenox Hill Hospital Auxiliary for their early recognition of the need for the Women's Heart Program and their continued support for it. I also thank the Jacob and Valeria Langeloth Foundation and Brenda and Ken Carmel for their support for my research on women and heart disease.

Special thanks to my friend Mirabai Holland for collaborating with me to create the Women's Heart Program, always offering a balanced assessment of life, and being there for me. I also thank Mary Ann Mackenzie, R.N., for sharing both the program's successes and the bumps along the road. Mary let me use her office whenever I needed to change location to complete the manuscript, never asking, "When are you going to be finished?"

Thanks to Jane Chesnutt who not only has been a supportive friend but has given voice to the movement for improved awareness of cardiovascular disease in women from her forum at *Woman's Day* magazine.

Thanks to Allison Dunn, P.T., Catherine Green, Hemavathi Umamaheswar, Debra Lauer, Lena Sanders, and all the other women who keep the spirit of the Women's Heart Program alive every day.

Thanks to my other colleagues and friends who contributed their support and expertise to this manuscript: Donna Capolla, Michael Collins, M.D., Neil Copian, M.D., Marguerite Corda, Nancy Craig, Doreen De Vivo, Jane Farhi, M.D., Catherine Flanagan, Ph.D., William Frumkin, M.D., Ellen Gabriel, Barrie Guise, Ph.D., Noelle Langhan, M.D., Sandra Lewis, M.D., Laura Keriakos, Stuart Orsher, M.D., Marlene Mason, Rose Marie Robertson, M.D., Breena Solomon, V. A. Subramanian, M.D., Melissa Weistock, and Julie Wityk.

Thanks to my "family" at the 92nd Street YM-YWHA, Sol Adler, Stacey Eisler, Helaine Geismar-Katz, Cathy Marto, Marissa Scotti, and David Schmeltzer, for "coaching" me through this and many other projects. Thanks to my personal trainer, Rose Tirado, for keeping me strong.

I cannot thank enough Michael Weamer and his staff at the American Heart Association for their help. Special recognition must be given to Alice Austin, Susan Bishop, Mark Hurley, Debra Mason, Tedd Smith, and Cathy Wilkens at the AHA affiliate in New York City and to Carol Bullock, Robyn Landry, Karen Hunter, and Darcy Spitz at the AHA's national center, for their extra efforts in helping me research this book. And for those hours when they were unavailable, I am thankful for the AHA website, www.americanheart.org.

Thanks to Richard A. Stein, M.D., a great teacher who acknowledged that the system is not always fair and encouraged me to make a difference (and for proving that my mentor did not have to be a woman).

Thanks to my parents, Minda and Leonard Goldberg, and to my mother- and father-in-law, Gerald and Leona Shapiro, for supporting me through this book and in all my professional endeavors. Thanks to my sister Cindy and my nieces Ashley and Sarah for being my cheering section.

A very big thanks to my agents, Janis Donnaud and Ling Lucas, for keeping me focused and guiding me through the manuscript process. And to my editor, Leslie Meredith, for her superb editing and her commitment to making sure that the message on women and heart disease is clearly communicated, heartfelt thanks.

PART I

Understanding Your Heart

1

Women's Hearts Are Different

As a woman and a cardiologist, I've written this book to help you improve the health of the most important muscle in your body—your heart. Knowing that heart disease has taken over the lives of 8 million women in the United States, I want to show you how taking care of yourself *today* will help you to have a stronger heart and a healthier life for years to come. You *can* prevent a heart attack from happening to you—even if it runs in your family—by following the Women's Healthy Heart Program that I present in this book. If you've had a heart attack already, this program will show you how to keep it from happening again. I have designed this unique cardiac prevention and treatment program specifically for women.

Until very recently, no book like this could have been written, because all the knowledge, research, and treatments concerning heart disease were based on findings in men. For too many years, the medical establishment was ignorant of women's unique needs and physiology and looked upon women as simply "small men."

But women are *not* small men. It is now understood that our physiology is very different from that of men, especially when it comes to heart disease. Our hearts are proportionately smaller, and when we develop the first signs and symptoms of heart disease, we are usually ten years older than men. Consequently, to be effective, heart disease prevention and treatment programs for women must be different from those for men.

If you're like most women, you probably have a Pap smear every year and, especially if you're over forty, a mammogram every year or two. I'm sure you've heard all the scare stories about breast and cervical cancer, and you know that these two simple tests can reduce your risk for them. But you may not realize that heart ailments disable and kill more women than all cancers combined.

Five years ago I established the Women's Heart Program at Lenox Hill Hospital in New York City to deal with that reality. Now that baby boomer women are entering menopause—the heart disease years—by the millions, I want to spread the word that *heart disease is a woman's greatest health threat.*

I'm not interested only in the condition of your heart; I want to help you become healthier as a whole person: healthier in your mind and entire body as well. That means you need to learn better ways to deal with stress, which takes a toll on your overall health and can set you up for heart disease as well as high blood pressure. As a woman working almost exclusively with female patients for over a decade, I know that we often tend to put off seeing to our own health needs in favor of seeing to the needs of those close to us. In this book, I'll help you figure out some ways you can make time to take care of yourself, which will help you have a stronger heart and a healthier life in general. You'll also learn to recognize unhealthy behaviors and replace them with healthy ones.

Perhaps you've already been diagnosed with heart disease, and you're feeling overwhelmed and frightened. This book is for you too. I'll tell you about the latest research on how to keep your disease under control and even—in some cases of high cholesterol—reverse its course. And if you've already had a heart attack, this book is for you too because following my program step by step can make your heart healthier and reduce your risk of further heart damage.

Sometimes it's hard for women to relate to heart disease unless they're already suffering from it. It's a silent and initially a painless killer, doing its dirty work in secret and over time. Heart disease can start early in life, even before the age of twenty. In its earliest stages, you can't see it or feel it—it has no symptoms.

Sometimes physicians have difficulty conceptualizing coronary artery disease in women too, even though they have been to medical school and seen the life-threatening waxy buildup of cholesterol on the insides of the coronary arteries—the atherosclerosis that lies at the root of heart disease. When I was training during the 1980s, doctors didn't even believe women got heart disease. In fact, when I was a resident, anytime we saw a woman with chest pain, a familiar symptom of heart attack, everyone said, "Oh, this is so unusual!" In my first month of internship, I examined a thirty-eight-year-old woman who worked at the hospital and was suddenly having chest pain. At first no one believed me when I said that she was having a heart attack. Yet she smoked two packs of cigarettes a day, and everyone knew that smoking put men at risk for heart disease. Even though heart disease was right there in front of them, the doctors couldn't see it in a woman!

Doctors now know that heart disease is so deadly for women that their chances of dying from it are one in two. That means basically that either you or your best girlfriend is likely to die of a heart attack, stroke, or related heart problem. By contrast, the odds of getting breast cancer during the course of your life are approximately one in eight, and your chances of dying from it are one in twenty-five.

The younger a woman is, the less likely she is to have symptoms of heart disease. Until the age of fifty-five, men are much more likely than women to develop symptoms. But after menopause a woman's risk goes up sharply. In fact, if you don't take steps to reduce the risk, your chances of having a heart attack after you reach sixty are as great as a man's.

In over a decade's practice helping women patients, I have learned a lot, and now through this book I want to help as many women as I can to recognize the prevalence of heart disease and to teach them how to be proactive in preventing it. I want you to see how improving the health of your heart will improve the health of your entire body. I want you to be able to recognize the signs and symptoms of heart disease and to know what to do if you should become affected. I want to show you how to demand the proper treatments if and when you need them. Above all, I want to keep you from ending up like a patient I will call Teresa.

At forty-seven, Teresa was a successful hospital administrator. She was a single mom and active in her church. Although she smoked, was overweight, and was often short of breath, she believed these habits and discomforts were due to her stressful job. One evening after a delicious restaurant meal, Teresa experienced a burning sensation in the lower part of her chest. The pain became so worrisome that she called her doctor, who assured her that it was just indigestion. "Take some Maalox," he advised. "And Teresa, next time don't eat so much."

The following day Teresa went to work, but the burning never stopped. When she finished work at the end of the day, she paged one of my colleagues, a cardiologist. He recognized from her symptoms that she needed to get to the coronary care unit. There she was given medications. I spoke with Teresa the next morning; her blood tests showed that she had *not* had a heart attack. But it was clear to me that she was at high risk and that anxiety alone was not the cause of her symptoms. In the past few months, she said, four doctors had told her to take a vacation or sign up for a yoga class to relieve her symptoms. I ordered a stress test to evaluate her heart, which, given Teresa's health history, should have been done days or even months earlier. (In a stress test, as the patient walks on a treadmill at a slightly increasing speed and elevation, her heart is monitored and its rhythm is recorded.)

Later that day, while Teresa was on the treadmill for her stress test, she got the burning feeling again, and the test had to be stopped. This is usually an indication that the patient has an obstruction in her coronary arteries, the blood vessels that supply the heart. Yet when I reported my findings to Teresa's doctor, he couldn't believe she had heart disease. "After all, she's a woman," he said to me. But Teresa *did* have heart disease; her stress test as well as other cardiac tests showed that one of the major arteries supplying her heart muscle had a near-total blockage. That was what had made her short of breath, a common symptom of heart disease in women. Teresa's specific heart disease was coronary artery disease, one of the first steps on the road to a heart attack.

Had her doctors been negligent? Maybe not—like many doctors, they simply didn't recognize Teresa's specifically female signs of heart attack. Except for her weight and smoking habit, Teresa had always been relatively healthy. She had never experienced the "classic warning signs" of heart disease; nor had her heart attack appeared to be a classic (that is, male) heart attack.

Women Have Different Symptoms from Men

Teresa didn't experience the "classic" signs and symptoms of heart disease, precisely because she is a woman. The guidelines upon which her doctor relied had been developed from clinical experience only with men. In short, Teresa's doctors treated her as a "small man." And because her heart disease did not conform to the male norm, it wasn't recognized for what it was.

Heart disease has too often been characterized by the stereotypical image of the middle-aged businessman turning red or pale, sweating, and clutching his chest. But for women, the picture is often very different. For women, the symptoms of heart disease or an incipient heart attack may resemble indigestion (as in Teresa's case), or backache, or a vague feeling of malaise. Twelve years ago, during my cardiology fellowship, different women who had had heart attacks told me this same story over and over: "I noticed that I felt breathless even during my usual activities." "Occasionally I'd feel a pressure in my upper abdomen, and there would be numbness in my jaw." "I'd get a strange numbness in my arm."

For other women, heart disease first shows up as unusual fatigue, dizziness, or palpitations. One patient, a relatively young woman in her mid-forties, experienced back pain whenever she walked up the hills in her Bronx neighborhood. Not until she went to a hospital in the middle of having a heart attack did she learn that her back pain had actually been the sign of that impending heart attack.

Because fatigue, shortness of breath, back pain, and the like were not known to be "classic" signs of heart attack, no doctors thought to test or treat these women for heart disease. Even today many women go from doctor to doctor knowing that something is wrong but being told that the problem is "just" their "nerves," fatigue, indigestion, or stress. But these problems *are* female symptoms of heart disease. Attention must be paid!

How did this life-threatening situation come about, and what can women do about it? Above all, we have to educate ourselves about the risks and learn how to protect ourselves and get the best care, if and when we need to see a doctor. This book is my attempt to help you with that education.

Prevention, diagnosis, and treatment of heart disease in women have all lagged behind that in men for a very long time. Until recently, as I mentioned, *all* clinical research on heart disease was based on studies conducted *only* on men: the commonly accepted symptoms, the risk factor evaluations, the types and dosages of medications, the surgical treatments, and the rehabilitation recommendations were *all* based on what was found to be true for men. As a medical student, I was taught that all medical care is based on what was normal for a 165-pound man. This particularly annoyed me, since I am a five-foot-one-and-a-half-inch, hundred-pound woman. How could a drug dosage for someone who weighed sixty-five pounds more than I did be correct for me? How could that drug act the same in my smaller female body? For too long, most researchers have assumed that women's reactions were exactly like those of men, except on a smaller scale.

My firsthand clinical and research experience underscores the important fact that women's heart disease is in fact *very* different from men's. I first became interested in this issue in 1990, when I began my own career as a full-time academic cardiologist at SUNY's Health Science Center in Brooklyn, where I ran the Heart Exercise and Imaging Laboratory. There I could not help but notice that fewer women than men were even referred for stress testing. Perhaps the reason was that stress tests tend to produce a higher rate of false positives for women than for men—that is, they more often indicate the presence of heart disease when none is actually present. As a result, many doctors avoided referring women for stress tests at all, even when it was the best option for helping them diagnose what was wrong. Later, improved techniques for stress-testing women, such as stress echocardiography (the use of ultrasound to visualize the heart during exercise), became available, yet even then women were still greatly underreferred. Today more women are referred for stress-testing than ever before, but they are less likely to be referred for follow-up tests if the results confirm a problem.[1] This is particularly true for minority women, who often have to insist on further testing to uncover the particular form of heart disease they have.

I still remember the day I delivered my first medical grand rounds on heart disease in women at SUNY's Medical Center. Grand rounds is a time-honored form of continuing medical education for physicians: here an invited expert in a field lectures on recent developments in that field, updating his or her fellow doctors. That day I learned that my lecture was the first time—ever—that the topic of women and heart disease had been addressed in that facility at medical grand rounds. Imagine how shocked I was!

This picture has begun to change—in the last five years, more research has started to be done on women. But the word still isn't out widely enough about women's high risk for heart disease. Most women, and many of their doctors, still don't recognize the risk. Even today, eleven years out of my specialized training, I still encounter a lot of women who have had the warning signs of heart attack, yet neither they nor their doctors recognized what was going on.

As I progressed through medical school and training, I became more and more aware that heart disease in women was vastly underdiagnosed and poorly treated. Finally, about seven years ago, I received the wake-up call that made me into a strong advocate in the fight against this silent killer.

The year was 1994, and I was sitting in my office reviewing charts when the phone rang. The caller, an internist and a good friend of mine, was barely audible because she had laryngitis and a sore throat. (Yes, doctors do get sick!) She was slated to speak that evening at a dinner conference for members of the American Medical Women's Association. Would I fill in for her? I eagerly agreed.

The audience consisted of more than fifty women, most of them medical students. Another cardiologist, a gentleman who was my senior, shared the podium with me. He started off the symposium by lecturing on heart attacks, and I followed with a discussion on risk factors and testing for heart disease.

Then came the question-and-answer session. One young woman raised her hand, introduced herself as a third-year medical student, and asked my colleague, "Doctor, do you think it is more difficult to take care of women than men?"

To this day I find his reply startling and yet revealing of how many doctors view women. He said, "Well, women *are* difficult. For some reason, they never seem to get to the point when we're taking their medical history. They never come right out and say they're having chest pain."

I could hardly believe his reply—he had totally missed the point—and was visibly outraged. I stood and was about to interrupt and say, "Women *are* different," when the medical student beat me to the punch. She told him that women don't necessarily have chest pain, which is why they don't "get to the point" of saying it! At that moment I became acutely aware of my life's mission. I had to let women and their doctors know that heart disease is different for women than for men, but just as fatal.

We women have unique needs and a unique physiology. We cannot be treated simply as "small men," particularly when we have heart disease. Traditional medicine is only now "getting to the point" of recognizing that heart disease manifests itself differently in a woman's body, making our typical symptoms "atypical" compared with men's, resulting in misdiagnosis and delayed treatment (see "Warning Signs for Women's Heart Attacks" on page 35). Often women's typical symptoms are misdiagnosed as anxiety-related or an upset stomach, and if a woman is considered anxious or even hypochondriacal, her symptoms may be ignored altogether. When it comes to heart disease, however, ignoring symptoms or misdiagnosing them can be deadly.

Women's hearts are biologically different from men's. Not only are our hearts and arteries proportionately smaller, but heart attacks manifest in us in different ways. For example, women more commonly get symptoms of heart attack about ten years after menopause, indicating that estrogen provides some protection from heart disease. While heart attacks are less frequent in women under fifty, those women who do get them have twice the death rate of men the same age.[2] Perhaps some women patients have coexisting medical conditions, such as high blood pressure, diabetes, or heart failure, that can complicate care. Women with heart attacks are more likely than men to have these chronic conditions, which worsen the prognosis. A stroke may also happen during a heart attack or immediately afterward. Some women have had diabetes for ten years before having a heart attack, making their treatment more difficult.

But many women often do not recognize the warning signs of a heart attack, and they get to the hospital too late or not at all.[3]

In many cases, a heart attack is the tip of the iceberg. It's the most serious and obvious manifestation of coronary artery disease, but as with an iceberg, more than three-quarters of the heart attack's mass is out of sight. For women who have no idea what their blood pressure or cholesterol is, a heart attack may be the first outward sign of coronary artery disease. In fact, it may be the first time they learn that they have high blood pressure and high cholesterol and that these conditions have put them at risk. It may be the first time they are confronted with the sad reality that smoking really did affect their health and put them at risk for heart attack. Though a heart attack is a dramatic event, the stage is gradually built for it over years, maybe even decades, in ways that are largely invisible.

Women's heart attacks also unfold differently, from the first symptoms through the actual heart attack and into recovery. Women's hearts appear to create different pains than men's. Doctors do not know why yet, but our symptoms are more varied: men get chest pain, while women get, for example, upper abdominal or back pain.

Because symptoms are so different from men's, doctors themselves don't always associate them with a heart attack, and many times life-saving treatment is delayed because women are not diagnosed as quickly as men. In addition, many women who suffer a heart attack delay going to the hospital because they are unsure of the symptoms. The problem with waiting to get professional help is that any delay in medical treatment means increased chances of losing heart muscle. The tragic result is that statistics show that women are twice as likely as men to die within the first few weeks following a heart attack.

Women also have different issues when they are recovering from a heart attack or surgery: Who will manage the household? Who will care for aging parents or young children? Some women worry about lost income and returning to work after an illness, while widows may be concerned about how they will pay their medical and medication bills.

Because of these various realities, a woman's program to prevent heart disease must be tailored to fit her individual life. It must take into account that she probably fills many roles, as supportive wife or significant other, as mother or grandmother, often in addition to holding a full-time job. In Chapter 5, I will suggest ways you can put your own health first and still fulfill your other obligations. Many of my patients have done this successfully, and I'll share their stories in hopes that their examples will give you a model for your own self-care—or catalyze other ideas for how you can change your schedule. Gloria Steinem once said, "I have yet to hear a man ask for advice on how to combine marriage and a career," but as women we can benefit from one another's knowledge and experience and share information.

I hope to help you understand your personal risk of heart disease so you can take necessary actions to reduce that risk—and live longer. Among the many things you will learn are:

- The unique symptoms of heart disease in women
- The specific factors that put women at risk, and the steps you can take to control most of them and keep your heart healthy
- How heart disease is diagnosed
- The most effective medications and surgical treatments that can help heal your heart
- How diet, exercise, and mind/body therapies can help you prevent or treat heart disease
- The role of hormones and supplements in healing (and hurting) the heart
- How to recover actively from a heart attack, so it does not happen again

Even with all this information, don't use this book in place of your physician's advice. Rather, use it in addition to your regular medical care.

The Women's Heart Program at Lenox Hill Hospital

When I started the Women's Heart Program at Lenox Hill Hospital in 1996, I wanted to accomplish several things. First, and most obviously, I wanted to establish a program that would focus all its resources on women and their special needs. Too many women, I knew, simply ignored their own health problems because they were so busy taking care of others. I wanted our program to help them recognize their own needs, so now we help women give themselves permission to take care of those needs, and we provide them with a structure and daily plan for doing so.

Second, I wanted a program that both doctors and patients could use as a resource. At the Women's Heart Program, we make use of the latest research for both prevention and rehabilitation of women's heart disease. All our treatments, including medications, are based on the most up-to-date research *in women*, not just in men. We teach patients to make the sorts of lifestyle changes that work best *for women*. Since 1996 the program has helped many hundreds of women. The doctors who refer their patients to us for outpatient heart disease prevention and cardiac rehabilitation now know that we help their patients organize a healthy recovery.

Finally, and perhaps most importantly, I wanted a program that would recognize women as unique individuals. One thing I have discovered is that most women do far better in a program that treats a woman as a whole person, with brains and a life as well as a heart. So our program offers women emotional support and a choice of options to change their lifestyles.

In the Women's Heart Program we treat the whole woman, not just her heart disease. Many women who come into the program have been diagnosed with coronary artery disease: They've had a heart attack, have had bypass surgery, or are on medical treatment for chronic stable angina (a condition in which narrowed coronary arteries cause chest discomfort or shortness of breath on exertion). Yet many other women join the program because they know they are at risk for heart disease and want to do what they can to prevent it.

No matter what a particular woman's reasons for enrolling in the program may be, my first goal is to learn as much as I can about her and to determine where she needs the most help. During the first interview, if she is looking for a prevention program, I explain how she can assess her own risk for heart disease. We discuss her personal risk factors, such as high blood pressure, smoking, physical inactivity, family history, high cholesterol, and diabetes. I also teach her about associated risk factors such as stress and obesity, which she also has to manage in order to keep her heart healthy or improve its health.

If she's already been diagnosed with a heart condition, we review her medical history, including hospitalization, and make sure she understands what puts her at risk for further or worse problems and what she definitely can do to prevent them from developing. We go over the kind of exercise that is best for her at this stage of her healing and the best eating plan. Next, whether she's preventing a heart attack or recovering from one, we formulate a treatment plan that fits her way of life as much as possible. So we take a good look at the whole picture. Is she working? Is she raising children or caring for aging parents? What are her leisure activities? What does she do to take care of herself? How does she relax?

What kinds of emotional and social support does she have? Social interaction has only recently been recognized as a very important factor in recovery from heart disease; I have personally found that degree of social support is directly correlated to a woman's survival from heart disease. By *social support*, I don't necessarily mean a support group. Social support is usually a social network that can include family, co-workers, friends, church members, and even health care professionals. It's important for you to identify all your possible sources of support. I'll have more to say on this topic and on ways you can maximize your own network in Chapter 5.

When I devise a treatment plan, I first work with the patient on identifying and changing the risk factors that she *can* change, such as the way she eats, how much she weighs, and the amount of exercise she gets. As I point out to my patients, a healthy lifestyle does not have to be a burden. But too many women have had the experience of going to the doctor and having him or her rattle off, "Cut down on fat in your diet. Go to the gym. Do this. Do that," without giving them any *specific* instructions.

So instead of shoving a general to-do list at my patients, I see if they actually are ready to change the things that put them at risk. Most women, no matter how sick, are usually *not* ready to change everything all at once. Sometimes a woman is ready to go on a diet; sometimes she's ready to start an exercise program or quit smoking. Sometimes she's so scared or confused, she doesn't know where or how to start. So I work with the individual and identify which risk factor she's most willing to change, and we go from there. That's how you and I are going to work together in this book too.

It's important to focus constantly not on what a patient is doing wrong but on what she's doing right. So I take a complete history of her physical activity. You may consider yourself sedentary, but you may actually be more active than you think. Perhaps you walk your dog every day, or use the stairs at home or at work, or vacuum your house every few days. Maybe you spend your early-morning hours working in your garden, bending and stooping. Every little bit of activity counts toward fitness. I like to find out first what the patient's level is and then start to build on it.

Eventually and gradually I will try to get you to make at least some changes in four basic areas:

1. Add more activity to your life.
2. Begin to eat in a more heart-healthy way.
3. Find ways to reduce the stress in your life.
4. Quit smoking, if you're a smoker.

Again, each woman is different, and her prevention or treatment plan must reflect that individuality. Despite these differences, however, every prevention or treatment plan helps women achieve much more than a healthy heart. For example, the eating plan for your heart's health will also improve the health of your other bodily systems. It may also improve the health (and weight) of everyone else in your household. A weight-bearing exercise program will also help to protect you, no matter what your age, against osteoporosis and some forms of cancer.

There's no magic pill that will prevent or cure heart disease. If you're out of shape or stressed out, it took you a long time to get that way, and it will take you time and effort to become healthier. But it's not beyond you, and it's not even as devastatingly difficult as you might think. The rewards are enormous: you'll have a healthy, vigorous life, and you'll be able to do the things you want to do longer. No matter what your age, you'll feel better, you'll look better, and you'll have more energy.

Your Personal Heart Consultation

My methods for reducing risk, factor by factor, have been proven to work. In the five years that I've directed the Women's Heart Program, we've had many successes. We've learned what works and what doesn't. I will share it all with you in the pages of this book.

This book is the next best thing to meeting with you in person. Woman to woman, I want to educate you about the very real dangers of heart disease. So as your first step, I want you to take the risk factor test ("Assess Your Risk for Heart Attack") and evaluate your own risk factors. If you're already suffering from heart disease, this test will help you see what you need to do to recover as fully as possible and to prevent the disease from recurring.

This self-test will help you begin to evaluate your own risk for heart attack and identify those areas you can work on to improve your heart health.

Assess Your Risk for Heart Attack

Take a few moments to identify your own personal risk factors for heart attack. The following questions are very similar to the ones I ask women who come into my office for an evaluation.

1. How old are you?
- a. 25–35 (1 point)
- b. 36–45 (1 point)
- c. 46–55 (2 points)
- d. 56–65 (3 points)
- e. 66–75 (4 points)

2. Do you have a family history of early coronary artery disease (a mother or sister who was younger than sixty or a father or brother younger than fifty when he or she had a first heart attack or symptoms of a heart attack)?
- a. no (0 points)
- b. yes (2 points)

3. Do you have high blood pressure (blood pressure equal to or higher than 140/90)?
- a. no (0 points)
- b. yes (1 point)
- c. don't know (1 point)

4. Do you have diabetes or elevated blood sugar?
- a. no (0 points)
- b. yes (3 points)

5. Are you physically active?
- a. I accumulate approximately thirty minutes of moderate aerobic activity (walking, going up stairs, vacuuming, dancing, gardening, aerobics, swimming, cycling, spinning, or jogging) almost every day. (0 points)
- b. I exercise only occasionally; I accumulate thirty minutes of aerobic activity one or two days per week. (1 point)
- c. I rarely engage in regular moderate aerobic physical activity. (2 points)
- d. I never engage in moderate physical activity. (3 points)

6. Which of the following best describes your total cholesterol?
- a. less than 200 mg/dL (0 points)

b. 201–239 mg/dL (1 point)

c. greater than 240 mg/dL (2 points)

d. don't know (2 points)

7. Which of the following best describes your HDL (good) cholesterol?

a. less than 45 mg/dL (2 points)

b. 45–49 mg/dL (1 point)

c. 50–59 mg/dL (0 points)

d. greater than 60 mg/dL (-1 point)

e. don't know (1 point)

8. Which of the following best describes your LDL (bad) cholesterol?

a. less than 100 mg/dL (1 point)

b. less than 130 mg/dL (0 points)

c. greater than 160 mg/dL (1 point)

d. don't know (1 point)

9. Which of the following best describes your triglyceride level?

a. 150–199 mg/dL (1 point)

b. 200–250 mg/dL (1 point)

c. greater than 250 mg/dL (2 points)

d. don't know (1 point)

10. Do you smoke?

a. yes (3 points)

b. smoked previously, stopped within the last year (2 points)

c. smoked previously, stopped five years ago (1 point)

d. smoked previously, stopped ten or more years ago (0 points)

e. no (0 points)

11. Are you a postmenopausal woman without a history of heart disease or stroke?

a. Yes, and I am not on hormone replacement therapy. (2 points)

b. Yes, and I am currently on hormone replacement therapy. (1 point)

c. I am not postmenopausal. (I am still having periods regularly.) (0 points)

12. Look at the chart on page 20. Find your height in the row on the left. Read across the row till you come to the column that equals your weight. The box where the row and column cross represents your BMI, or body mass index, which is considered a better indicator of "fatness" than weight alone.

What is your body mass index (BMI)?
    a. 18–22 (0 points)
    b. 22–24 (1 point)
    c. 25–30 (2 points)
    d. 31–35 (3 points)
    e. higher than 35 (4 points)

13. How would you describe the way you handle anger?
    a. I avoid getting to the breaking point. (0 points)
    b. I yell or slam doors. (1 point)
    c. I always hold my anger in. (2 points)

Interpreting your score:

1. 0—Great! You are presently healthy, and following the suggestions in this book should make you even healthier.

2. 1–10—You have a low risk, but it pays to investigate the areas where you amassed points and modify your lifestyle accordingly. You should find Part III particularly helpful.

3. 11–20—You have a moderate risk. This book will help you understand why it's important to begin changing your lifestyle *now*. I suggest paying close attention to Chapter 2.

4. Greater than 20—You have a high risk for heart disease. Though you may feel well now, I suggest that you get a complete physical as soon as possible. In the meantime, reading this book will help you understand more about your heart and how it works, and you'll learn what changes you need to make to begin reducing your risk.

Now that you have some idea of your own risk for heart attack, you're ready to discover the hows and whys of prevention. In the rest of Part I, you'll learn about women's symptoms of heart attack, in-

BODY MASS INDEX TABLE

BMI	19	20	21	22	23	24	25	26	27	28	29	30	31	32	33	34	35
Height (inches)	Body Weight (pounds)																
	Normal Range						Overweight						Obese				
58	91	96	100	105	110	115	119	124	129	134	138	143	148	153	158	162	167
59	94	99	104	109	114	119	124	128	133	138	143	148	153	158	163	168	173
60	97	102	107	112	118	123	128	133	138	143	148	153	158	163	168	174	179
61	100	106	111	116	122	129	132	137	143	148	153	158	164	169	174	180	185
62	104	109	115	120	126	131	136	142	147	153	158	164	169	175	180	186	191
63	107	113	118	124	130	135	141	146	152	158	163	169	175	180	186	191	197
64	110	116	122	128	134	140	145	151	157	163	169	174	180	186	192	197	204
65	114	120	126	132	138	144	150	156	162	168	174	180	186	192	198	204	210
66	118	124	130	136	142	148	155	161	167	173	179	186	192	198	204	210	216
67	121	127	134	140	146	153	159	166	172	178	185	191	198	204	211	217	223
68	125	131	138	144	151	158	164	171	177	184	190	197	203	210	216	223	230
69	128	135	142	149	155	162	169	176	182	189	196	203	209	216	223	230	236
70	132	139	146	153	160	167	174	181	188	195	202	209	216	222	229	236	243
71	136	143	150	157	165	172	179	186	193	200	208	215	222	229	236	243	250
72	140	147	154	162	169	177	184	191	199	206	213	221	228	235	242	250	258
73	144	151	159	166	174	182	189	197	204	212	219	227	235	242	250	257	265
74	148	155	163	171	179	186	194	202	210	218	225	233	241	249	256	264	272
75	152	160	168	176	184	192	200	208	216	224	232	240	248	256	264	272	279
76	156	164	172	180	189	197	205	213	221	230	238	246	254	263	271	279	287

cluding the latest research into hormones, stress, and emotions. In Part II, you'll find a symptom guide to various kinds of heart disease, along with a detailed description of the Women's Healthy Heart Checkup. In Part III you'll find detailed, step-by-step instructions on using the Women's Healthy Heart Program to maintain or improve your own heart health. I'll help you discover which parts of the program are likely to be most beneficial to you. You'll find complete, step-by-step instructions for achieving your goals in all the areas of risk that are relevant to your individual situation.

If you've already had a heart attack or heart surgery, Part IV presents your survival guide, a must-read. Here I'll explain all about recovery from heart disease, medications that may save your life, and cardiac procedures that are on the front lines.

Throughout these pages you'll meet many of my patients who have been through the Women's Heart Program. You'll see exactly how they've changed their own risk factors and successfully recovered from heart disease.

My goal is to help you recognize your personal risk factors for heart disease and motivate you to make the necessary lifestyle changes to keep your heart healthy. Your goal is to change the risk factors *you* can control, so that *you* reduce greatly the chance of having a heart attack.

Now please turn to the next chapter, to learn about the distinctive symptoms of heart disease that we women can have and what to do if you experience any of them.

2

Women's Symptoms of Heart Attack

If you started to have a heart attack, would you know what symptoms it would produce? Or, like many of my patients, would you be familiar only with the symptoms typical of men's heart attacks—severe pain in the chest, a numbness in the left arm, and shortness of breath? As a woman, you *might* have these symptoms, but you also might have very different ones.

Cindy, a fifty-eight-year-old shop owner, had a slight pain in her upper back for more than two weeks. She went to see her internist for a physical, and he noted that her blood pressure was unusually high, yet she still ended up having a heart attack. "Neither my doctor nor I connected the back pain with my heart," she said.

"My daughter was getting married, and I was having a big year-end sale at my boutique. The stress was overwhelming. So when my back began to hurt, I thought I had lifted too much preparing for the sale. I had had some disk problems several years before, so I thought they were flaring up again.

"When I saw my internist, he took my blood pressure and found that it was 150/90. He also noted that my weight was up, and he handed me a pamphlet about a diet that his office typically recommends. He said if I lost twenty-five pounds, my blood pressure would drop and my back pain would resolve. He never mentioned any concern about my heart!"

A week after this doctor visit, however, Cindy realized that the problem was more than a recurring back injury. The pain was relentless, and as she recalled, "I was very dizzy and couldn't catch my breath." After suffering for a few hours, she called 911 and was taken to the coronary care unit of her local hospital, where she was diagnosed as having a heart attack.

Contrast Cindy's story with that of my patient Connie, age fifty-one, who knew she was at high risk for a heart attack. An energetic stockbroker with a fifteen-year history of diabetes, she knew her abdominal pain was unusual when Maalox did not relieve it. Instead of calling 911, however, she took a taxi to the emergency room. When the ER doctor offered her more Maalox, she announced that she was not taking any medicine until someone did an electrocardiogram (ECG), a test that measures the electrical activity of the heart. She knew that her pain could indicate a heart attack and wanted to make sure it was diagnosed and treated quickly.

Connie's ECG showed some abnormalities, but blood tests indicated that she did not have heart muscle damage. She was admitted to the coronary care unit and had a coronary angiogram, a procedure that shows blockages in the arteries. All three coronary arteries proved to be seriously blocked, and Connie was referred to a heart surgeon for coronary artery bypass surgery.

Because Connie knew the atypical warning signs of a woman's heart attack, she saved herself from a delayed diagnosis. But she did make a mistake in hailing a taxi instead of calling 911. If you have any of the risk factors described in Chapter 3 or any of the warning signs listed on page 35, do not second-guess your heart's status. Call your doctor. Call for an emergency vehicle. Go to the emergency room. Don't be like my patient Lydia, age fifty-seven, who, while having signs of a heart attack, straightened up her home before she allowed her husband to call 911, because she wanted to "make sure her house was clean before leaving for a few days, in case relatives stopped by." This delay could have been fatal.

When you get to the hospital and report your symptoms, the hospital personnel may not think, given your atypical symptoms, that a heart attack is possible, so you want to insist, as Connie did, that they check. Trust me, this happens more often than you might think. In fact, one 1996 survey found that 88 percent of primary physicians surveyed thought that women's symptoms of a heart attack were the same as men's. Sometimes you have to be your own advocate.

Many active, vital women are totally unaware that they have any heart problems. Signs and symptoms unique to women, such as Cindy's upper back pain or Connie's abdominal pain, are frequently ignored or written off as pulled muscles, arthritis, or gastrointestinal problems. To show you how pervasive this problem is, the box on this page shows statistics from a recent American Heart Association poll of 1,004 women.

THE PERCEPTION

1. Fewer than 1 in 10 women believes she is at risk for heart disease.
2. Sixty-two percent of women believe that cancer is a woman's greatest health threat.
3. Women between the ages of twenty-five and thirty-four are least likely to identify heart disease as a major health threat—a dangerous attitude that may contribute to unhealthy habits and set the stage for heart disease as they get older.[1,2]

THE REALITY

1. One of every two women will die of heart disease. Currently, eight million women in the United States have heart disease.
2. More than 500,000 women die of heart disease each year.
3. Nearly 250,000 women die of heart attack each year.
4. Heart disease is the leading cause of death in women over the age of thirty-five.
5. Heart disease begins in women under twenty, many years before they have symptoms.[3]

My mission as a cardiologist is to close the gap between perception and reality and increase women's awareness about their very real risk for heart disease. I want *you* to know what puts *you* at risk. Lack of awareness is one of the largest hurdles women have to overcome in order to start their prevention programs and live "heart healthy" their entire lives.

While it took the medical community decades to realize that women—as a group—are at risk for heart disease, the fact that you are reading this book shows that you do not want to be a victim, and that's the first step to successful prevention and treatment. In this chapter, I want to teach you when you should call a doctor when you have an unusual symptom that may be related to your heart, and which symptoms must be treated quickly so as to avoid further danger to your heart.

It's important that you understand *all* of the symptoms that can warn you about coronary artery disease and heart attack. Again, if you receive proper medical treatment early on, you have the best chance for avoiding heart muscle damage and for living a normal, active life.

An awareness that heart attack can happen to you—to any woman—is important to your long-term health. Just as with breast or ovarian cancer, early detection and effective treatment are vital with heart disease, since many of the potential complications can be prevented, including the first heart attack—which is the most important one to prevent. You can protect yourself by understanding how a heart attack manifests itself—the signs and symptoms—and how to seek immediate treatment should this happen to you.

Are Women at Higher Risk for Heart Attack Today?

Some of my patients ask, "Why are women at such risk for heart attack today? Didn't women die of heart attacks in the past?" Women's heart attacks are not new, but only in the last ten years have medical researchers studied heart disease in women. Today physicians know more about how serious a problem heart disease is for women, and they are able to diagnose it—and treat and prevent it—more frequently than in the past. That's part of the reason you hear about it now more often than before.

During the late 1940s to late 1970s, medical data collected on chest pain, called *angina,* in men and women concluded—wrongly— that it was a benign symptom in women. This conclusion was based on the fact that in the study more men than women with chest pain went on to have heart attacks.[4] Today physicians believe that researchers arrived at the inaccurate conclusion that angina was a benign symptom in women because the women in the study were premenopausal. At the time all women who got their periods were thought to have the natural, hormonal protection of estrogen against heart attacks. But as the researchers continued to follow the women into their menopausal and postmenopausal years, their symptoms of heart attacks increased. We now know that the majority of heart attacks in women occur about ten years after menopause.

Angina is a typical symptom of coronary artery disease in men, but *women do not normally get chest pain,* even though the same factors that cause men's coronary artery disease also cause ours. Still, chest pain in women should *not* be ignored. For some, it can be a symptom of underlying heart disease. Angina is caused by decreased circulation of the blood to the heart muscle. This decrease is most often caused by *atherosclerosis,* or the buildup of cholesterol in fat-containing cells in the walls of the blood vessels. Instead of chest pain, women with atherosclerosis usually get angina-equivalent symptoms of coronary artery disease, including shortness of breath, left arm discomfort, and/or lower chest discomfort.

The Anatomy of a Heart Attack

Besides causing angina, atherosclerosis—the narrowing and hardening of the arteries—is also the basic problem that leads to most heart attacks. Atherosclerosis also causes heart and kidney failure and strokes—the most common sources of serious illness and death in America. I've treated women in their twenties who have risk fac-

tors for atherosclerosis and whose blood tests show them to be already developing it. By midlife, almost everyone has some degree of
atherosclerosis.

Atherosclerosis Can Cause Heart Attacks

Atherosclerosis begins when the inner layer of the artery walls, the *endothelium*, becomes damaged. Possible causes of endothelial damage
include elevated cholesterol and triglyceride, high blood pressure,
and smoking.

Cigarette smoking more than doubles a woman's risk for developing heart disease and appears to speed up the development of atherosclerosis greatly, particularly in women under fifty who have been
diagnosed with heart disease. Smoking also raises blood pressure, restricts the amount of oxygen that the blood supplies to the body, and
stimulates the production of blood-clotting factors, resulting in an
increased risk that blood clots will form in the coronary arteries.

In atherosclerosis, some of the cells in the endothelium accumulate fats, cholesterol, cellular waste products, calcium, and other
substances that together are called *plaque*. As these plaque deposits
enlarge, they cause minor injuries or wear and tear on the endothelium. Any such injury causes a reaction in some of the blood cells,
which gradually makes the area of injury larger, causing scarring and
calcium deposits. A large area of plaque, or *atheroma*, is an inflammation in the inner lining of an artery.

Once plaque forms, three different reactions may occur:

1. *The plaque stabilizes and calcifies.* Calcified plaque narrows the
artery. At rest you may not have any symptoms, but when you exert
yourself, you may feel tightness in your chest or shortness of breath.
You may become short of breath, say, after climbing three flights of
stairs, but after you rest, the shortness of breath is relieved. Or you
may notice that while you are vacuuming, you must rest after doing
only one room. One of my patients, a teacher, said she was exhausted just getting ready for work each day—and actually teaching
was becoming almost impossible. This condition is called *stable
angina* (see page 38).

2. *The plaque ruptures, resulting in partial blockage of the blood vessel.* Rupturing the plaque initiates a series of reactions that leads to clot formation and spasm. This process, called *unstable angina* (see page 40), is very serious. The symptoms—*chest tightness* and *shortness of breath*—are more pronounced and might occur at rest or even wake you up from your sleep. With unstable angina, you may be able to walk only a few steps before the symptoms occur. Or the symptoms may come and go for no reason. Unstable angina may be the first warning of a heart attack, but it can be stopped with rapid intervention, hospitalization, and medication. Your doctor will use certain tests to diagnose the location of the obstruction and may recommend procedures to open up the obstruction.

3. *The plaque ruptures with clot formation that totally obstructs the blood vessel.* If the plaque ruptures and a blood clot is formed, it may obstruct the artery so that blood flow is severely reduced or totally obstructed. When the blood supply to the heart is blocked, the heart muscle that the blood supplies with oxygen is damaged. *This is a heart attack.* If treatment is not immediate, life-threatening heart muscle damage or sudden death can result.

Arterial Spasms Can Cause Heart Attacks

In one study of men and women who had had heart attacks, researchers did angiograms (a dye test to evaluate the arterial system discussed in Chapter 16) to study their arteries.[5] They found that fewer of the women's vessels were diseased with plaque deposits than the men's! This finding has led researchers to believe that in addition to clot development, a spasm in the coronary artery may be a key mechanism in women's heart attacks. Spasms may be a particular problem in younger women who don't have atherosclerosis or other risk factors but—inexplicably—get heart attacks.

A spasm causes the artery to narrow, decreasing or stopping blood flow to part of the heart muscle. Researchers are unsure of the causes of spasms; they may occur in normal-looking vessels without large amounts of plaque, but they may also occur in those blocked by atherosclerosis. A severe spasm blocks blood flow to the heart muscle, resulting in a heart attack.

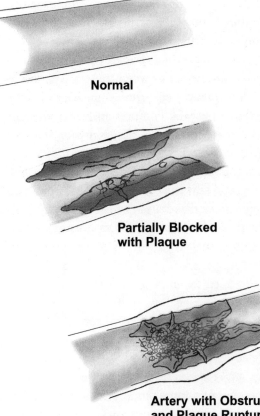

Normal

**Partially Blocked
with Plaque**

**Artery with Obstruction
and Plaque Rupture
(Heart Attack)**

**Figure 2.1
Atherosclerosis Causes Heart Attacks**

After a woman has had a heart attack caused by a spasm, her doctor can put her on a medication called a calcium channel blocker (see Chapter 14) to prevent future ones. Her doctor will also look for her other risk factors and work to reduce them. Because we don't know yet why these spasms happen or what triggers them, we don't know for sure how to prevent them. But following the Woman's Healthy Heart Program (presented in Part III) to prevent a first or second heart attack *will* help.

Studies have shown that women over fifty who have had heart attacks have diseased arteries and other risk factors that are similar to men's, meaning that their arteries are narrowed by plaque lining the walls.[5] Yet a host of comprehensive studies also reveal that *women younger than fifty are twice as likely as men of the same age to die from their heart attack.*[6] The reason may be that younger women are less likely to recognize early the atypical warning signs of heart attack or unstable angina, and they may also be less likely to be accurately diagnosed since they may not have chest pain or a typical electrocardiogram (a measurement of heartbeat changes that indicate an attack). As a result, they may not be given medication that reduces heart muscle damage during a heart attack or that prevents a recurrent attack. Younger women have a more serious time when they have heart attacks. A revealing 1999 study[7] found that upon testing, women under fifty were more likely than men to have more severe abnormalities with their heart attacks. For instance, they more frequently have lower systolic blood pressure levels and higher pulse rates, which signal shock—an additional life-threatening condition.

Heart attacks in young women are more commonly the result of large clots or spasms in their arteries, even though the arteries of these women do not look as bad as those in men or older women.

Your Heart's Plumbing

Heart attacks range greatly in severity. For example, severe heart attacks usually cause heart muscle damage due to an occluded blood vessel to the heart muscle.

To explain how a heart attack affects the function of your heart muscle, I like to use the analogy of household plumbing. Think about the water pipes in your home or apartment. If the main water pipe at the entry of your home were blocked with debris or corrosion, you would have no water in the entire house. But if the obstruction were in the pipe leading to the kitchen sink, you would still have water in your bathroom or basement sinks, even with no water flowing into your kitchen sink.

Now consider how this plumbing analogy relates to your heart. Your heart muscle's main job is to keep blood pumping through your body, while the heart valves work to make sure the blood moves in a forward direction. The blood vessels are like pipes, circulating blood all around your body. If an artery in one part of your heart is blocked, you lose function in that part. For example, if the beginning of the left anterior descending artery (see Figure 2.2) is obstructed, you lose the function of the front portion of your heart. This type of obstruction is quite serious and will severely compromise the pumping action of the heart. An obstruction farther down the vessel, as shown in Figure 2.2, results in less muscle damage.

DETERMINING THE LOCATION OF HEART DAMAGE

Obstruction occurs here	Damage occurs here
left anterior descending artery	➡ the front of the heart
right coronary artery	➡ bottom and back of the heart
left circumflex	➡ the left side of the heart

Because a heart attack can result in damage to the heart muscle, the heart attack you want to prevent is the first one.

Heart Damage Leads to Abnormal Rhythm

Once you've had a heart attack and have damaged your heart muscle, you have an increased risk for heart rhythm problems, such as ventricular tachycardia and ventricular fibrillation (see page 135),

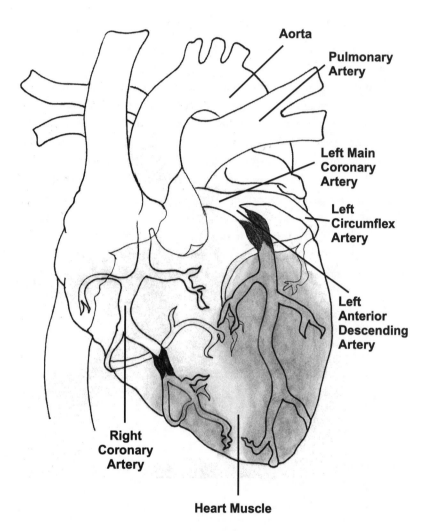

Aorta

Pulmonary Artery

Left Main Coronary Artery

Left Circumflex Artery

Left Anterior Descending Artery

Right Coronary Artery

Heart Muscle

Figure 2.2
Heart Muscle Damage Due to Obstruction

a rapid, irregular heartbeat that is fatal if not treated immediately. Patients who have had a first heart attack and don't immediately start a prevention program, such as the Women's Healthy Heart Program, are at higher risk for a second heart attack. Losing a large portion of your heart muscle places you at risk for heart failure.

The biggest concern in a heart attack is losing heart muscle, because it decreases your ability to pump the blood out of your heart to the rest of your body. As you can imagine, the more muscle you lose from the heart, the less able your heart is to pump. When the heart can't pump normally, blood accumulates greatly in the heart, and pressure rises in the heart chambers and blood vessels. This forces fluid from the blood vessels into the lungs and lung tissue, resulting in a condition called *pulmonary edema*. (*Edema* means fluid accumulation.) The accumulation of fluid in the lungs due to reduced pumping action by the heart is also called *congestive heart failure*.

Sudden Cardiac Death

Unfortunately, death can happen suddenly in coronary artery disease. The most common cause is ventricular fibrillation, the rapid, disordered heart rhythm that essentially stops the heart and its pumping action. Sudden death by definition is death that occurs within one hour of initial symptoms. Usually with ventricular fibrillation, the cardiovascular system collapses rapidly and suddenly.

Because so many deaths occur within the first twelve to twenty-four hours of a heart attack, time is of the essence! Heart attacks have a 50 percent death rate if they happen outside of the hospital. But ventricular fibrillation can be treated if discovered. If you are at home, these rapid rhythms cannot be effectively treated and may lead to sudden death. They can be controlled by medical treatment— once you get to a hospital, the danger of dying from a heart attack is reduced.

Understanding Your Symptoms

Women and their doctors simply have to change their perception of heart attack symptoms. Before reading this book, would you have thought that back pain could be related to a heart attack? By now I hope you realize that many women experience "atypical" symptoms. If you are having a heart attack, you might indeed have chest tightness or discomfort, but *you may not be having chest pain.* Some women, especially elderly women and diabetics, experience *no* symptoms at all and suffer so-called silent heart attacks. They have not even had the atypical symptoms for women of back or abdominal pain, shortness of breath, or dizziness. If you're elderly or diabetic, please get to know your particular risks for heart attack. Diabetic women, for instance, should have an LDL or "bad" cholesterol level (see page 57) of under 100 to help prevent heart attack.

The box below shows the most common symptoms of heart attack in women. If you have these symptoms and they persist for more than a few minutes—or come on when you're asleep or resting—they may indicate you're *having* a heart attack. You may get these symptoms when you're exerting yourself by walking, working, or lifting. But you can also get them while you're resting. They can appear while you're reading a book or sitting on the couch watching TV. Sometimes they occur after a large meal. You may feel symptoms when you are least active, especially at night, and they might awaken you from sleep. The key is that when you're having a heart attack, they don't go away.

If you have any of these symptoms occasionally, and they go away if you stop what you're doing, you may have an underlying condition, like atherosclerosis, that *leads up to* a heart attack. Some women have told me that their first symptoms occurred during ordinary daily activities such as picking up a package in the mail, mopping the floor, or walking upstairs to their bedroom or office, but they went away when they stopped what they were doing. Please pay attention to these symptoms too, because they can lead to a heart attack.

WARNING SIGNS FOR WOMEN'S HEART ATTACKS

The following symptoms are the more common for heart attack in women. Most doctors still refer to them as "atypical," even though for women they are typical. I have worded them in a slightly different way than most doctors do because I want you to know what to look for.

- Unusual fatigue
- New, unusual shortness of breath during everyday activities (or at rest)
- Nausea
- Dizziness
- Lower chest discomfort
- Back pain
- Upper abdominal pressure or discomfort

"CLASSIC" WARNING SIGNS FOR HEART ATTACK

These symptoms apply more often to men than women, but they *can* appear in women.

- Pressure, fullness, squeezing pain in the center of the chest, spreading to the neck, shoulder, or jaw
- Chest discomfort with lightheadedness, fainting, sweating, nausea, or shortness of breath

WHAT YOU MAY FEEL

According to the American Heart Association, almost a third of all women age forty-five to fifty-four have cardiovascular disease—but most don't know it. If you have a new feeling in your chest or stomach and you've never felt it before, then call your doctor or get to the closest emergency room.

Some of the feelings that you might have with a heart attack include pressure or a burning sensation in your lower chest. Or you could have palpitations or shortness of breath. No matter what the symptom or "odd" feeling, you really don't know if it is heart-related until you get it checked out.

"What if I think it's a heart attack, but I'm wrong? I'd be so embarrassed to bother the ER doctor to be told it was just gas or a pulled muscle." Forty-five-year-old Alicia's fear of being wrong is common among many women, and sadly it is especially common among those who overlooked or ignored the feelings of an impending heart attack.

Patients have called me in the middle of the night with "odd" symptoms, when they were actually suffering from acid indigestion, severe heartburn, or palpitations from high anxiety or stress. Others have had severe pain in the ribs, and it turned out to be arthritis of the cartilage or a rib separated by a bad cough. In all these cases, I was glad to be able to congratulate them for being in touch with their bodies and for knowing the "atypical" symptoms of heart attack for women. I was happy *not* to have to diagnose a heart attack.

My greatest concern is that you may fail to connect warning signs like these with your heart. If you experience any of them, get a professional opinion right away. Even if you aren't having a heart attack, *anytime you have unusual signs or symptoms, seek medical help quickly.* If a doctor can start treatment in the early stages of unstable angina or a heart attack, the chances of saving your heart muscle are great. I'm sure you'll agree that it's better to be wrong and alive than to face possible heart damage.

HOW IS HEART ATTACK DIAGNOSED?

The standard diagnosis of heart attack is made by taking a personal health history, doing a comprehensive physical examination, and running blood tests, an electrocardiogram (ECG), and other tests discussed in Chapter 7. In some women, the electrocardiogram may reveal permanent changes in the configuration of the heart's electrical impulses that indicate they have already had a heart attack.

The problem with ECGs, particularly for women under fifty, is that even if they have had a heart attack, the ECG may not indicate the changes typical to the aftermath of a heart attack—the test result may look as if the woman has no heart problems at all. For this reason, giving an accurate account of your symptoms and personal history to your doctor is important—it may be the only way he or she can determine that you have a problem and need treatment. For example, suppose you have symptoms of upper abdominal pain, along with dizziness and nausea. If you tell your doctor that you smoke cigarettes and have a family history of early heart disease, it may give him or her a clear signal that a heart attack is imminent. If it doesn't occur to him or her, I want you to say, "I think I'm having a heart attack."

Coronary Artery Disease and Women

Heart disease can appear in several different forms in your body. Heart attack is perhaps the most dramatic, but another serious form of coronary heart disease is angina, or angina pectoris (Latin for "chest pain"). Angina is a symptom of coronary heart disease in which circulation of the blood to the heart muscle is decreased (see page 26). Ironically, *in women, angina does not always mean chest pain.* While decreased circulation to the heart muscle triggers pain in men, in women it usually produces other symptoms (called *angina-equivalent symptoms*), such as shortness of breath or fatigue on exertion. Again, even though most doctors are taught that these are "atypical" symptoms, for women they are typical!

Just as atherosclerosis is at the root of a heart attack, atherosclerosis also causes angina. Both angina and heart attack are related to reduced blood flow through the coronary arteries. But *angina is different from a heart attack, even though it can lead to a heart attack.* With angina, the blood flow is reduced particularly when your heart is working harder, as when you're exercising or walking up a flight of stairs or running for the bus. Because the blood flow is reduced, your heart is getting less oxygen and fewer nutrients, so as your body tries to get more oxygen to your heart, you get short of breath. For example, Liz can walk six blocks before developing shortness of breath and chest pressure. When she rests, the pressure goes away, and she continues walking. What is going on in Liz's heart is a simple supply-demand problem. The narrowed artery cannot widen to allow the increased blood flow to the heart muscle required by exercise, so it hurts or she gets short of breath. This predictable pattern is referred to as *stable angina*.

Angina is a peculiar phenomenon because it is both a symptom of a condition and a label for a condition. When doctors talk about stable and unstable angina, for instance, they're talking about a heart condition, not chest pain. In *stable angina*, the symptoms are predictable and related to exertion. But *unstable angina* is a very serious condition that may precede a heart attack. It is a life-threatening warning sign that can alert you to take immediate action—and to seek medical help. Let's look more closely at both these conditions.

Stable Angina

WHAT YOU MAY FEEL

"I've had chest pain a few times. But it only lasted for two or three seconds, and when I turned my body to the left, it went away. Is that the same as angina?" Katherine's concern is one I hear from many women. When it comes to your heart's health, you need to know what's normal and what's not, so let me explain.

Just because a pain comes from your chest does not necessarily mean it is angina. If the pain lasts for just a few seconds, or if it goes away when you move or drink something and does not recur, the chances are great that it is not angina. If you have chest discomfort or other "atypical" symptoms for heart attack (listed in the box on page 35) that last longer than a few minutes and do not go away if you rest or change positions, this may signal a heart attack. Especially if these pains are accompanied by other symptoms such as sweating or nausea, you should seek immediate medical treatment and call 911.

With stable angina, at least one of the coronary arteries is narrowed. The narrowed artery allows only enough blood (and oxygen) to supply the heart muscle when it is at rest. With more activity, the heart increases its work level and needs more blood, but the narrowed vessel limits the supply of blood, and angina symptoms develop. When the person is at rest, the need for more blood supply lessens, and the symptoms diminish.

THE "AGITA" OF ANGINA

As with a heart attack, the risk of angina is increased if you have diabetes, obesity, hypertension, high cholesterol, or if you smoke, and if you have a family history of heart disease (all of which we'll discuss in Chapter 3).

If you have coronary artery disease, the following emotions and activities can increase the demand on your heart, because blood flow cannot increase in response to the increasing heart rate and blood pressure:

- Anger
- Emotional upset or "agita"
- Excitement
- Increased walk intensity
- Exertion of arms or upper body
- Uphill walking
- Walking after a heavy meal
- Exercising in cold weather

Some prevention measures include:

- Stop smoking cigarettes.
- Exercise daily.
- Lower your LDL ("bad") cholesterol and raise your HDL ("good") cholesterol.
- Eat a low-saturated-fat diet.
- Get your blood pressure checked regularly.

HOW STABLE ANGINA IS DIAGNOSED

Angina does not damage your heart muscle as a heart attack does, and you can have angina without ever having a heart attack. It can lead to a heart attack, though, and you can also have angina *after* a heart attack, which would indicate that you need angioplasty, a procedure that locates and opens the exact site of a blockage (see page 398). Angina is a serious condition, and its symptoms can be missed or misdiagnosed even by doctors, so it's important to tell your doctor about your symptoms and your suspicion of underlying heart disease. Describe their frequency, duration, and what precipitates them. Let your doctor know that you also have risk factors for heart disease, and be specific in telling him or her what they are (which you'll know after reading Chapter 3).

If your doctor diagnoses angina, he or she will do a physical examination and run tests, such as a resting electrocardiogram (see page 181.) In many women with angina and in women who have symptoms such as shortness of breath or fatigue on exertion, the ECG reading will be normal in the absence of symptoms. Therefore, if your ECG is normal, your doctor may recommend further testing with an exercise electrocardiogram, sometimes called a stress test (see page 187), to evaluate the symptoms under exertion. Your doctor may also recommend an exercise imaging test with thallium or sestimibi (see page 190) or a stress echocardiogram (see page 192).

HOW STABLE ANGINA IS TREATED

For stable angina, I prescribe medications that treat the symptoms and lower cholesterol. These effective drugs decrease the heart rate and blood pressure, reduce the work of your heart, relax and widen the arteries, and reduce further plaque buildup. Lifestyle changes— diet, exercise, and stress management—are also important to treat stable angina symptoms. In some cases, if medication does not work to stop the symptoms, an interventional procedure, such as angioplasty with stenting, or a surgical procedure, such as bypass surgery (both are described in Chapter 16), may be necessary.

Unstable Angina

Unstable angina occurs when angina symptoms become more frequent or longer lasting or occur at rest. This is important to understand because unstable angina means danger and a higher risk of a heart attack.

WHAT YOU MAY FEEL

In unstable angina, you may feel the symptoms more frequently than in stable angina or while you are doing less activity or exerting yourself less. Unstable angina may happen even while you are resting and awaken you, or it may occur when you awaken. These are signs that a stable angina pattern has become unstable and very serious. The symptoms can also occur after a heart attack if you have been diagnosed with coronary artery disease.

WHAT CAUSES UNSTABLE ANGINA?

Even when you have done everything as prescribed to keep your angina stable, unstable angina can arise suddenly for no apparent reason. Researchers have found that plaque may rupture and start a series of reactions, leading to clot formation in unstable angina. This can happen from a small crack or fissure in the wall of the artery, as discussed on page 27. The fissure causes a reaction nearby, resulting in a clot in the artery that blocks the blood flow. The actual event that causes the crack or fissure is not known.

TAKE SYMPTOMS SERIOUSLY

If you have any of the warning signs listed in the box on page 35, or any discomfort that lasts longer than twenty minutes, then I want you to treat this as unstable angina or a heart attack and call 911 to get to an emergency room. You will not know what is going on until you get there and the blood tests and ECGs are done.

Variant Angina

Variant angina is an angina-related condition that is more common in women than in men. While the symptoms are the same as angina, their cause is different. In angina the symptoms are caused by plaque buildup; but with variant angina the symptoms are caused by a spasm of the artery (see page 28). About 25 percent of women with variant angina have a history of migraine headaches or Raynaud's phenomenon, a condition in which sporadic blood vessel spasms interrupt the blood flow to the fingers, toes, ears, and nose. Raynaud's phenomenon is caused by exposure to the cold or strong emotions.

The diagnosis is made by an ECG while symptoms are present. Treatment consists of calcium channel blockers (see Chapter 14).

Other Serious Causes of Chest Pain

Syndrome X

Syndrome X is a heart condition in which chest pain and ECG changes suggest narrowed arteries, yet the angiogram shows no obstuctions. People with Syndrome X also have lipid abnormalities.

Fifty-six-year-old Martha, the wife of one of my medical school professors, had all the classic signs and symptoms of Syndrome X. As an office manager at a law firm, she had a fairly active lifestyle, and she took an aerobics class in a local community center. During her class, when she progressed from the warm-up to the exercise interval, she began to notice chest tightness. The symptoms lessened when she stopped using her arms for the exercise and completely went away when she stopped exercising. Her husband urged her to see me.

When I first met Martha, she was overweight and tended to carry her weight around her middle, which is known to increase the chance of heart disease. She had no family history of coronary artery disease and had never smoked. She was postmenopausal but was not on hormone replacement therapy. She had elevated triglycerides.

I gave Martha a stress test in which she exercised for ten minutes. As soon as she started to develop ECG changes and chest tightness, I stopped the test. The stress test showed an area of a potential blocked artery, so I referred Martha for a coronary angiogram. The results thankfully showed no obstruction in the coronary arteries.

I started Martha on a long-acting nitroglycerin preparation and a calcium channel blocker. Together we reviewed her diet. Like many women, she was a "carb craver," eating mostly pasta, breads, and sweets. I recommended reducing portion sizes and replacing simple carbohydrates with whole-grain products, fresh fruits and vegetables, fish, lentils, and nuts. I'm thrilled to say that eight years later Martha is still healthy and very active.

Syndrome X is much more common in women than men and is

believed to result from an abnormal flexibility of the arteries. The symptoms are similar to those of angina, showing ECG abnormalities on treadmill testing, and abnormalities on a nuclear exercise electrocardiogram or an exercise echocardiogram (see Chapter 7). But the coronary angiogram shows no abnormalities, and the arteries are not obstructed by plaque.

Once Syndrome X is diagnosed, the symptoms are treated with nitroglycerin and calcium channel blockers or beta-blockers. Once treatment is under way, the prognosis is quite good, but you should get a handle on all your risk factors and work to reduce them (see Chapter 3). If you are postmenopausal and are taking hormone replacement therapy (HRT), you may choose to continue taking it, but be aware that HRT has no demonstrable benefit on your heart's health. Please review the information in Chapter 3 carefully. HRT can help prevent osteoporosis and reduce menopausal symptoms, but it cannot prevent heart disease.

Pericarditis

Sometimes recurrent chest pain stems not from a blocked coronary artery but from pericarditis, an inflammation of the sac that surrounds the heart. This condition may develop after open-heart surgery, such as a coronary artery bypass or a valve replacement. It may also arise a few days after a heart attack. In some cases, infection is a possible cause of pericarditis.

With pericarditis, you may feel sharp chest discomfort when you are lying down, and it is relieved when you sit up and lean forward. You'll also feel discomfort when you inhale.

Your doctor will do an echocardiogram to see if there is fluid in the pericardial sac. If pericarditis is diagnosed, the treatment is aspirin or ibuprofen. In more severe cases steroids may be prescribed. Even though the treatment is simple, this problem should never be self-diagnosed.

Pulmonary Embolism

WHAT IS PULMONARY EMBOLISM?

A pulmonary embolism is a blood clot that originates in veins in the legs or pelvis and travels to the lung, where it obstructs blood flow to the lung tissue. The obstruction deprives the lung and other vital organs of oxygen.

WHO IS AT RISK?

Several factors may put women of all ages at risk for a pulmonary embolism. One factor is a genetic predisposition toward blood clotting.[7] This predisposition often goes undetected until acquired conditions help precipitate the blood clots. Some of the factors that can stimulate the blood clots that lead to a pulmonary embolism include:[8]

- Immobilization
- Obesity
- Cigarette smoking
- High blood pressure
- Pregnancy and postpartum
- Oral contraceptives
- Hormone replacement therapy
- Cancer

SIGNS AND SYMPTOMS

Pulmonary embolism is sometimes referred to as a "masquerader" because its symptoms are so similar to those of heart attack or anxiety. And just as the diagnosis for women's heart attacks is often delayed, so too is the diagnosis of pulmonary embolism. The symptoms of a pulmonary embolism include shortness of breath, anxiety (induced by the shortness of breath), rapid heart rate, and chest pain. The chest pain is sharp and often increases in intensity when you take deep breaths. It differs from the chest pain associated with a heart attack, which is an intense pressure that does not change with breathing.

These symptoms often come after the patient has had severe pain and swelling in the legs due to another blood clot called a *deep vein thrombosis*. This blood clot, if it goes untreated, can break apart and travel to the lung. It is often the original source of the pulmonary clot.

THE DOCTOR'S QUESTIONS:
Your doctor will ask you questions like these:

1. Have you had recent surgery or been bedridden?
2. Do you smoke or have high blood pressure?
3. Do you take oral contraceptives?
4. Are you on hormone replacement therapy?
5. Do you have a history of blood clots?
6. Do you have a family history of blood clots?

TESTS YOU MAY NEED
Often the first test that a doctor orders is an ECG, because the symptoms of a pulmonary embolism can mimic those of a heart attack, and the ECG helps to make the diagnosis or rule it out. Other diagnostic tests are a lung scan and a CT scan. These tests will show if the blood clot has traveled to the lung. A sonogram of the leg veins may also be done, to see if the blood clot originated there or in the lung.

YOUR ACTION PLAN
If you have any of the symptoms of pulmonary embolism, you should get emergency medical care because this condition is life-threatening. Once the diagnosis is made, you will be started on an intravenous blood thinner. After a few days, you will be started on warfarin (also called Coumadin, a blood thinner taken orally), and you'll stay on it for three to six months to make sure the clot dissolves.

In some instances, a pulmonary embolism causes shock, in which case clot-busting medications may be prescribed to dissolve the clot. Should you develop a painful, tender, and swollen leg, have it checked out early so you can prevent the clot from becoming dislodged and traveling to the lung. If you have a known history of blood clots, you should avoid oral contraceptives and hormone replacement therapy.

Be Smart! See Your Doctor

If you have any of the symptoms discussed in this chapter, you should talk to your doctor or get to an ER immediately, particularly if you are having them for the first time or if they last for more than a few minutes. If you already know that you have coronary artery disease, and the discomfort lasts longer than usual or comes on more often than usual, you should immediately pick up the telephone and call your doctor or dial 911.

Timing Is Crucial

The optimal time to get medical treatment is within six hours of the first sign of a heart attack. With clot-dissolving medicine or an angioplasty (see page 396), a doctor can open up the clogged artery and save the heart muscle. If you ignore these symptoms, you may be ignoring a heart attack, which can permanently damage your heart.

Do Not Treat Cardiovascular Symptoms Yourself

As a doctor, I know from experience that when chest pains or other symptoms occur, most women are reluctant to dial 911. Many women think they have no risk of a heart attack and suspect the chest pain is the result of severe heartburn. They assume that popping a few antacids or even aspirin will stop it. But antacids and aspirin will not stop a heart attack!

Stop a Heart Attack Before Damage Occurs

Whatever you do, don't ignore your heart. You do not have to be a victim of a heart attack. Using the new clot-busting drugs that are now available, physicians can stop a heart attack even *after* it's begun and *before* it causes serious damage—*if* you get to the hospital promptly. Remember, the warning signs listed on page 35 may be the only ones you ever have! So follow these life-saving rules:

- Don't ignore or deny chest pains or other "atypical" feelings.
- Don't be embarrassed to tell your doctor about what may seem like trivial or meaningless signs or feelings.

Understanding heart disease and its unique manifestations in women is crucial. You may be wondering what you can do right now to prevent heart disease altogether. Keep reading! In the next chapter, I will teach you about your own risks for heart disease—some serious, some not so serious. Then we'll go into the advantages of different prevention methods in the Women's Healthy Heart Program. By the time you finish this book, you will have all the tools necessary to make positive lifestyle changes to ensure your heart's health.

3

Are You at Risk?

"So when will I have a heart attack?" Jennifer said sarcastically, after I'd explained that she had several serious risk factors for heart disease. Then she added, "Isn't heart disease a problem my father should worry about—not a forty-one-year-old woman?"

Let me answer Jennifer's second question first. While it is more common for women to suffer from their first heart attacks about ten years after menopause, the disease process begins much earlier. The stage is set for a woman's heart disease as early as her teenage years. Studies of the blood vessels of adolescent girls who died in car crashes show the early buildup of plaque—the fatty substances, cholesterol, cellular waste products, calcium, and other inflammatory substances that clump in the inner lining of an artery.[1] These girls all had something in common: they all smoked and ate a high-fat, fast-food diet. They also had heart disease. Yet they didn't know it because they didn't feel it. That's why the American Heart Association refers to heart disease in women as a "silent epidemic."

I've treated women between the ages of twenty and ninety, and the younger my patients are, the less likely they are to believe they are at risk. Maybe you're the same way and feel that you're not old enough to have heart disease. Or maybe you believe—mistakenly—that heart disease is a natural part of the aging process. But heart disease is not natural, and it can be prevented.

I've shocked many patients who are under age forty when I've pointed out that they have serious risk factors. Some of these risk factors exert their effects earlier than others, but the longer a woman allows them to continue, the greater the likelihood that she will have heart disease. That's why identifying your risk factors early in life is your first step to staying healthy and preventing heart disease.

Now I'll address Jennifer's first question.

When my patients ask me "if" or "when" they will have a heart attack, I always tell them that I can't predict the hour, minute, or second that it could happen, but I *can* identify the things they do or health conditions they have that put them at risk for heart disease. And when they stop doing these things and improve those health conditions, I explain, they'll lessen the chance that they'll have that first heart attack. So, to some extent, when or if you'll have one is up to you.

Understanding Your Risk Factors

Risk factors are the habits or histories that put a person at greater likelihood of developing a medical condition—in this case, heart disease. Some of these factors may be inherited, such as a family history of heart disease. Others may be the result of a less-than-healthy lifestyle, such as lack of exercise, a high-fat diet, or smoking cigarettes. No matter what they are, risk factors often do their damage in silence. *Even if you don't have any noticeable symptoms of heart disease, if you have any of the risk factors we discuss, you* are *at risk of developing heart disease.*

Early Recognition May Save Your Life

The good news is that if you recognize your risk factors and act to change the ones you can control, you may save your life.

My patient Caroline, at age forty-five, had smoked cigarettes since age seventeen to keep her weight down. A wife and the mother of a ten-year-old daughter, she was also an accountant with a high-stress job. One weekend while hiking she noticed that as she walked up hills, she developed back pain, but when she rested, the pain would disappear.

The next morning Caroline was so fatigued that she could hardly climb the stairs to her office, and her back pain was worse. So she rushed to a nearby hospital emergency room, where she was given an electrocardiogram. This reading revealed the cause of her back pain—she was in the middle of a heart attack. Caroline was shocked; after all, she was female and relatively young, and she subscribed to the prevailing belief that these characteristics kept her safe from heart disease. The first thing she wondered, while lying on the stretcher in the ER, was how could she be having a heart attack. The second was who would pick up her daughter from elementary school.

Caroline was lucky. Once the diagnosis of heart disease was made, her cardiologist referred her for an angiogram, which revealed that a clogged artery was causing the heart attack. After undergoing a procedure to open the artery, she was given medication to lower her cholesterol. Caroline now takes her heart health seriously and has made several changes in her eating and exercise habits to prevent further heart disease. Most significantly, she stopped smoking. If she had stopped smoking twenty years before, her heart attack most likely would not have happened.

Some Risk Factors Are Age-Specific

Every woman's risk and experience with heart disease is different, but some risk factors are age-specific. Taking oral contraceptives, for example, is more common for women under forty. As you age, other risk factors become more common, such as becoming sedentary after the kids go off to school, or entering menopause, which most women do in their forties and fifties. These risk factors add up, and having three risk factors is definitely worse than having one or two. No matter what your age, the more risk factors you address, the more you reduce your risk for heart disease.

I cannot stress enough that the risk for heart disease is not limited solely to our sons, fathers, and grandfathers. It is also about our mothers, daughters, and grandmothers. This disease strikes whole families, but because women are usually the family caregivers, they identify risk factors for heart disease in other family members before they see them in themselves. In my practice, the greatest challenge has been to get women forty years and under to believe they are at risk and to act on those risk factors they can change. For that reason, I developed a system by which women can learn about their risk by age. Not only does this system allow you to personalize your risk, to see how close to home heart disease may be, it also helps you see how and when you can act to alter your risk factors.

Start by finding your age and the corresponding risk factors on the "Age-Specific Risk Factors" chart. Then you can continue reading about these factors in this chapter. I don't want you to feel pressured to know or memorize all the ins and outs of these risk factors and their treatments. But I do want you to be familiar with what may be putting you and your heart at risk. Please pay particular attention to the facts about each of your specific risk factors, and also notice that for each one I've set up an action that I've called "Your Next Step." Then make a plan to take those steps.

You may want to take some notes on what risks apply to you and what you need to discuss further with your doctor. You'll particularly want to discuss the "next steps" that I recommend.

AGE-SPECIFIC RISK FACTORS

Risk Factors	Age		
	30–40	40–50	over 50
Family history	♥	♥	
Smoking	♥	♥	♥
Oral contraceptives	♥	♥	
Polycystic ovary syndrome	♥	♥	

Elevated LDL or "bad" cholesterol	♥	♥	♥
Low HDL or "good" cholesterol	♥	♥	♥
High triglycerides	♥	♥	♥
Diabetes	♥	♥	♥
Perimenopause		♥	
Obesity		♥	♥
Hypertension		♥	♥
Sedentary lifestyle		♥	♥
Age			♥
Surgical Menopause	♥	♥	
Menopause			♥

Common Risk Factors for Women Under Forty

"My mother and her sister both had heart attacks in their late for-ties," thirty-seven-year-old Lauren said. "I'm the oldest daughter, and I worry that I'm next in line for a heart attack. As I get near forty, I just keep hoping it never happens to me."

Even if your family history is a risk factor for heart disease, you can do more than just hope you don't get a heart attack. You can actu-ally predict your own chances of getting one, using the "Age-Specific Risk Factors" chart. Check out the common risk factors for women under forty. Are you smoking? Are you on the pill? Do you eat fatty foods? Do you know if your cholesterol is too high? If you answer yes to any of these questions, your chance of developing heart disease is higher. You may already have it in its early stages. But if you avoid these risk factors, you *reduce* the chance of following in your family's medical footsteps. Control the ones you can. (Please keep in mind that while risk factors such as hypertension and a sedentary lifestyle may be more common in women over forty, if you already are over-weight or hypertensive, you are increasing your risk even as a younger woman.)

If you had a hysterectomy in your thirties or forties, and are on hormone replacement therapy, HRT will not keep you safe from de-veloping heart disease if you have other risk factors, as we'll discuss in Chapter 4. Hysterectomy and surgically induced menopause may actually increase your risk of developing heart disease.

Family History

THE FACTS

Your family history is strongest as a risk factor for heart disease if first-degree relatives like your father, mother, sisters, or brothers were stricken at a young age. If your father or brother was younger than fifty when he had his first symptoms of heart attack or heart surgery and if your mother or sister was younger than sixty, then you have a 25 to 50 percent risk of being in a similar situation when you reach the same age. If your grandparents were also affected early, this factor also increases your risk. If one or more of your parents' siblings had heart disease, the risk is not as great, but it's still reason enough to as-sess your other risk factors, including the new or emerging risk ones discussed on page 35.

Family history is my own major risk factor for heart disease. My father had his first symptoms when he was forty-seven years old and heart surgery at age fifty-two. His mother, my maternal grandmother, also had early symptoms of heart disease.

This genetic predisposition may be due to an inherited abnor-mality in how the body produces cholesterol, such as an overproduc-tion of cholesterol or a low level of protective HDL cholesterol. It may be due to some of the risk factors that we're only just beginning to identify and understand. While you cannot rewrite your family history, you should remember that families often share habits (which doctors call environmental factors), such as diet, smoking, or lack of exercise. You *can* change all of this and by doing so rewrite your medical future.

YOUR NEXT STEP

Talk to your parents and grandparents. Ask them about your family health history. If your father, mother, or both have heart disease, then you need to take action to improve your own health. Bring up these risk factors with your doctor at your next visit, and pinpoint which risk factors need medical attention, such as high blood pressure and cholesterol. Your blood pressure and cholesterol should be checked more than once a year. Keep track of these risk factors. You might even want to invest in a blood pressure monitor that you can use at home. Have your doctor show you how to use it and what to look for. If you do not identify with any of the other common risk factors in the "Age-Specific Risk Factors" chart, be sure to discuss with your doctor whether you might have any of the new or emerging risk factors (page 35).

Smoking

THE FACTS

The most common lifestyle risk factor that I see in young women under forty is cigarette smoking. In fact, the fastest-growing group of smokers in the United States is girls between the ages of twelve and eighteen.

Younger women are more likely to smoke in response to stress and anxiety or to lose weight. But smoking raises blood pressure, causes the arteries to constrict, and increases the likelihood of clots to form and obstruct the arteries. Smokers also have higher levels of LDL ("bad") cholesterol and lower levels of HDL ("good") cholesterol. Most dangerously, *smoking more than triples a woman's chance of having a heart attack.* Secondhand smoke increases a woman's risk of heart disease too. And—still more bad news: women who smoke go through menopause two years earlier than nonsmokers. They also develop premature wrinkles, especially around the mouth.

YOUR NEXT STEP

Stop smoking. I know you've heard it before, and it's easier said than done. Still, the benefits from stopping smoking—whether cigarettes or cigars—are enormous. After two years, your risk of heart disease will be cut in half; after ten years, your risk will be the same as for a nonsmoker. Please check out Chapter 13 for my highly effective smoking cessation program.

Oral Contraceptives

THE FACTS

In the early days of oral contraceptives, heart attack and stroke increased in women who took birth control pills. But the newer low-dose oral contraceptives do not increase your risk. What does increase your risk of heart attack and stroke, however, is to be on oral contraceptives, to be over thirty-five, *and* to have other risk factors, particularly smoking and high blood pressure.

In some women, oral contraceptives cause abnormal levels of lipids (cholesterol and other fats that increase your risk for heart disease). One of my patients, Elaine, brought her daughter Britt in for a consultation. A young woman in her late twenties, Britt had been on birth control pills for several years and had had an abnormal cholesterol test. Her gynecologist gave her a prescription for a cholesterol-lowering medication, explaining that she might need to take it for the rest of her life. When Britt came to me, she had not filled the prescription because she was understandably concerned about going on a medication for so many years. I suggested that she discontinue her oral contraceptive and have a repeat cholesterol test. Three months later Elaine called me to report that Britt's cholesterol test was greatly improved. My patient also announced that she was going to be a grandmother! Both women were thrilled. If you have high total cholesterol and are taking oral contraceptives, talk to your gynecologist about a different method of birth control.

YOUR NEXT STEP

A trip to the gynecologist for oral contraceptives is an opportunity for an evaluation of risk factors for heart disease. But too often this opportunity is missed. Many younger women use their ob/gyn as their primary physician, yet they are rarely counseled on techniques to help them stop smoking or improve their diet and exercise. *Before* you go on oral contraceptives, *especially* if you have a family history

of early heart disease, you should have your blood pressure and cholesterol checked. If you're a smoker, it's best to avoid oral contraceptives and use a different method of birth control until you have quit
smoking. After you start taking oral contraceptives, if your blood
pressure goes up, stop taking them. Use an alternative means of
birth control—one that will not put your heart health at risk.

Oral contraceptives can increase the likelihood of blood clots,
which can obstruct blood flow. Blood clots are more likely to develop in the blood vessels in the legs and the lungs. If you have a
history of these types of blood clots, you should avoid oral contraceptives. If you develop blood clots while on an oral contraceptive,
quit taking it and use a different method of birth control.

Polycystic Ovary Syndrome (PCOS)

THE FACTS

Polycystic ovary syndrome is an endocrine (hormone) disorder that
is often recognized in women of childbearing age who are having
trouble conceiving. PCOS occurs when there is a period of time
without normal ovulation. Women with PCOS do not have the normal cycling of hormones during the menstrual cycle. Women with
PCOS may have similar characteristics including obesity, an apple-
shaped body, excessive or thinning hair growth, acne, and abnormal
menses. PCOS is associated with higher levels of circulating male
hormones, insulin resistance, carbohydrate intolerance (which makes
you prone to gaining weight), low levels of HDL ("good") cholesterol, elevated triglycerides, high levels of LDL ("bad") cholesterol,
obesity, and high blood pressure. As women with PCOS get older,
the presence of these risk factors increases their chances for heart
disease.

YOUR NEXT STEP

If you have been diagnosed with PCOS, your should get a medical
evaluation of all your heart disease risk factors. This includes a check
of your blood pressure, a lipid profile (a blood test for cholesterol,

triglycerides, LDL cholesterol, and HDL cholesterol), and a blood test for glucose (blood sugar).

Women with PCOS may benefit from the dietary guidelines in Chapter 10 as well as regular aerobic exercise.

Abnormal Lipids

THE FACTS

The higher your cholesterol levels, the greater your risk of coronary heart disease. This fact was discovered by the Framingham Heart Study, a federally funded study that has tracked 5,209 adults in Framingham, Massachusetts, since 1948 to find out about the epidemiology of cardiovascular diseases.[2] Likewise, when total cholesterol levels are low (below 200 mg/dL), heart disease is less common.

Cholesterol is a fatlike substance that your body needs in order to function properly. There is "good" and "bad" cholesterol, and too much of the "bad" cholesterol puts you at a higher risk of heart disease. Abnormal lipids (high cholesterol) are "blood fats" and include total cholesterol, LDL cholesterol, HDL cholesterol, VLDL cholesterol, and triglycerides.

Cholesterol is carried around the body on lipoproteins. The cholesterol attached to LDL (low-density lipoprotein) is the "bad" cholesterol. HDL (high-density lipoprotein) is the "good" cholesterol. VLDL (very-low-density lipoprotein) cholesterol is composed of triglycerides, which are broken down by your metabolism into free radicals, products that promote the development of atherosclerosis.

ELEVATED LDL CHOLESTEROL INCREASES RISK

Levels of LDL ("bad") cholesterol in the bloodstream may be increased when the body overproduces it. Elevated LDL levels result in the formation of plaque in the walls of the arteries. The more LDL cholesterol in the bloodstream, the greater the chance it will be oxidized, which leads to plaque rupturing from the artery walls.

SECONDARY CAUSES OF
ELEVATED LDL CHOLESTEROL

- Hypothyroidism
- Diabetes
- Oral contraceptives
- Steroids
- Liver disease
- Chronic kidney failure

If a clot forms at a plaque site and blocks the blood flow to a portion of the heart muscle, the result is a heart attack (see page 27). If a clot blocks the blood flow to part of the brain, the result is a stroke.

So you can see that it's important to prevent plaque formation. Diets high in saturated fat result in too much LDL cholesterol and put you at risk for both heart attack and stroke.

ELEVATED HDL CHOLESTEROL DECREASES RISK
High levels of HDL ("good") cholesterol in the bloodstream help to *protect* you from heart disease; conversely, low levels put you at risk. HDL cholesterol travels away from the arteries and helps remove LDL ("bad") cholesterol, reducing your risk of heart attack. Usually women have higher HDL cholesterol levels than men because in premenopausal women estrogen tends to keep HDL cholesterol higher. After menopause HDL levels may remain the same or decrease. So it's important to know what your HDL and LDL cholesterol levels are and to take steps to keep them in the right proportion.

ELEVATED TRIGLYCERIDES INCREASE RISK
Some new studies confirm that triglycerides (another type of blood fat) are a greater risk factor for heart disease in women than in men—even when the levels are low.[3] Triglycerides are crucial for good health, but when they get too high and HDL cholesterol gets too low, your arteries become unhealthy. Women with elevated triglycerides also often have high total cholesterol, high LDL choles-

terol, and low HDL cholesterol. Even if your blood cholesterol is normal, an elevated triglyceride level sharply increases your risk of heart attack.

YOUR NEXT STEP

I recommend that all women age twenty or older have a *fasting lipoprotein profile*, which measures total cholesterol, LDL cholesterol, HDL cholesterol, and triglycerides. If your profile is normal, then you do not have to recheck it for five years. If it is abnormal, then it needs to be brought down, and the abnormal components need to be further evaluated. If necessary, your doctor will prescribe appropriate steps such as a change in diet, an exercise regimen, or medications.

If you have a family history of abnormal cholesterol, a condition known as *familial hypercholesterolemia*, you should have a profile taken before age twenty. Familial hypercholesterolemia, an inherited disorder, rings up cholesterol levels of 350 and above. It is uncommon, but it can increase a young woman's risk for heart disease. If your family has this condition, be sure to have your children tested for it too. If you are forty or under and have abnormal cholesterol but no family history of abnormal cholesterol, you should be evaluated for other possible causes.

Cholesterol may become elevated during pregnancy, but it is not treated until afterward. It happens as a side effect of the higher levels of progesterone necessary to maintain a normal pregnancy. While this condition usually goes away after delivery, have your doctor do a repeat cholesterol test a few months after the pregnancy is over to make sure it is gone.

Treatment for any elevated cholesterol starts with a diet and exercise program (which I give in Chapters 9 and 10). The medical treatment you get will depend on your particular cholesterol abnormality (as we'll discuss in Chapter 14).

INCREASING HDL CHOLESTEROL

If your HDL ("good") cholesterol is low, you need to change your diet and increase your physical activity to reduce your risk of heart disease. Diet and exercise are the first steps to improving HDL cholesterol. For women who have a combination of elevated triglycerides and low

HDL cholesterol, there are medications that can lower triglycerides. But there are currently no specific medical recommendations to raise HDL cholesterol levels. Estrogen replacement therapy and niacin increase HDL, but before you take either, read the information on hormone replacement therapy in Chapter 4, as well as the material on supplements in Chapter 11, and discuss it with your doctor to make sure these are all right and appropriate for your body.

ELEVATED TRIGLYCERIDES

Because elevated triglycerides may result from diabetes, oral contraceptives, or alcohol excess, your doctor will order a test called a *fasting lipid profile* to check them out. You can effectively lower your triglyceride levels with lifestyle changes, including losing weight, lowering intake of dietary cholesterol and saturated fat, decreasing alcohol intake, and starting a regular exercise program. Some women may need to use medications to reduce their triglyceride levels.

Diabetes

THE FACTS

Diabetes is a serious risk factor for heart disease, and more women than men have it. A condition that keeps the body from regulating blood sugar, "type 1" or juvenile diabetes usually begins early in life, while "type 2" diabetes is directly linked to age, obesity, inactivity, and genetics. Recently in the United States there has been an epidemic of type 2 diabetes in adolescent children, most likely because of obesity, and statistics show that diabetes is on the increase in our country in general. Women with type 1 diabetes have a primary insulin deficiency due to the destruction of insulin-producing cells in the pancreas (autoimmune process), and they must take insulin to maintain their glucose levels in the normal range. In type 2 diabetes, the body does not make enough insulin, but the reason is unknown. In most cases, particularly if the woman is obese, the insulin that is made is not used properly. Changes in the body's metabolism with age, made worse by obesity and inactivity, may contribute to type 2 diabetes.

Women of color have a higher risk of type 2 diabetes, especially

Native American, Latina, and African American women. In fact, African Americans are twice as likely to have diabetes as the general population, and the rate of diagnosed diabetes in the African American community has tripled in the past thirty years. Latinas and Native Americans have a higher risk for diabetes than African American women.

TYPE 2 DIABETES MELLITUS

You are at risk if you:
- are more than 20 percent over desirable body weight
- have a first-degree relative with type 2 diabetes
- are in a high-risk ethnic group (African Americans, Native Americans, Latinas)
- are inactive
- delivered a baby weighing more than nine pounds or had previous gestational diabetes

How is it diagnosed?
- a test called fasting plasma glucose

The problem with diabetes is that it can produce many serious complications, such as kidney damage, atherosclerosis and coronary heart disease, stroke, and peripheral vascular disease (blockage of the arteries to the legs). Peripheral vascular disease can damage the nerves, especially those that supply the legs and feet, and can lead to chronic inflammation, wounds that don't heal, and even gangrene and amputation. Diabetes also makes treatment of a heart attack and heart disease more difficult.

YOUR NEXT STEP
Early detection for diabetes will let you get proper treatment and prevent complications before there are serious problems. The American Diabetic Association encourages all people over age forty-five to have a blood glucose test every three years.

If your doctor says that you are a *borderline* diabetic, you *can* control the complications, including those that lead to heart disease, if you control your weight, exercise regularly, eat a reasonable diet, and take medication, if needed, to control blood glucose. (See Part III for lifestyle measures to help control blood glucose.)

In a recent study in the *New England Journal of Medicine*, researchers calculated that when patients were counseled on how to lose weight, change their diet, and increase their exercise, their risk of diabetes was reduced by 58 percent, compared with those who received only general advice.[4] In chapters 9 and 10, I give you specific advice on how to lose weight through diet and exercise.

Common Risk Factors for Women Forty to Fifty

My patient Jess just turned forty and appears to be the picture of health, but her risk for heart disease is actually unusually high. She is heavyset, has a high-stress job as a trial attorney, and had an early menopause from a hysterectomy in her mid-thirties. Jess has elevated LDL ("bad") cholesterol, high triglycerides, and high blood pressure. Also, her father was diagnosed with heart disease early in life (at age forty-five), which increases Jess's own risk for developing heart disease at midlife.

For most women, menopause is a normal life transition, starting with perimenopause in their forties. Contrary to what you may hear, neither perimenopause nor menopause is a medical condition. They are natural times during which your body undergoes a number of changes in metabolism, hormone production, and the length and frequency of periods, among other things. But during these times you will tend to gain weight more easily if you don't watch what you eat or exercise, so you need to adjust your health habits.

As you read about specific conditions that increase the risk of heart disease in women age forty to fifty, remember also to review the common risk factors for women under forty. Many of these risk factors are common in women of all ages. If a risk factor pertains to you, then make changes now to get in control.

Perimenopause

THE FACTS

Perimenopause is the ten-year transition period before menopause, when estrogen levels first begin their decline. During these years, physiological changes start occurring, and you may have a rise in cholesterol, increased blood pressure, and weight gain—all separate risk factors for heart disease. Having more than one of them increases your risk of heart disease even more. While these risk factors may not cause immediate symptoms, left unchecked they will put you at a higher risk for heart attack after menopause. So it's best to attend to them when they first appear.

THE NEXT STEP

The earlier you start to control these risk factors, the greater protection you will have against heart disease later in life. The Women's Healthy Heart Plan in Part III lays out the steps you need to take: increase your physical exercise; follow the healthy-heart diet plan; and stop smoking. The sooner you address these risk factors for heart disease, the more benefits you will enjoy—for the rest of your life.

Weight Gain and Obesity

THE FACTS

Women who have excess body fat, especially in the waist area, are more likely to develop heart disease and stroke, even if they have no other risk factors. Excess weight increases the work of the heart, raises blood pressure, boosts LDL ("bad") cholesterol and triglyceride levels, and lowers HDL ("good") cholesterol levels. It can also make diabetes more likely to develop.

It isn't the "spare tire" itself that makes apple-shaped bodies at higher risk for heart disease. It's the visceral fat, the deeper layer of adipose tissue (the medical term for fat) that cushions your abdominal organs. Visceral fat is linked to an elevated blood sugar count (glucose), lower levels of HDL cholesterol, and higher levels of LDL cholesterol. The elevated glucose is a result of insulin resistance (which we'll go into in more detail on page 72).

Here's a way to figure out whether you need to do something

about your weight: measure your "fat point." Grab your measuring tape, and follow these steps:

1. Measure your waist just above the navel.
2. Measure your hips at the widest part.
3. Divide your waist measurement by the hip measurement.

For example, if your waist is 30 and your hips are 40, the ratio will be 0.75. A safe waist-to-hip ratio is anything less than 0.8.

YOUR NEXT STEP
If your waist-to-hip ratio is above 0.8, it's important to get it down by losing weight with proper diet, exercise, and even drug treatment if necessary. I have lots of recommendations for helping you manage your weight in Chapters 9 and 10.

Recommended Waist-to-Hip Ratio
Women   less than 0.8

Hypertension

THE FACTS
In women, hypertension (high blood pressure) increases the risk of heart attack and coronary heart disease by about *25 percent*. More than half of all women over age forty-five have it. High blood pressure makes your heart work harder than it should, putting stress on the heart muscle and arteries and setting them up for possible injury. Not only does hypertension increase the pressure inside the left ventricle (the pumping chamber of the heart), but this elevated blood pressure causes your heart to work harder just to pump the same amount of oxygenated blood to your tissues and organs. The heart initially attempts to compensate for the increased pressure by thickening the heart muscle. A thickened heart muscle predisposes you to arrhythmias or irregular heartbeats (see pages 130–137).

So if your blood pressure remains high and goes untreated, your heart enlarges, and the heart muscle is weakened. Upon exertion, you may get short of breath. Often this is an early symptom of heart disease or hypertension. If you get short of breath when you exert yourself, don't ignore it. Make certain your doctor knows about it. If your physician does *not* have your blood pressure recorded in your chart (or if you don't know whether it's there), make an appointment today to be tested for high blood pressure, and make sure the result is in your file.

The effect of hypertension on the arteries is a reduction in elasticity. Healthy arteries are supple so that they can help push blood through the body. When they stiffen up or become less flexible with hypertension, circulatory problems result. High blood pressure is also a trigger for atherosclerosis, the mechanism by which it causes heart attacks and most strokes. It may also cause a hemorrhagic stroke, which results in bleeding in one of the blood vessels to the brain.

THE NEXT STEP

Keep regular tabs on your blood pressure. Your doctor can decide if medications might be needed, but simply making healthy dietary changes and adding regular exercise helps many women to lower their blood pressure. Losing weight, stopping smoking, and de-stressing will improve your heart health too. You'll particularly want to read Chapters 9, 10, and 11, as well as Chapter 14 if medications are needed.

FACTORS ASSOCIATED WITH
HIGH BLOOD PRESSURE IN WOMEN

- Family history (heredity)
- Race (African Americans are at higher risk)
- Age (Blood pressure tends to increase with age. Women seventy-five and older are more likely to develop high blood pressure than men the same age.)
- Salt sensitivity
- Excess weight and obesity

- Heavy alcohol consumption (more than two drinks daily)
- Inactivity
- Medications
- Diabetes
- Kidney disease

Sedentary Lifestyle

THE FACTS

Like many New Yorkers, I'm used to walking everywhere I need to go, and I'm proud to say that I don't have a driver's license. I consider owning a car one of the biggest risk factors for heart disease, as lack of regular, moderate-to-vigorous exercise eventually catches up with you and your heart. Women who participate in regular physical exercise are leaner and have higher levels of beneficial HDL cholesterol and lower blood pressure than women who do not. Other heart benefits are more flexible blood vessels and resistance to plaque formation. Regular physical activity reduces very-low-density lipoprotein (VLDL) levels, which in turn leads to reductions in triglycerides, raises HDL cholesterol, and lowers LDL levels. It can reduce insulin resistance and positively influence endurance. It also reduces your risk for diabetes and obesity, two key risk factors for women.

YOUR NEXT STEP

I recommend that you do moderate aerobic physical activity every day for at least a half hour. Perhaps this is where my Women's Healthy Heart Program differs from other highly touted programs. Many physicians recommend making dietary changes *first* to prevent heart disease, but I disagree. I believe that starting a regular, individualized exercise program, as outlined in Chapter 9, can give you the most benefits, including weight loss, reduced blood pressure, lower cholesterol, and less chance of diabetes—all risk factors for heart disease. These benefits begin virtually immediately, as soon as you start moving around. You don't have to wait for the changes. Once you've gotten regular in your personal exercise practice, some new evidence shows, your muscles will "remember" to burn fat, depending on your level of fitness. With habitual athletes, even the thought of exercise may turn up their "burners" or metabolism. If you're moderately fit, you need at least fifteen minutes of exercise to burn fat; and if you're out of shape, you need thirty minutes.

So I want you to increase the amount of moving around you do, and increase your exercise, by doing something active that you enjoy. Knowing you're doing something to improve the health of your heart will allow you to enjoy it even more.

Common Risk Factors for Women Over Fifty

You may think that the older you get, the greater are your chances for heart disease, but that's simply not necessarily the case—especially if you reduce your risk factors early on. My patient Elizabeth, age fifty-nine, has few risk factors for heart disease, even though she is post-menopausal. A nonsmoker, she has normal blood pressure and high HDL ("good") cholesterol. She has no family history of heart disease and has maintained a normal weight for most of her adult life. She race-walks several miles each day at a neighborhood track. Elizabeth knows that the more risk factors you have, the greater your challenge to stay healthy. She made a commitment early on to make her heart's health a priority as she aged.

Still, aside from the key risk factors of age and menopause, women age fifty-five and up have the greatest risk of heart disease. Be sure to reread all the risk factors discussed in the sections for younger women. They are relevant to older women as well.

Age and Menopause

THE FACTS

Before age sixty, men die of heart attacks at six times the rate that women do. By age seventy, however, the rates are virtually even. After menopause many women gain weight, and as their estrogen levels go down, their blood pressure increases. Studies show that many postmenopausal women have higher levels of triglycerides, overall cholesterol, and LDL ("bad") cholesterol than women before menopause.[5] So you do have to pay attention to these changes in your body to keep yourself and your heart healthy.

YOUR NEXT STEP

If you haven't already done so, now is the time to get serious about checking your cholesterol regularly. The treatment of abnormal cholesterol in women has changed dramatically in the last three years. In the past, women were prescribed hormone replacement for cholesterol abnormalities. Now we know that hormone replacement is *not* always the best option for every woman. In Chapter 4 you'll learn how to weigh the risks and benefits of hormone replacement for your personal health situation. If your triglycerides are up, for instance, hormone replacement may not be for you; you may need to make the lifestyle changes explained in Part III and take a cholesterol-lowering medication. The Women's Healthy Heart Program shows you excellent ways to make the lifestyle changes that are especially important during menopause, when estrogen levels decline.

Once you have the results of your cholesterol test, discuss them with your doctor. The treatment you receive will depend on the nature of the cholesterol abnormality (if any). Is your LDL cholesterol elevated? Do you have low HDL cholesterol? Are your triglycerides 300 or more? As I'll explain in Chapter 14, statins are a very effective medication that can lower LDL cholesterol. Depending on the cholesterol abnormality, your treatment will be a combination of things. Aided by the information in this book, you and your doctor should be able to figure out the best choices for your heart health and your overall health.

Special Considerations for Women of Color

Race

THE FACTS

Heart disease is the greatest health threat to women of color, of *all* racial and ethnic backgrounds. Consider the following differences:

- African American women are 28 percent more likely to die of a heart attack than white women, and 78 percent more likely to die of a stroke.
- From ages thirty-five to seventy-four, the death rate from coronary artery disease for African American women is nearly 69 percent higher than for white women.
- For the forty-five-to-fifty-four group, the death rate from cardiovascular disease for white women is 8.1 percent, while the death rate for African American women is more than tripled, at 25.2 percent.
- African American women have a higher prevalence of diabetes, hypertension, and obesity—all strong risk factors for heart disease.

Risk factors such as high blood pressure, diabetes, and obesity begin at an earlier age in African American women than in Caucasian women, often as early as the mid-thirties. This means an earlier exposure to these risk factors and a predisposition to heart disease.

Heart disease is also a great health threat to Hispanic women. More than 50 percent of Hispanic women are overweight and sedentary, and 17 percent have total blood cholesterol levels that are too high, greater than 240 mg/dL. (To understand what this measurement means, see the chart on pages 176–177.) More than 11 percent of Hispanic women have been diagnosed with diabetes; in fact, the risk of diabetes for Mexican Americans and non-Hispanic blacks is almost twice that for non-Hispanic whites.

While awareness of heart attack risk for African American and Hispanic women is increasing, this awareness needs to be translated into greater action by health care providers and *by each woman of color.* Women patients need to know how sedentary lifestyle, obesity, high blood pressure, and diabetes contribute to their increased heart attack rate and understand how their diet and other health habits affect their hearts.

YOUR NEXT STEP
Review the risk factor chart on pages 51–52 and learn which apply to you. Make sure you have regular physical examinations that include an evaluation of your blood pressure, cholesterol, and blood glucose, since hypertension, obesity, and diabetes are prevalent among women of color and at an earlier age. Act upon the risk factors you can control—and do so well before menopause—using the Women's Healthy Heart Program outlined in Part III. If you're already menopausal, it's not too late to take these steps. Whatever your age, talk to your doctor about any medication you might need to control your high blood pressure or cholesterol, and learn more about effective medicines in Chapter 14.

Emerging Risk Factors

Some women have no apparent risk factors for heart disease and yet still have a heart attack. My patient Louise, age fifty-six, was one such woman. "Active and on the go" is how everyone described her. Louise ran several miles most mornings, went to kick-boxing three times a week, and even worked with a personal trainer. It never occurred to this trim wife and mother that she would be at risk for a heart attack.

Yet one evening at a dinner party, she mentioned to a friend that she had been having a funny feeling in her chest during her morning run for the last month. Luckily for Louise, her friend was a cardiologist, and he referred her for a stress echocardiogram. Her exercise tolerance was good, but her test was markedly abnormal. As she ran on the treadmill, the ultrasound revealed that a large portion of her heart stopped contracting; with rest it went back to normal. Louise needed treatment to open the artery. After the procedure, she returned to her normal aerobic exercise and activities. Her husband asked why this had happened to Louise and not him. "I smoke. I drink. I eat red meat all the time, and Louise does everything right," he said. "How did this happen to her?"

As I explained to Louise and her husband, even in the absence of any obvious risk factors, it's still possible to have heart disease. There are a number of new or what we call emerging risk factors that are not routinely measured and that may be the cause of heart attack even in someone who does everything right. Louise had one such risk factor: an elevated homocysteine measurement.

Emerging risk factors are newly defined risk factors thought to be associated with an increased risk of heart attack and stroke. In many cases, while scientists have identified these new risks, they are not yet certain if treating or reducing them will lower the risk of heart disease. Specifically, in cases where a woman has a family history of early heart disease but none of the traditional risk factors we just discussed, I check out her emerging risk factors to see if they can complete the picture.

Read on to learn more about what homocysteine is, as well as about other emerging risk factors that might affect you. While the jury is still out on how much credence should be placed on these factors, I think it's a good idea to understand why they are now being considered. Depending on your situation, you may want to have your doctor evaluate them for you and, if needed, take precautions.

Homocysteine

THE FACTS

Homocysteine is a product derived from the metabolism of methionine, an essential amino acid predominant in animal protein. Studies show that at high levels homocysteine damages artery walls, which can cause cholesterol to build up and block the vessels.[6] For women who have heart disease but don't have the traditional risk factors or who have family history of early heart disease, homocysteine levels are usually checked nowadays.

YOUR NEXT STEP

In some cases, taking supplements of the B vitamins folate, B6, and B12 may be necessary to lower elevated homocysteine levels. But I believe that, in many cases, homocysteine levels can be managed with diet, including the following foods:

- *Folic acid,* which is abundant in green leafy vegetables, oranges, and fortified cereals
- *Vitamin B6,* found in baked potato with skin, bananas, and fortified cereals
- *Vitamin B12,* found in potatoes, bananas, and fortified cereals

Do not start taking vitamin B supplements without talking to your doctor first.

WHAT INCREASES HOMOCYSTEINE LEVELS?

- Deficiency of B vitamins (folic acid, B6, B12)
- Estrogen deficiency
- Smoking
- Hostility, stress
- Low thyroid hormone levels
- Organ transplant
- Kidney failure

Insulin Resistance Syndrome

THE FACTS

I'm seeing insulin resistance more and more in my patients. Insulin is a hormone released by the pancreas that promotes the storage of calories, increases fat stores, and regulates glucose levels in the blood. The insulin resistance syndrome happens when your body steadily becomes less responsive to the actions of insulin. In the insulin resistance syndrome, blood sugar levels rise despite high levels of insulin, and eventually type 2 diabetes results.

Women who are insulin resistant tend to gain fat in the waistline, around the belly. If you put women with insulin resistance syndrome on a very-low-fat, high-carbohydrate diet, they tend to develop higher blood sugar or diabetes and have elevated cholesterol, higher LDL cholesterol, lower HDL cholesterol, and increased triglycerides, because insulin-resistant people are ineffective at metabolizing carbohydrates.

YOUR NEXT STEP

If you are insulin resistant and also have this triad of symptoms of increased blood sugar, abnormal cholesterol, and obesity—all risk factors for heart disease—talk to your doctor about getting a glucose tolerance test. Then avoid very-low-fat or high-carbohydrate diets, or those with less than 20 percent fat (as I'll explain in Chapter 10), and be sure to get plenty of aerobic exercise. The chart below may give you some clues to your risks for insulin resistance.

CLUES TO THE INSULIN RESISTANCE SYNDROME

- BMI greater than or equal to 30
- More apple than pear shape
- Elevated triglycerides
- HDL less than 50 mg/dL
- Blood pressure greater than or equal to 130/85
- Blood sugar greater than or equal to 110 mg/dL

Lp(a)

THE FACTS

Lp(a) is a problematic lipoprotein with a chemical structure similar to that of LDL ("bad") cholesterol and one of the blood-clotting proteins. Lp(a) levels increase at menopause; estrogen and combined estrogen and progesterone lower Lp(a).[8]

A groundbreaking study identified Lp(a) as an independent risk factor for atherosclerosis in women.[7] Although how increased Lp(a) contributes to disease is not understood, levels of Lp(a) greater than 30 mg/dL are associated with premature coronary heart disease, peripheral vascular disease (plaque buildup in the arteries to the legs), and cerebrovascular disease in women (plaque buildup in the arteries to the brain).

YOUR NEXT STEP
While testing for Lp(a) is not routinely done, your doctor may order a test if you have heart disease with no traditional risk factors or if you have a family history of heart disease and have not been diagnosed with it. While the levels of Lp(a) usually remain steady in individuals, a level higher than 30 mg/dL may increase the risk of heart disease, particularly in younger women who appear to have few risk factors.

There is no specific treatment for Lp(a), although studies have shown that both estrogen and niacin can help to lower levels. But don't run out to buy niacin or start HRT, because *no* studies have shown that lowering Lp(a) with these agents reduces heart disease risk. In my practice, I prescribe statin drugs, which you'll read about in Chapter 14, for women who have elevated LDL and Lp(a). This medication helps reduce some of the risk of heart disease by lowering LDL cholesterol.

C-reactive Protein

THE FACTS
C-reactive protein is a marker of inflammation. During infections levels of C-reactive protein are elevated, and elevated levels have also been found in men and women with heart disease. Elevated C-reactive protein is also predictive of the development of future heart disease. It is elevated in people who have heart disease and heart attacks. Sometimes blood levels of C-reactive protein may be elevated years before a first heart attack or stroke. In one study, elevated levels of C-reactive protein in women actually predicted their risk of heart attack even when LDL ("bad") cholesterol levels were less than 130 mg/dL.[9] This is important because *half of all heart attacks occur in people who don't have elevated cholesterol.*

High cholesterol, cigarette smoking, high blood pressure, and diabetes can also cause inflammation in the blood vessels, which can lead to heart attack. Some researchers speculate that upper respiratory tract infections may boost this inflammatory process. They are investigating the role of antibiotics in stopping the process.

YOUR NEXT STEP
While the most effective medications and duration of treatment for C-reactive protein have not been determined, studies have shown that aspirin and statin medications lower its levels. One study showed that treatment with pravastatin, a cholesterol-lowering medication, reduced levels of C-reactive protein in men and women with heart disease. It's also been found that estrogen replacement actually increases levels of C-reactive protein, although it has not been determined if these elevations are harmful. (This is another reason to consider alternatives to hormone replacement therapy.)

Fibrinogen

THE FACTS
Fibrinogen is a blood-clotting protein whose levels are increased in response to inflammation.[9] Elevated levels of fibrinogen are seen in women and men who have an early family history of heart disease. Fibrinogen levels are also elevated in the presence of elevated LDL ("bad") cholesterol and triglycerides and low levels of HDL ("good") cholesterol, high blood pressure, and in smokers.[10] Elevated levels of fibrinogen may promote the formation of blood clots.

YOUR NEXT STEP
Fibrinogen levels are measured with a blood test. Although not routinely checked, they should be considered in women with early family risk or those women who have heart disease with no obvious risk factors. Fibrinogen levels subside with weight loss and when smokers stop smoking. Postmenopausal estrogen replacement also brings them down.

Control Your Risk Factors

The more risk factors you have, the greater your chance of heart disease. But the sooner you start to control your risk factors, the healthier you will be for the rest of your life.

Once you have identified your risk factors, you can start to reverse or even eliminate them by making small, gradual changes over a period of weeks, using the Women's Healthy Heart Program in Part III. You will become more active each day, as you start an exercise program tailor-made for your lifestyle. Once you begin exercising several days a week, you will review your diet and include heart-healthy foods from the Mediterranean-style diet (see page 259) and foods low on the glycemic index (see page 270). Then, once you are automatically choosing fresh salmon instead of fatty beefsteak for dinner and opting for fresh fruit instead of New York cheesecake, you'll take a personal inventory of the stress in your life and learn some new techniques for relaxing. Lastly, if you need to, you'll stop smoking. My goal is for the program to become an enjoyable part of your daily routine for the rest of your life, as you prevent, reverse, or halt heart disease.

Now as you get ready to take control of your heart's health, let's see what role hormones play in your risk of heart disease.

4

The Hormone Connection

I f you are forty or under, you have some natural immunity against heart disease in your natural estrogen, as long as your other risk factors don't outweigh its benefits. If you're a post-menopausal woman on hormone replacement therapy (HRT), you may feel you're protected too, but research now shows that HRT does not help keep your heart healthy. In fact, in August 2001 the American Heart Association revised its position on HRT and heart disease and announced that:

1. HRT should not be prescribed for women who have already had a heart attack or been diagnosed with a blood vessel disease.
2. HRT should not be prescribed specifically to prevent heart disease in women.
3. Women who were taking HRT before being diagnosed with heart disease should talk to their doctors about whether to continue taking it.

These new guidelines represent a major departure from previously held beliefs that HRT was effective in preventing heart and blood vessel disease.

In this chapter, I want to tell you about the female hormone estrogen and its effect on our hearts at different ages. I'll also give you some guidelines to help you decide with your internist or ob/gyn whether HRT is right for you, and for how long you should take it for menopausal symptoms and osteoporosis prevention.

From the time of the onset of menstruation (menarche), the estrogen that women's bodies produce gives us some natural protection against heart disease. This protection is most easily seen in our cholesterol levels: young women have higher levels of protective HDL cholesterol and lower levels of damaging LDL cholesterol and triglycerides. Estrogen also keeps the LDL cholesterol that exists inside the plaque from becoming excited or oxidized and breaking off to cause a heart attack. As women approach menopause, however, total and LDL cholesterol and triglycerides levels rise, increasing your risk of heart disease. At the same time, levels of HDL cholesterol may remain the same or go down.

Until menopause, women's arteries maintain their flexibility because of this natural hormone protection. The endothelium, the wall of the artery, helps the artery dilate and contract. Some studies show that estrogen widens the blood vessels, reducing the chances that a clot will lodge in a narrowed artery.[1] When estrogen protection is reduced after menopause, these vessels become less flexible, and their function is impaired, which contributes to the increases in blood pressure commonly seen in postmenopausal women. The arteries also become more susceptible to the buildup and breakup of plaque as they lose the protection of estrogen, which appears to act like an antioxidant.

Because of the reduction in estrogen and the resulting cardiovascular changes, women are commonly ten years younger than men when they develop their first signs and symptoms of heart attack, which is about ten years after menopause. While a woman's heart is proportionately smaller than a man's heart, the biggest difference between men and women's hearts is in the timing of the onset of heart disease.

Understanding the Hormone-Heart Connection

Although estrogen helps to keep the cardiovascular system working smoothly, younger women do have heart attacks. Fewer premenopausal women have heart attacks than postmenopausal women, yet they do occur in the presence of normal estrogen levels. Younger women's heart attacks are actually even deadlier than older women's. We physicians and researchers don't always know why younger women have heart attacks, but it's been speculated that their arteries may be less responsive to the estrogen that their bodies produce. It's a particularly disturbing problem, because these younger women may have fewer risk factors for heart disease than many older women, and when their arteries are examined, they show less plaque buildup (as we noted in Chapter 2). Yet even though they may be healthier overall, something triggers a clot or an arterial spasm that leads to the attack.

No matter your age, the best way to prevent heart disease is to practice healthy habits. This includes eating the right kinds of food, getting enough exercise, keeping your weight down, and not smoking. I'll talk more about how to do this in Part III. For now, keep in mind that while treatments for heart disease can include expensive, high-tech medications, the low-tech concept of *prevention* can keep you from developing heart disease in the first place. And if you've already had a heart attack or other indication of heart disease, the Women's Healthy Heart Program will definitely help you heal and prevent additional problems.

Concerns of Childbearing Years

By themselves, the current low-dose oral contraceptives do not increase a woman's risk for heart attack. But if you take them *and* smoke *and* have high blood pressure, they do increase your risk. Any young woman who has a family history of abnormal cholesterol or a personal history of high cholesterol should get her cholesterol checked *before* starting on oral contraceptives.

Recently Merri, age twenty-nine, came to see me because of sudden pain and swelling in her left leg. Merri, a heavy smoker, had been on oral contraceptives since she was eighteen and had recently been diagnosed with hypertension. She was concerned because of the severe pain in her leg and also because her own mother had died at the age of forty-two from a heart attack. Blood clots are a complication of oral contraceptives, so I ordered an ultrasound of Merri's leg, which showed a blood clot in the vein of the left calf. Merri's hypertension and family history indicated that another form of birth control would be a better choice for her, and she quit taking the pill.

Perimenopausal Changes

As the saying goes, thirty-five is when you finally get your head together and your body starts falling apart. New evidence suggests that, to ensure a healthier heart after menopause, women of all ages should focus on their risk factors well before menopause.[2] During perimenopause, which begins about ten years before menopause, physiological changes already start occurring: because of the slow decline of estrogen, blood pressure, weight, and cholesterol may begin to increase. In a recent study published in *Circulation*, researchers found that the presence of elevated levels of LDL ("bad") cholesterol, low HDL ("good") cholesterol, and high blood pressure five years before menopause helped to predict plaque in the carotid arteries, which puts women at risk for a stroke.[3] (The carotid arteries are arteries in the neck that supply blood to the brain. When plaque builds up in these arteries, it increases the risk for stroke.)

Menopause

Just a generation ago, menopause was most commonly referred to as "the change of life" (if it was spoken about at all). The media ignored the topic, for the most part, and even close female friends rarely talked about its onset. Fortunately, attitudes toward this physiological and psychological passage have changed. Still, the new education and openness about menopause have been accompanied by a downside: a preoccupation with menopausal symptoms as a disease, and a tendency to label menopause as a medical condition. Menopause itself does not require medical treatment. It is a process of physical change that goes on for about ten years before you finally have your last period.

AN ONGOING PROCESS

Fifty-four-year-old Marian described menopause as something that happened to her suddenly. In reality, the multisystem transformations in her body had been going on for some time, even if she hadn't noticed them. Menopause occurs naturally at an average age of fifty-one. In some women, it occurs earlier; in others, later. The most noticeable parts of menopause are the skipped periods, hot flashes, night sweats, and vaginal dryness, among many other symptoms, which vary greatly among women. You probably won't even notice the age-related cardiovascular changes—higher blood pressure and hardening of the arteries—that occur simultaneously.

Common Menopausal Changes That Increase Risk for Heart Disease

Increases in:

Weight	Homocysteine
Blood pressure	Glucose intolerance
Total cholesterol	Blood-clotting proteins
LDL ("bad") cholesterol	

HEART DISEASE IS NOT INEVITABLE AT MENOPAUSE

Before you call your gynecologist to order a lifetime supply of estrogen to keep your heart healthy, I need to tell you the whole story: *the loss of estrogen is not a surefire cause of heart disease.* Heart disease is not inevitable at menopause. Despite the hormonal fluctuations, many women who take good care of themselves—mind and body—will likely have healthy hearts. That is why I tell women to *get healthier before menopause* by improving their diet and exercise regimen. When they do, their hearts will stay healthy after menopause. In many women, estrogen loss merely "unmasks" vulnerabilities that previously existed, such as atherosclerosis. While some of these vulnerabilities may be related to genetics or a family tendency, most are caused by smoking, a sedentary lifestyle, and other risk factors.

In short, the cardiovascular vulnerabilities—the problems that often surface during menopause—do not just happen but develop over the course of decades. Heart disease doesn't just spring into existence on the last day of your period, as one of my patients concluded! It takes years and years to develop. That's why prevention is so important. Please start working on the Women's Healthy Heart Program as early as you can to keep heart disease at bay, now and in your later years. As Bette Davis said, "Old age ain't no place for sissies." This program will keep you strong for all sorts of challenges that you'll face.

Remember the studies of young adolescents who died in car crashes and already had early signs of atherosclerosis.[4] Possibly by their early to mid-thirties, if these young women had kept on eating and smoking the way they had been, they would have been heart attacks waiting to happen—even though they were premenopausal.

ESTROGEN LOSS IS JUST ONE RISK FACTOR

The estrogen loss of menopause by itself does not cause heart disease. If it did, we would see major increases in deadly heart disease just as women were entering menopause, but I have seen no evidence of any such trend. Instead, we see the evidence ten years afterward, which indicates that something else is going on. Estrogen loss is just one factor that interacts with many others.

Hormone Replacement Therapy

For years, gynecologists gave their patients prescriptions for post-menopausal hormone replacement therapy, presenting it as "one-stop shopping"—a single solution that cured menopausal symptoms and at the same time prevented osteoporosis and heart disease. Today, the benefits of HRT for the heart are in dispute. In fact, the research to date shows us that *HRT may not be good for all women.*

About three years ago while I was attending a national scientific meeting, I read the AHA meeting catalog of research papers and found that one of the papers to be presented that afternoon was on research comparing the role of soy and estrogen on blood-vessel flexibility in females. I very much wanted to be at the presentation because a number of women I treat use soy to relieve menopausal symptoms, believing that it also helps their heart, even without much research to back up the heart benefits. I rushed to the room where the paper was being delivered and literally got the last seat. Obviously, a lot of my colleagues were interested in the same information. But as soon as the speaker was introduced, I could tell I wasn't going to be able to help my patients with the information, because the researcher was a veterinarian and she was presenting a paper on female monkeys, not women. It hit home to me then that just as HRT is not best for all women, not all research studies give results that are relevant for all females. Some research is news that you just can't use. So please keep that in mind as you go read about studies in the next pages and as you hear of future studies that are published.

Estrogen Therapy

From the early 1940s until around 1985, doctors gave women estrogen replacement at menopause to compensate for their natural decline of this hormone. From this therapy, however, women developed an increased risk of uterine cancer. To try to prevent this risk in women who have not had hysterectomies, progestin, a form of the other female hormone, progesterone, is now added to estrogen replacement therapy. This combination medication is known as *hormone replacement therapy*, or HRT. The added progestin, an *estrogen antagonist*, negates not only the risk of uterine cancer but also some of the beneficial effects of estrogen on the heart. The big concern with HRT is that for some women it may increase their risk of developing breast cancer. Although not conclusive, studies suggest that the incidence of lobular breast cancer is increasing nationwide and that the use of postmenopausal HRT may be contributing to this increase.[5] And women who have their uterus intact still have the increased risk of uterine cancer with HRT.

For many women, bothersome side effects of HRT, such as post-menopausal bleeding, bloating, and weight gain, are unacceptable. HRT may also cause an increase in C-reactive protein, one of the new, emerging risk factors for heart and blood vessel disease (discussed in Chapter 3). The increases in C-reactive protein seen in women on HRT may result not from inflammation but rather because estrogen stimulates the liver to increase production of C-reactive protein. We still do not know the significance of this elevated C-reactive protein in women on HRT, but ask your doctor to test you for it, and if you have it after taking HRT, you may want to consider discontinuing the therapy and finding an alternative.

The Role of Progesterone

During the childbearing years, progesterone works together with estrogen to maintain normal sexual and reproductive function. While estrogen promotes cell growth (preparing the lining of the uterus, for example, to receive an implanted embryo), progesterone stops that growth, which eventually results in a menstrual period. Progesterone is also the hormone that helps to maintain a normal pregnancy.

Your body curtails production of both estrogen and progesterone at menopause, yet estrogen never disappears completely from your system; your ovaries, adrenal glands, and fatty tissues continue to manufacture small amounts of other hormones that your body converts to forms of estrogen.

When progesterone is added to estrogen replacement therapy in HRT, it helps to prevent uterine cancer. But progesterone alone can raise your total cholesterol and LDL ("bad") cholesterol—two numbers you want to *reduce*, not increase. You should not take progesterone alone, without estrogen. Scientific findings show that in heart disease prevention there is no role for progesterone (natural or not) alone, and that includes progesterone creams. Taking estrogen alone raises triglycerides (a possible risk factor for heart disease), and yet when progesterone is taken with estrogen, the combination appears to prevent the rise. That's the upside of estrogen-progesterone therapy. The downside is that progesterone opposes some of estrogen's positive effects on blood-vessel flexibility and cholesterol and may also increase your risk of breast cancer.

Should You Take HRT?

Let me share with you some of the latest information on HRT, so you can make an informed decision with your own doctor for your individual needs.

Doctors used to think that HRT replaced estrogen in a way that reduced the risk of heart attacks in some women. Estrogen may actually give your heart some protection by keeping cholesterol in normal ranges and blood vessels healthy, and studies show that estrogen or HRT lowers cholesterol by 12 to 20 percent.[6] Cholesterol-lowering medications (statins) also reduce cholesterol by 25 to 35 percent, and for cholesterol reduction they (not HRT) are now the preferred treatment. Yet keeping your cholesterol low is not the only thing you need to do to prevent a heart attack or heart disease. A recent study published in the *Annals of Internal Medicine* showed that some women on HRT who had been tracked by another study went on to have heart attacks.[7] The affected women appeared to be those who had been on the HRT for less than one year. This is why the American Heart Association no longer recommends HRT as a medication for preventing heart disease.

Benefits of Natural Estrogen	Potential Problems of Estrogen Therapy
Reduces LDL ("bad") cholesterol	Increases triglycerides
Acts as an antioxidant	Increases C-reactive proteins

Improves blood vessel flexibility	Increases risk of blood clots in veins
Lowers Lp(a)	Possible increased risk of breast cancer
Reduces levels of blood-clotting proteins	

Deciding whether to go on HRT is not easy, primarily because of the side effects and risks. What is clear is that you should *not* take it to reduce your risk of developing heart disease.

I realize that's not much help, especially if you are approaching menopause or have experienced it. Although I can't give one general answer for everyone regarding HRT, I'll provide some questions later in this chapter to help you and your doctor decide whether HRT is right for you (see "Risk/Benefit Evaluation for Taking HRT"). Review these questions before making your decision, and consider the current scientific data, being aware that it may change, depending on the latest studies.

Three Major Studies

Two early studies of HRT and heart disease in women led doctors to believe that HRT is beneficial for prevention.

THE NURSES' HEALTH STUDY

The best-known recent study relevant to heart disease is the Nurses' Health Study, an observational study that followed 121,700 nurses, ages thirty to fifty-five, from 1976 to 1994. Their lifestyle practices and health problems were tracked by means of a questionnaire mailed biennially, and for each of the 3,637 who died during the study period,[8] the cause of death was noted.

The Nurses' Health Study revealed a 40 percent *reduction in heart disease risk* in women who took HRT. Yet the hormones failed to reduce the risk of stroke. In fact, *the risk of stroke increased 30 percent in women on hormones. And some women who were on HRT for less than one year had an increased risk of heart attack.*[9] This same study also showed that women who took estrogen for five or more years had a 30 to 50 percent elevation in breast cancer risk; those who used it for ten or more years had a 40 percent risk. The women with the highest risk were those over sixty-five, which is also the age when women most at risk for coronary heart disease begin to have symptoms.[10] Although this study's results were mixed, it and the next study formed the basis of the recommendation that HRT be used for heart attack and heart disease prevention.

THE PEPI TRIAL

While not as large as the Nurses' Health Study, the Postmenopausal Estrogen Progestin Intervention (PEPI) trial evaluated 323 women on the effect of HRT on heart disease risk factors, such as cholesterol and blood pressure. In the study, women were separated according to the different hormone preparations and a placebo. Researchers showed that all hormone groups were better than placebo in reducing cholesterol.[11] They also found that in women with a uterus on estrogen alone, the stimulation of the uterine lining was increased, which may predispose women to uterine cancer, and uterine bleeding increased.[12]

While the PEPI trial was not designed to answer the question of whether HRT increases breast cancer or heart disease risk, researchers did conclude that all estrogen-progestin combinations were significantly better than placebo in reducing the risk factor of high cholesterol. But it was a third study, the HERS trial, that awakened the medical community to the dangers of HRT for women who already have heart disease.

THE HERS TRIAL

Published in the *Journal of the American Medical Association* in August 1998, the HERS trial (Heart and Estrogen/Progestin Replacement Study) gave women who already had heart disease HRT of different kinds or a placebo for four years. It was the first large clinical trial to examine the effect of HRT on women with heart disease, studying 2,763 postmenopausal women. The results were surprising. The researchers expected to find that HRT reduced further heart disease. Instead, *they found no dramatic benefit at all from HRT for women who already had heart disease.*[13] More specifically, *the women on*

HRT in the first year of the study actually had a higher rate of recurrent heart attack and death than women who were taking the placebo. Over the three remaining years of the study, no statistical benefit was noted in those on the medication. Furthermore, the women who did take HRT had a slightly higher occurrence of gallstones and blood clots in their veins.

I want to point out that these studies looked at very different groups of women, so their findings are different. The Nurses' Health Study participants were healthy when the study began. In addition, they were predominantly Caucasian, educated, and knowledgeable about health, and they followed heart-healthy lifestyles. As health care professionals, they were more likely to follow up with their annual gynecological checkups and regular mammograms, which are vital for all women on HRT or estrogen. The women in the HERS study were older and already had diagnosed heart disease and the identified risk factors. The difference in the findings shows that you cannot assume that HRT will be effective in preventing heart attack.

Frequently Asked Questions

It's partly because of these different findings that I wanted to write this book, so that you would have your own prevention plan to follow should HRT *not* be right for you. Here are some of the most commonly asked questions that I get about HRT, along with my brief responses:

Q. Is it safe to take estrogen or HRT for menopausal symptoms?
A. *Yes. From what the research indicates, HRT is safe for treating menopausal symptoms. But it does have side effects.*
Q. How long should I take HRT to prevent osteoporosis?
A. *You have to take HRT or an alternative for the rest of your life to maintain the protection.*
Q. Does HRT increase my risk for breast cancer?
A. *Research suggests that there is an increased risk with long-term therapy, and that this risk increases after five years.*
Q. If I've had a heart attack, should I take HRT?

A. *If you were recently diagnosed with heart disease, you should not initiate HRT therapy.*

Q. Can I keep taking HRT if I've had angioplasty or bypass surgery and took HRT before the procedure?

A. *Here is where the problem lies, as there is no set answer. If you took HRT for years and then were diagnosed with heart disease, you may not have to discontinue it. Keep in mind that the HRT did not prevent you from having heart surgery or angioplasty.*

Estrogen Is a Bone Booster

In making your decision, you need to know that HRT may be helpful for menopause-related symptoms such as vaginal dryness and hot flashes. Replacement estrogen is also a bone booster. Without estrogen, osteocytes, the cells necessary for keeping bones strong, die off. In fact, bone loss in women starts to occur between age thirty and forty, even while a good amount of estrogen is still naturally working in your body. During this time, the removal of bone begins to equal the building of bone. After a woman reaches forty, the total amount of bone becomes less. Then over a period of several years, bone loss continues at a much faster pace than bone building. As all this happens, there are usually no signs or symptoms to alert you to the possibility of osteoporosis.

Around ages forty-five to fifty-five, bone loss increases, coinciding with the period when estrogen levels decline. You may lose bone faster or slower than other women, depending on the following factors:

- Calcium intake
- Family history
- Activity level
- Medications
- Lifestyle habits, such as smoking or drinking alcohol (which speed bone loss)
- Time of menopause
- Estrogen replacement therapy after menopause

After menopause, if estrogen is not replaced, your bones may continue to decrease in density until they become thin enough to break or fracture. Left untreated, fractures may continue, with often a great deal of resulting pain and disability. Deformities in the spine and other areas may also become much more obvious. HRT slows bone loss. If you stop taking the HRT, the protection against osteoporosis stops as well.

If you do not opt to take HRT, however, you do have other options to maintain bone density. For strong bones and a healthy body, the National Institutes of Health recommend that postmenopausal women ingest 1,500 mg of calcium per day; premenopausal women should ingest 1,000 mg daily. Calcium is not only necessary for strong bones as women age, but it may also help to keep blood pressure low and play a role in preventing colon cancer. (You can easily boost bone strength the natural way, by eating low-fat dairy products, calcium-enriched foods, and calcium-containing vegetables such as artichokes, broccoli, brussels sprouts, cabbage, carrots, snap beans, spinach, and Swiss chard.)

If your diet is not high in calcium, use calcium supplements or add more soy products (which also contain calcium) to your diet. Also be sure to do weight-bearing exercises such as walking, running, or aerobics to boost your bones' health. If you do have osteoporosis, ask your doctor if you should take a medication, such as Fosamax, that can actually build bone strength.

Making Your Decision

Even the best doctors who pore over all the studies are unsure about the long-term outcome of HRT or estrogen therapy. And even though some of this information sounds hopeful, the *studies to date have not proven that HRT prevents heart disease in all women*. In fact, it's believed that the progestin can have different effects on cholesterol, depending on which type you take. Also, research indicates that estrogen patches do not have same lipid-lowering effect as estrogen taken orally.

My personal conclusion is that if you are a healthy woman and need help reducing menopausal symptoms, hormones may be beneficial in the immediate short term. *I would recommend you use them for only up to five years, no longer.* Over the long term, findings on HRT suggest an increased risk of breast cancer. And if you have had a heart attack, HRT raises the risk of a recurrence. *For now, HRT is not a guarantee against heart disease.*

As you consider whether to use HRT for menopausal symptoms and to prevent osteoporosis, please also take into account your risk of getting breast cancer and blood clots. If, after reviewing the risks and benefits, and the types of hormone replacement, you decide to take HRT, be sure to get yearly mammograms and make the other lifestyle changes in Part III for heart disease prevention. If your cholesterol is not controlled, you may need to consider anticholesterol medication, along with the HRT.

If you choose not to take HRT, you need to follow a healthy lifestyle to keep your heart healthy: eat right, get regular aerobic exercise, and stop smoking. These better lifestyle habits, combined with anticholesterol medications if needed, and good control of blood pressure, can give you a heart benefit without increasing your risk of certain cancers or blood clots.

Look again at the risk factors chart on pages 51–52, then talk with your doctor, and let the decision you make together be one that you can live with without regrets or fears.

Alternatives to HRT

Keep in mind that HRT is one choice. You do have other options. Here is an alternative that you might consider.

Selective Estrogen Receptor Modulators (SERMs)

Raloxifene (Evista) is a selective estrogen receptor modulator (SERM) used to build bones for those who have osteoporosis. This medication, called an *anti-estrogen*, was developed to block the effect of estrogens in breast cancer.

SERMs do not increase the risk of breast cancer or cause uterine bleeding, breast tenderness, and irregular menstrual periods, as estrogen treatment can. (Irregular menstrual bleeding is a big reason why many women don't stay on estrogen treatment.) Raloxifene can provide the benefits of estrogen replacement treatment for the bones without the annoying side effects. One beneficial side effect is that it may help lower blood cholesterol.

Still, raloxifene does have its own annoying side effects, as my patient, Maria, experienced. Maria, age sixty-nine, recently started raloxifene after having some side effects from HRT, including bloating and breast tenderness. A healthy woman who has never had a heart attack, Maria takes medication to control her otherwise high blood pressure and exercises on her treadmill regularly. When Maria stopped the HRT, her gynecologist prescribed raloxifene. Yet when she started the medication, she got leg cramps and began to notice spider veins on her skin. Her doctor recommended that she consult with me about the leg pain, because he did not feel it was related to the medication.

I examined Maria and carefully listened to her medical history. I did think the symptoms might have been caused by the raloxifene, and she agreed to discontinue it. Within days, the leg cramps went away. I told Maria to continue what she was doing to prevent heart disease and gave her another medication, Fosamax, for her osteoporosis. (Fosamax is not a SERM.) Maria's story confirms the importance of your doctor listening to your medical history. Now that Maria's medication has changed, she feels great and has even added more time to her daily treadmill exercise.

Natural or Herbal Preparations

Many natural supplements, foods, and creams are on the market, claiming to be effective "estrogen alternatives" at menopause. While some of these preparations are safe and may have some health benefits, many are unsafe and may cause you serious problems. I recommend generally that you talk to your doctor before taking any "estrogen alternative," just to get a medical viewpoint. Also keep in mind that the FDA does not regulate supplements. What you get in that bottle may not be what you paid for. You need to be very wary of anything that claims to be a natural cure or alternative treatment, because in many cases, the claim will be false.

ESTROVEN

Among the many natural supplements on the market touted to ease menopausal symptoms, one in particular, Estroven, has gotten a lot of media attention. Estroven contains vitamin E, riboflavin, calcium, purified isoflavones, folic acid, vitamin B6, kava root, and black cohosh. While the vitamins are within safe supplemental ranges, the calcium content is quite low. Isoflavones are phytochemicals found in soy that act in the body as phytoestrogens (plant estrogens that are close in structure to the body's form of estrogen). The isoflavone dose in Estroven is small. Black cohosh contains estrogenic sterols and is widely touted as the cure-all for menopausal symptoms. Although black cohosh is basically a phytoestrogen and acts like estrogen, its phytoestrogens are very different from those of soy products, and their long-term safety has not been established. Nor has Estroven been tested for its effect on existing heart disease or been shown absolutely to provide any protection against it.

ANGELICA

Other herbs are often used to ease the symptoms of menopause without scientific substantiation to back up their safety, and we have no evidence that they can help reduce the risk of heart disease. One such herb, angelica, is taken to treat symptoms of menopause—hot flashes, dry skin, memory loss, mood swings, and irritability. *Angelica cannot be used with warfarin (Coumadin) or other blood thinners;* it can have potentially dangerous interactions and cause excessive bleeding.

CHASTEBERRY

Another herb highly touted by naturalists is chasteberry, which is said to normalize fluctuating hormone levels and ease menopausal symptoms. Again, the proof of safety is just not there.

KAVA AND ST. JOHN'S WORT

During menopause, some women find kava and St. John's wort helpful to ease anxiety, irritability, and sudden mood swings. Kava, a member of the pepper family, is a sedative and muscle relaxant. This herb has been reported to help insomnia, anxiety, and the stresses of daily life, and many proponents enjoy its "mellowing" effect. Still, most people do not know that *long-term use of kava may lead to hypertension, reduced protein levels, blood cell abnormalities, or liver damage.*

St. John's wort is another popular choice at midlife to relieve mild depression without some of the common side effects of prescription antidepressants. While the drug seems safe, check with your doctor before taking it, as symptoms of depression can be serious. St. John's wort should not be used concurrently with antidepressants.

NATURAL PROGESTERONE

Some of my patients ask about progesterone cream, which is sold at health food stores. The ingredients in this over-the-counter hormone cream are usually made from wild yams. Although claims are made for its efficacy, scientific studies do not support its use in preventing heart disease.

Phytoestrogens

I will explain more about the heart-healthy benefits of soy foods in Chapter 10 and of isoflavone supplements on page 95. But for now, let's look at the direct effect soy has on your health after menopause, when it is used as a natural hormone substitute.

For years, soybeans have been an integral part of Asian diets, and they have identifiable positive health benefits. Japanese women have blood levels of phytoestrogens that are ten to forty times higher than those of their Western peers. In fact, breast cancer (and prostate cancer) rates in Japan are four times lower than in the United States.

In one study of 104 postmenopausal women in Bologna, Italy, one group took 60 gm of isolated soy protein and reported significantly fewer hot flashes compared with the placebo group.[14] A very short-term study of 145 menopausal Israeli women concluded that the 78 women who ate a phytoestrogen-rich diet had significantly fewer hot flashes and less vaginal dryness than the 36 women in the control group, who ate their normal diet. These researchers concluded that soy isoflavones may be an anti-estrogen in premenopausal women, reducing circulating ovarian steroids and adrenal androgens and even lengthening the menstrual cycle of premenopausal women.[15]

But the research on soy's ability to alleviate menopausal symptoms, such as hot flashes, and to act as a natural hormonal supplement is not conclusive. At this writing, all the studies have been short term (twelve weeks), not nearly long enough to determine either harmful side effects or long-term benefits.

While consumption of soy whole foods may be directly associated with a reduction of breast, prostate, and colon cancer in populations where soy is prominent, newer studies show that adding one serving a day of soybeans may increase bone strength. Recent guidelines also show that adding 25 gm of soy daily can reduce cholesterol, giving an added heart-protective benefit.

ISOFLAVONES

There are three main categories of phytoestrogens: isoflavones, lignans, and resorcyclic acid lactones. Soy products, chickpeas, and other legumes are high in isoflavones, but isoflavones are much weaker than human estrogen, about five hundred to one thousand times weaker. In one study, participants took nearly 50 gm/day of isoflavones, resulting in decreased levels of total and LDL ("bad") cholesterol.[16]

While isoflavone supplements are available over the counter, there are no human studies on the long-term effects of taking large doses of purified isoflavones. Long-term benefits of isoflavones with regard to fracture prevention, prevention of hormone-dependent cancers, reversing memory loss, and prevention of cardiovascular disease are currently unknown. Even though some research concludes that isoflavones can help prevent the rise in serum cholesterol associated with declining estrogen levels, there is no proof that these phytochemicals can help to prevent heart attack.

If you want to try isoflavones to help alleviate menopausal symptoms, I recommend that you stick with the whole soy food—tofu, soybeans, and other variations. Soybeans contain 2 to 4 mg of isoflavone per gram of protein. Soy milk and tofu contain about 2 mg of isoflavone per gram of protein. Isoflavone content varies among soybean products and manufacturing. The chart is an estimate of isoflavone content of commonly used soy preparations.[17]

ISOFLAVONES, SOY SUPERSTARS

Soy Product	Serving Size	Isoflavones (mg)
Roasted soy beans	½ cup	167
Tempeh, uncooked	4 ounces	60
Regular tofu, uncooked	4 ounces	38
Soy milk	1 cup	20

LIGNANS

Lignans are also phytoestrogens and are found in flaxseed, whole grains, beans, and vegetables. Flaxseed, a tiny brown seed that looks like a sesame seed, is the richest known source of omega-3 fatty acids. Nutritional studies show that lignans have a more obvious estrogenic effect than isoflavones.

Like most vegetable oils, flaxseed oil contains alpha-linolenic acid, an essential fatty acid (EFA) needed for survival. Alpha-linolenic acid is also found in fish, pumpkin seeds, and walnuts. EFAs help keep your skin, vaginal tissue, and other mucous membranes healthy. You can purchase flaxseed and flaxseed oil at most natural food stores. They can be added to smoothies or other heart-healthy recipes. Be sure to keep them in the refrigerator, as they can go rancid. Use a spice or coffee bean grinder to grind up the seeds before adding them to smoothies or other recipes, or your system cannot absorb them.

GENISTEIN AND DAIDZEIN

Genistein and daidzein are two components of the soybean that have been shown to have beneficial effects in prevention of cancer, heart disease, and osteoporosis, along with reducing the signs of menopause. In particular, genistein blocks several of the key enzymes that tumor cells need to grow and thrive.

In osteoporosis research, genistein and daidzein have been shown to inhibit bone breakdown in animals because of their estrogenlike actions. Studies show that eating animal protein can weaken bones, as it causes the body to remove calcium faster. Soy protein also causes less calcium loss in the urine than animal protein, helping your bones to stay calcium dense and strong. Because Japanese women have half the rate of hip fractures of women in the United States, preliminary studies suggest that soy may be the key factor in helping to retain bone mass.[18]

Risk/Benefit Evaluation for Taking HRT

To get an idea of your own risk/benefit profile, review the following questions and answer them completely and honestly. Discuss your answers and the subsequent recommendations with your own doctor.

1. *Have you had a recent mammogram?* If not, then you should have one before you consider going on estrogen therapy or HRT. If you decide in favor of hormone therapy, you should have yearly mammograms.

2. *Have you ever been treated for breast cancer?* If yes, then you should not go on HRT.

3. *Does breast cancer run strongly in your family? (Did your mother, grandmother, or sister have breast cancer?)* If so, then HRT is not the best option for you. Your heart disease prevention program should be based on a healthy diet, exercise, smoking cessation, and cholesterol medication if necessary.

4. *Have you recently had a heart attack or been diagnosed with heart disease?* If you have had a heart attack or unstable angina within the past year, you should hold off on starting HRT. The HERS trial of women with heart disease (see page 87) showed that women on HRT had a higher rate of gallstones, blood clots, and deaths during the study's first year. Over the four years of the trial, there was no difference in death rate between women on a placebo and those on HRT. Ongoing studies may help to clarify the situation, but for the time being I advise women with recently diagnosed heart disease not to begin hormone therapy.

5. *Are you at high risk for heart disease?* It you have a number of risk factors for heart disease, including a family history of early cardiovascular problems (see page 53), and you do not have breast cancer, are not at a high risk for breast cancer, and do not presently have heart disease, you can take HRT for preventing osteoporosis or menopausal symptoms. But you cannot consider HRT as a heart disease prevention therapy. Use the Women's Healthy Heart Program in Part III to keep your heart healthy.

6. *Are you at high risk for osteoporosis?* If you are white and have a small frame, or your mother developed osteoporosis, and you do not have a high breast cancer risk, then you *may* be a good candidate for HRT. If you are postmenopausal and have not yet had a bone scan, you should get one. Keep in mind that you have other options besides HRT for preventing osteoporosis: you can eat a diet high in calcium and vitamin D, and do regular weight-bearing exercise. Other medications can also prevent osteoporosis, such as the biphosphonates.

7. *Have you ever taken estrogen therapy or HRT and stopped?* If so, why did you stop? If you stopped because of postmenopausal bleeding but were found to be free of uterine cancer, you can start HRT again, provided that you have regular checkups with your gynecologist. Taking progesterone daily, rather than alternating between progesterone and estrogen, may help prevent further bleeding.

If you stopped HRT because your menopausal symptoms stopped, and you don't have breast cancer or any current heart disease, starting back on HRT will protect your bones, if that is your concern. But again, I do not advocate HRT for heart disease prevention.

8. *Have you had a hysterectomy?* If you have had a hysterectomy and the other questions in this section indicate that you can benefit from hormone replacement, then you can take estrogen alone.

9. *Are you willing to put up with the risks and side effects of hormone therapy?* This is not as obvious a question as it sounds. Many patients who stop taking hormones do so because they are unwilling to live with the side effects. A woman in one of my discussion groups told me that her friend had stopped taking HRT because her breasts grew so big, she needed a bra for the first time in her life. Many women do not like the vaginal bleeding that frequently occurs.

I hope these questions have helped to clear up some of the confusion about hormone therapy and given you a basis for an informed discussion with your physician. Currently, it appears that the women who are most likely to benefit from this therapy are those who are at risk for heart disease (and osteoporosis) but do not yet have heart disease.

It's quite clear, however, that hormone replacement is *not* your only answer for preventing heart disease. While hormone replacement therapy works for some women, it is not a foolproof protection. It may help reduce the risk of heart disease in some women, but it does not totally eliminate it.

The bottom line is there are many factors to weigh, and the decision is different for every woman. What works for you may not be best for your colleague or your best friend. Whatever you decide— hormone replacement or not—do not be afraid to assert yourself and let your doctor know exactly how you feel. I've seen many women take HRT simply because it's the standard prescription that some doctors write when a woman complains of menopausal symptoms. Know the facts, and know your health history. You do have other options, if you need them.

No matter what you ultimately decide, remember that the proven heart disease prevention program is still a combination of lifestyle changes: diet, exercise, smoking cessation, and weight loss. If you already have high blood pressure and high cholesterol, and dietary or other changes do not help you, use medication to prevent the development of heart disease. You can be healthier, and I will help you find the ways that work best for you.

WHAT WE KNOW ABOUT HRT AND MENOPAUSE

For alleviating menopausal symptoms	HRT is proven.
For preventing osteoporosis	HRT is proven.
For preventing primary heart disease	HRT is unproven.
For treating cholesterol	If you are not already on HRT, choose statins over HRT. If you are on HRT, ask your doctor for statins instead.
For high triglycerides	Drop HRT; reduce the carbohydrates in your diet, exercise, and avoid alcohol excess; you may need medication.
For preventing secondary heart disease	Do not initiate HRT.

Your Best Bet at Menopause: Change Your Lifestyle

There is no one magic pill that will protect your heart, bones, and mind from disease. If there were, then there would be no need for this book! The most effective preventive measure you can take at menopause is to follow healthy lifestyle practices, including:

- Increase your physical and aerobic activity through the Exercise Prescription given in Chapter 9.
- Change the way you eat to include more fresh fruits and vegetables, fish, whole grains, and monounsaturated fat, through the Healthy Heart Eating Plan in Chapter 10.

- De-stress your life, using the Stress Reduction Program in Chapter 12; make only commitments that do not put too much pressure on you.
- Stop smoking cigarettes; the Stop Smoking Program in Chapter 13 can help. Stay away from those who do smoke.
- Know your lipid levels. If you have high cholesterol, talk to your doctor about cholesterol-reducing medications and lifestyle changes necessary to keep them in a healthy range.
- Stay on top of your blood pressure, and make sure it is controlled at a normal level.

5

The Truth about Stress, Emotions, and Your Heart

At forty-five, Lynn thought she was too young to have heart disease. Sadly, so did her doctors. This astute magazine editor and mother of two teenagers had worsening symptoms of strong heart palpitations, difficulty breathing, and unending fatigue. She went to three different doctors over a period of eleven months seeking diagnosis and treatment. Because she was a smoker, lived on caffeine, and was very nervous, all the doctors gave her the same advice: quit smoking and find ways to de-stress. One doctor told her to take a cruise so she could forget her troubles.

After her sudden death of a massive heart attack, Lynn's husband, Ron, spoke to me. "Lynn was adopted, so we had no clue about any family history of heart disease. If only the doctors had done some cardiac tests to find the problem, perhaps she would be alive today. Yet they all figured since she was a thin woman and had low blood pressure, she was exaggerating her symptoms, which they believed were all stress related."

Ron and the doctors learned from an autopsy report that, in fact, Lynn's symptoms were caused by blocked coronary arteries, which led to her sudden heart attack and premature death.

Because fatigue, shortness of breath, upper chest discomfort, dizziness, and palpitations can also be signs of anxiety and other disorders, female patients and their doctors often do not aggressively seek other answers besides anxiety. Frequently, as in Lynn's case, when women do see a doctor, their symptoms are misdiagnosed. Their stress is often written off as something that will go away with a vacation.

Stress simply is not taken seriously enough as a health threat to women. You may not know that *stress even affects your ovaries*. It can cause ovarian failure, which results in lower levels of estrogen in premenopausal women and increases their risk for developing atherosclerosis.[1] Women who have a lifelong history of menstrual irregularity, a by-product of stress, may also be at higher risk for developing heart disease.

I tell my patients that they *must* reduce their stress because it does create the risk for heart disease. Prolonged stress can lead to permanent feelings of helplessness and ineffectiveness, and it can produce physical changes in the body that can affect the heart. For example, an acute or prolonged state of tension can cause your heart rate and blood pressure to increase. You may have dry mouth, enlarged pupils, sweaty palms, and fast, shallow "chest" breathing. Talk with your doctor or a professional therapist about ways to identify your stressors. You can also try to reduce stress triggers on your own by using the suggestions in Chapter 12; they have helped my own patients a great deal.

Are You All Stressed Up with No Place to Go?

I treat many women like Lynn, who exhibit the signs and symptoms of stress and have other risk factors for heart disease. Many of these women are actually young mothers; some are trying to balance the challenge of raising children with other family demands or with working in high-stress careers. Others are older or middle-aged women who care for aging or ill parents and their husbands, and are also the only breadwinner in the family. No matter what the source of your stress may be, too much of it can increase your risk of heart disease.

Many women today are so busy caring for others that they ignore their own health. As Lynn's husband told me after her death, "Lynn never exercised because she was so busy trying to make our home perfect or carpooling the girls to activities and working hard to help pay our mortgage. Instead of watching her diet, she usually made sure the girls and I ate healthy food, but then she'd eat some crackers, cheese, and wine. She would relax for the evening by smoking cigarettes and watching old movies on television."

Lynn didn't make her health a priority, but *you* must do so to keep your heart healthy. In this chapter, we'll explore some ways to manage life's demands so that you—not they—rule your self-care. I know this can be difficult. Another patient, Emily, age thirty-six, also found it tough to take time for herself; she told me she needed a "wife" to keep her organized each day and to remind her to eat right, de-stress, and exercise. At the time, Emily was pregnant with twins and was having some problems with irregular heartbeats. She felt overwhelmed by the demands on her as a wife and mother-to-be who also worked in a highly competitive retail consulting job.

I empathized with Emily. The demands of being a woman today are incredible, and the term *working mother* is redundant. For most women, the message we get from society is that we should not only be highly educated and develop our talents as professionals, we must have bright children who are competitive in sports and academics, and our homes must pass the white glove test. No real woman is capable of meeting all of the nurturing or caregiving feats that are expected of her without inflicting real wear and tear on her physical well-being. We all have a great deal of stress from family and other obligations, and we try to do it all—even though it eventually will have a negative impact on our health. And when we do get sick, it creates even more stress.

"I used to think I was immortal," Shelly, age forty-four, told me, "until I started having health problems. And I think they all came just from the ongoing stress of daily life." This young mother of four came to see me when she experienced ongoing palpitations and shortness of breath, even with little exertion. She also reported an unshakable fatigue. Although she was very petite, Shelly's blood pressure was surprisingly high. After she gave me a rundown of her "typical day," it was apparent why she was short of breath and exhausted.

Shelly got up at five A.M. every day to make school lunches for her children. She then did two loads of wash and a few household chores before the children awakened. While the children ate breakfast, Shelly took a quick shower and got dressed for work. She then wiped mouths, piled all four kids into the van, and picked up a few more children in their school car pool.

Shelly worked full time as a nurse practitioner at a family planning clinic and was devoted to her patients. On many days, she worked without taking a break or even eating lunch, so she could help someone with a problem. At exactly four P.M. each day, Shelly got back in her van, picked the children up at school, then dropped them off at various extracurricular activities. Two days a week, she helped coach the girls' soccer team at her oldest daughter's school.

It was usually seven P.M. before Shelly picked up her brood and got home to greet her husband and start dinner. After dinner, she did the dishes, paid the bills, monitored homework, and more. Then Shelly washed more clothes, ironed school uniforms for the next day, and bathed the younger children.

Shelly could have told me much more about her daily responsibilities, but after hearing all of this, I too was exhausted! While Shelly had it all—family, career, and commitments—she, like so many women, simply did not have the energy to take care of her own health. She needed to start by getting some more control over her schedule to make time for herself. That would result in her actually having *more* energy to deal with the rest of her day. I've seen this happen time and again with my patients, and I want to show you how to do this for yourself too.

INDIRECT EFFECTS OF STRESS
ON HEART HEALTH

Chronic stress can result in unhealthy habits, such as the following, which increase your risk of heart disease.

- Smoking
- Sedentary lifestyle
- Overuse of alcohol
- Poor eating habits
- Social isolation

Lack of Control Adds to Stress

Empirical studies confirm that a strong sense of control is vital for our health and stability.[2] Yet studies also show that women tend to have to balance more life roles and responsibilities than men but have less control at home and in the workplace. The stress of having no control contributes to increased blood pressure and higher cholesterol, so it is not surprising that it is associated with a greater risk of heart disease. You might think that work outside the home is associated with a higher rate of heart disease, but that's not true. While women who have jobs with little control, such as clerical positions, are at higher risk for heart attack, women in managerial positions do not have increased risk. Other findings associated with a risk of heart attack include suppressed hostility (holding in anger) and not having a supportive boss.

A recent study done in Sweden showed that women with heart disease who also had marital stress had a threefold increase in recurrent heart attack.[3] In that study, work stress did not have an association with increased risk for a second heart attack, but anger and anxiety did increase the heart attack risk.

Stress levels measured among working mothers sometimes approach those of combat! Working women and mothers, juggling kids and career, are all greatly stressed from overwork, lack of time, or no energy. Some respond by becoming more sedentary, smoking cigarettes, eating or drinking too much, and becoming apathetic about their own health.

"Stress is nothing new to me," forty-six-year-old Mira said, accounting for her sudden rise in blood pressure. "In one week, my sixteen-year-old son had an accident with my car, my husband lost two major accounts at work, and my mother had a breast biopsy that was positive and is scheduled for surgery. On top of that, the washing machine broke, and our property taxes went up. What else do I need? My life is a roller coaster with no end in sight."

We can all easily relate to Mira's feeling of being on an unending roller coaster. I also try to balance caring for my patients with family responsibilities and caring for family members who are ill, doing volunteer work, giving speeches to women across the country, and researching and writing. I know it's not easy for you to find time for yourself, even when you have a family history of heart disease, which I also do. But my one sure de-stressor is my regular aerobic exercise. No matter how stressed I am with commitments and chaos, I never miss my regular time at the gym. It allows me to do something good for myself, and the heart-pumping exercise reduces all symptoms of stress. I want to work with you to help you find your best de-stressor and work it into your daily life.

How Stress Affects Your Heart

Your body and brain have a physical response to every stressful situation, from rebellious teenagers to importunate clients to the nonstop ringing of a telephone at the office. And no two women respond in the same way to all stressful events. What may be a source of emotional excitement for you may be a source of abject terror for your best friend. Although this response can vary in intensity, the physical symptoms characteristic for one woman will predictably happen again and again during "tense" moments. Yet you *can* learn to manage your response to stress and to lessen its negative, physical effect.

Many of my patients want to know how stress actually affects the heart. I explain that it starts with the autonomic nervous system, an unconscious part of the nervous system that has two branches, the sympathetic and parasympathetic. These branches work together to control some of the involuntary activities of the body, producing chemicals that direct those activities. The sympathetic branch normally releases adrenaline, but under unregulated stress it produces excessive levels, which cause your heart rate and blood pressure to soar. Most people have felt palpitations, a strong heartbeat or a racing pulse, at times, which indicate an increase in your blood pressure. When stress continues without letting up over a long period of time, your blood pressure stays elevated, and you may develop hypertension. Another silent form of heart disease, hypertension can become so serious that you need medications, along with a better diet and other lifestyle changes, to get your blood pressure back to normal. So it's better to prevent hypertension from developing.

If you are experiencing a few of the stress characteristics listed in the box, chances are good that your level of stress is excessive.

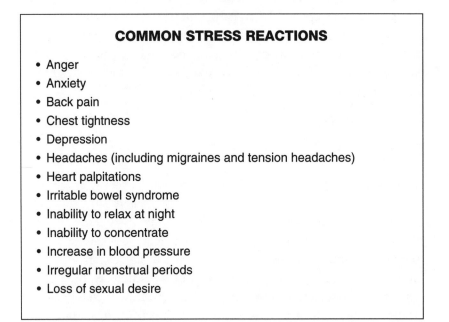

COMMON STRESS REACTIONS

- Anger
- Anxiety
- Back pain
- Chest tightness
- Depression
- Headaches (including migraines and tension headaches)
- Heart palpitations
- Irritable bowel syndrome
- Inability to relax at night
- Inability to concentrate
- Increase in blood pressure
- Irregular menstrual periods
- Loss of sexual desire

During stressful moments, adrenaline, the body's main stress-related hormone, is released by the autonomic nervous system. This adrenaline release sets up a whole cascade of reactions, including increased heart rate and blood pressure and stimulation of platelets (blood-clotting cells). Stress hormones can damage blood vessels by altering their flexibility and making them more vulnerable to plaque disruption.

Because every woman responds to life's stressors differently, our emotions profoundly influence our hormonal production. The way we perceive a problem, and the amount of control we have to change it, influences how we cope with it. The kind of personality we have also affects how our body and its internal systems respond. Let's look at how these factors dictate our unique stress responses.

Perception

Of the four contributing factors to stress, perception is absolutely the most important. If you perceive that something is a threat to you, it triggers an adrenaline surge that puts your body on "red alert." To some extent, a thing is a threat if it is perceived that way. For example, perhaps your best friend looks forward to going for a ride on her motorcycle. For her, this is a great experience and a form of emotional excitement. For you, the thought of being on two wheels in traffic may cause great anxiety. Your friend may also love speaking in front of people at work, while for you giving a talk or presentation is upsetting. The environmental trigger is identical, but you and your friend perceive the situation in entirely different ways.

Control

When you perceive that you no longer are in control, your emotional state can turn anxious. Quite honestly, the physiological line between positive emotional excitement and anxiety is very fine. I tell my patients that control is like a strong bridge that protects you from the turbulent rapids below. River rapids can be fascinating to watch when you are thirty feet above them, safe and sound, but if the bridge over them is shaky or has holes in it, they can become terrifying. In that case, your control is weakened, producing stress.

To some extent, being in control protects you from stress. If you feel you've lost control in your life, you feel helpless and anxious and can develop health problems. Knowing this, you can work to get more control over your life or at the very least over your perceptions and coping style.

Coping Style

Does the slightest irritation get you upset? Does your heart rate soar, and do you perspire profusely? When you are under pressure, does your breathing become rapid and shallow? These are all signs of your particular coping style, another psychological variable that can influence your heart's health.

Some people cope with life's stressors by staying cool and calm. Some become highly anxious, and some completely deny having any problem at all. Interestingly, when I ask some of my patients about how they cope emotionally, they often say that they are generally very calm—yet test results repeatedly show them to have signs of high anxiety. I interpret this to mean that these women are only outwardly calm and are repressing, denying, or "stuffing" their feelings.[4]

Suppressing hostility and anger is specifically associated with increased heart disease risk.[5] It is very hard on your body and will take a toll on your overall health. In addition, some studies show that an accumulation of the stress hormones may make blood vessels constrict and accelerate the formation of new blockages.[6] In Chapter 12, we'll work on how you can release these damaging emotions.

Personality Type

Finally, your personality type can affect your susceptibility to illness. For example, a woman with a type A personality is usually in a hurry—she is always racing the clock. She speaks quickly and impatiently finishes other people's sentences for them. She seldom takes time out to enjoy life, to relax or de-stress.

A type B personality gets the work done, but she also takes time out to smell the roses. She takes walks at lunchtime, allows time for a leisurely bath at night, and even reads quietly or does relaxing exercises like yoga or gardening.

PERSONALITY TYPE AND
SUSCEPTIBILITY TO HEART DISEASE

Type	Traits	Susceptibility to Heart Disease
TYPE A	Angry, hostile, driven (anger is disease risk)	High risk for heart disease, including hypertension and heart attack
TYPE B	Moves more slowly, takes time to "smell roses"	Less risk than "angry" type A
TYPE D	Negative, insecure, distressed. Depressed.	Increased risk of heart disease

Type D personalities are not as driven as type A, but they too risk heart disease due to their tendency to suppress or not deal with anger. They have a generally bleak, helpless view of themselves, their future, and the world.

The A and B personality types were identified in the late 1950s by Doctors Friedman and Roseman, who were looking for a correlation between behavior and heart disease. Although these categories came out of studies on men, they were later determined to be relevant for women through another study.[7] The type D category was identified some forty years later, in a study that looked at the effects of depression and social isolation on heart patients. In the past, experts said that type A people are most likely to succumb to heart attack, but researchers have since discovered that the time-pressured orientation is less associated with increased risk of heart disease than the anger and hostility components of this personality trait. These traits increase the amount of stress hormones that your body produces and reacts to both consciously and unconsciously. In other words, these traits may result in chronically elevated stress hormones.

For instance, you know you're angry when you're cut off by

a rude driver on the highway, because your pulse races. What you don't see is how high your blood pressure soars when this stress reaction occurs. So it's important to deal with these emotions and define them.

Managing Anger and Stress

Sustained mental stress is as likely as strenuous physical activity to precipitate heart attack in people with heart disease.[8] People with type A personalities have twice the likelihood of undergoing a repeat angioplasty than calmer patients.[9]

The bottom line is that you need to know how you react under stress. You have to recognize what triggers your anger and work rationally to lessen these feelings so that you are not in a prolonged state of stress. You may not be able to change your stressors, but you *can* learn to alter your response. You want to identify when, where, and why you get angry and then take steps to recognize and deal with your anger before it builds up over time and damages your heart. I'll help you do this in Chapter 12.

If you already know that you're living with a high level of anger, please try to avoid situations that drive up your anger thermostat. Go shopping during a slow time at the grocery store to avoid long lines, for instance, and avoid rush hour on the highway. If your anger is explosive, talk with a counselor about constructive ways of dealing with it before you hurt yourself or someone else. Exercise is an especially effective way to disperse stressful or angry thoughts. It's hard to stay angry if your mind is focused on pedaling uphill or keeping up in an aerobics class.

Besides exercise, one of the best ways I've found to manage my own stress is to follow the techniques devised by behavioral psychologist Dr. Barrie Guise, who teaches that while we cannot change our personalities or the stress that comes with living, *we can modify our response to stress.* For example, in any stressful situation, try to learn what you can and cannot control, and accept it. Then learn to change your response to situations that normally cause great stress such as deadlines, bills, or challenging children. I'll show you more specific ways to deal with chronic stress in Chapter 12.

SEVEN WAYS TO MANAGE
ANGER AND STRESS

1. Think rationally: break the stressful situation down into controllable components.
2. Behave assertively but not aggressively.
3. Find support for getting rid of your anger by talking to a friend, a loved one, or a counselor.
4. Learn a relaxation method that you like, such as meditation, prayer, exercise.
5. Make sleep a priority. When you're rested, you can see more options to and interpretations of any situation.
6. Increase your physical activity—exercise reduces stress hormones.
7. Seek out humor in your life—laughter also reduces stress hormones. Read humor books, collect jokes that you like, and watch funny videos with a friend.

Panic Attacks May Mimic
Heart Disease Symptoms

The symptoms of heart disease may be very similar to those of panic attacks. People who have panic attacks cannot predict them, and usually they occur at the most inopportune times. They may strike while you are sitting in a theater, working on a project at your job, or even while sleeping. During a panic attack, you may feel sweaty, weak, faint, or even dizzy. Your heart pounds, and your hands may tingle. Even if you aren't hypertensive and don't have heart disease, your blood pressure may rise. Some people have chest pain or difficulty catching their breath and think they are having a heart attack. Some recent studies show that panic attacks may restrict blood flow to the heart and result in chest pain in people who also have heart disease.[10]

The symptoms of panic attack resemble not only heart attacks but also cardiac arrhythmias and hyperthyroidism. So the symptoms need to be evaluated and not assumed to be a panic attack.

If you know that you have heart disease as well as panic attacks, you want to be sure you can distinguish between the two. Yet it's difficult even for a physician to know the difference without doing a complete physical, taking your personal health history, and ordering tests such as an ECG or electrocardiogram, if needed. That's why seeing your doctor is important, so that you learn which symptoms signal heart disease or a heart attack and mandate treatment, and which you may have to live with occasionally as part of a panic attack. Please remember that cognitive-behavioral therapies and medications are effective in treating most cases of panic disorder, so check with your doctor to get the most appropriate treatment for you.

Depression May Be a Risk Factor

Recently, depression has been isolated as a risk factor for the development of coronary artery disease. Patients who have had a heart attack and who also have a serious clinical depression are more likely to die earlier than heart attack patients who are not depressed. Depression appears to decrease a patient's compliance with medical advice and instructions, and she tends not to take necessary heart medications, or stick with a healthy low-fat diet and regular exercise program, or quit smoking. Biological factors that we have yet to discover may also affect the depression-heart link. For instance, depression's effect on the autonomic nervous system may result in lower immune function, and depression may coincide with other chronic illnesses, such as hypertension. Some studies show that depression stimulates platelet activity,[11] which makes them stickier, so that they tend to form blood clots, which is the trigger for a heart attack.

It's not surprising that a woman who has had a heart attack or who has high blood pressure would be somewhat depressed by her diagnosis. It is certainly a challenge to have to deal with a chronic ill-ness and to make changes in the way you eat and otherwise live your life in order to get healthier. It's scary, too, to know that you have a condition that may shorten your life. Coming face to face with your own mortality is always a sobering experience.

But please remember that there *are* things you can do to get bet-ter. You *do* have control over how you perceive your illness—you can view it as a call to take action to be healthier and live longer. See your heart and body as having sent you a message that it's time to take care of *you*. You can do things that make you feel better and im-prove your heart's health. Talk to a friend or relative, or a minister, rabbi, or counselor about your feelings so that you isolate what it is that's depressing you and act to heal that depression. If you have been depressed every day for more than two weeks, talk to your doc-tor or a professional counselor.

One of the best ways to improve your life and health is by being with other women. You can find new ways to exercise and more ac-tivities that you enjoy when you join a group. You can also ask advice for what to do of your doctors, physical therapists, and rehabilitative therapists.

The Importance of Social Support

Social Isolation Increases Stress Symptoms

It is our nature, as women, to need social support. Of the two sexes, we are the nurturing caregivers. We empathize with family and friends and do things for them. We communicate well with people around us, and we usually work compassionately with others to form strong relationships. While men lean toward having the "fight or flight" response during times of stress, women appear to have the "tend and befriend" response.[4]

Women who lack social support suffer greatly from the subse-quent loneliness and disconnection. Forty-eight-year-old Diane, a single mother and bookkeeper, lived in constant fear and isolation af-ter having a major heart attack. She was nervous about returning to exercise and a normal lifestyle and even became paranoid that her co-workers would feel she was too ill to be effective. Diane was even afraid to tell her new boyfriend about her heart attack, for fear he would think she was "too fragile to be much fun," and she actually considered breaking off the relationship. She stayed awake until the wee hours of morning, unable to sleep because fears of "what might happen" were racing through her mind. These fears all stemmed from how she interpreted having had a heart attack.

When such anxiety and fears go unrelieved, the overwhelming sense of isolation can keep you from trying to improve your health. Other symptoms, such as elevated blood pressure and heart rate, can also be magnified. When you're highly anxious, you may have difficulty sleeping, and being tired will of course make it harder for you to stay on your heart-healthy exercise and diet programs.

On the other hand, some women, like forty-three-year-old Marilyn, tell me that being with friends causes her more stress than being alone. Marilyn, a single woman and technical writer who works out of her home, said, "I can feel very calm and confident when I'm alone, then after being with a group of friends or colleagues and listening to their troubles, I cannot wait to find the exit door to go home." You just have to judge for yourself what is best for keeping *your* stress at a healthy, low level and for speeding your recovery.

Seek Support for Optimal Health

You can find or create a positive support system for yourself. Whether your main support comes from your friend, spouse, significant other, religious organization, or even the women at the beauty salon, support is available—and you can develop a network that works for you. Let's look at some of the ways that social support can help you to keep your heart disease in perspective and to feel whole and healthy.

SOCIAL SUPPORT GIVES YOU A SENSE OF CONTROL

While you may not be able to control some of the risk factors for heart disease or past health problems you've had, there are always some other things you can control. Creating a strong network of family, friends, and acquaintances is one of them. Years of research on heart disease reveal an important connection between longevity and social support. One recent study from the National Institutes of Health showed that women who have a family history of heart disease may have an increased risk of getting it themselves if they also are hostile and isolated.[12] Their risk of heart disease is actually even greater than that of high-risk men and men and women who have low to moderate risk. In this case, your risk is higher than any man's! Other comprehensive studies conclude that people with strong social support tend to fare better in every life situation, particularly when confronted with a serious illness like heart disease.[13]

SOCIAL SUPPORT HELPS YOU TO FEEL ACCEPTED

Feeling accepted is a basic emotional need. In years past, people lived close to their family and relied on parents and siblings for affirmation and emotional strength, even after marriage. They could turn to their family for comfort and support in times of trouble, illness, or other challenges. Today, however, most adults live hundreds of miles away from parents and siblings.

A connection to others is important for feeling accepted. No matter what we are facing in life, when we have an emotional tie to someone else, we can feel comfortable in letting out our fears and insecurity, or in communicating our interests and happiness. We can give and receive comfort from someone who accepts us—just as we are.

SOCIAL SUPPORT HELPS YOU TO BE RESILIENT

Research on stress-resistant personality traits has identified keys to staying healthy. They include:

- Involvement in work or other tasks that have great meaning
- The ability to relate well to others
- The ability to interact in a strong social network[14]

Especially for women, social support allows us to connect with others, nourish our minds, bodies, and spirits, and recharge ourselves after giving all to working our jobs and to caring for our kids and community. When you have strong social support, you have a greater weapon against all of life's problems.

SOCIAL SUPPORT KEEPS YOU ACCOUNTABLE

For any woman who is trying to lose weight or maintain a regular activity program, social support can help. The women who make—and keep—the commitment to come three days a week to the Women's Healthy Heart Program for exercise, nutrition guidance, and stress management tell me that they feel better. I see that they are healthier too, and they're definitely extending their longevity. Women who say that they will exercise or stay on a heart-healthy diet, yet have not developed a social network to keep them accountable to this commitment, often find that their good intentions fall by the wayside. I'm most impressed by the way the women in my program keep an eye out for each other. They call friends or acquaintances who are absent from class. They make lunch and movie plans and have fun getting and staying healthy together.

Numerous other support groups can help you to stop smoking, lose weight, and be more active. Ask your doctor for information on groups in your area, or call your hospital's physical therapy department or social services. Your local Y, senior or community center, or church or synagogue will also have information about a group that may appeal to you. Locate one, and try it out. I see women every day who are glad they did, including my patient Christine.

An outgoing, bright forty-seven-year-old with a successful computer consulting business, Christine initially came to see me about palpitations and shortness of breath. I ordered a series of tests for her that included an ECG, a stress echocardiogram, and a thallium stress test. The tests revealed that Christine had no evidence of blocked arteries or any heart rhythm problems.

Yet just looking at Christine, I knew that blocked arteries were inevitable. She was extremely overweight, at five foot two and 239 pounds, and her lifestyle was sedentary. She had hypertension that she was not doing anything about. We talked about all these items as risk factors for heart attack, and I suggested that she begin a heart disease prevention program. Initially Christine attended every exercise session, joined the support group, and changed her eating habits. I was thrilled by her enthusiasm and by how she always gave words of encouragement to new participants in the program. Then suddenly she dropped out completely, citing family commitments.

Christine didn't come back to see me for about a year. At that visit, she told me she had been having shortness of breath for three months and that these episodes were now waking her up in the middle of the night. She also had chest pressure and shortness of breath even after walking only three blocks. She admitted that the symptoms coincided with increased stress from some financial problems that had cropped up when she started a new business. Because of the additional workload, she had stopped exercising, gone back to her old eating habits, and gained thirty pounds. Even though she knew her heart health was declining, she had not been able to find the time to return to the program.

Christine's physical examination and ECG told the rest of the story. Her blood pressure was thirty points higher than it had been a year before, and her ECG showed that she may have already had a heart attack. I admitted her to the hospital, where testing revealed a 90 percent obstruction in one of her coronary arteries, with smaller obstructions in the other two. After she underwent a procedure to open up the blocked artery, I sat down with her, and we had a long heart-to-heart talk on how to prevent further heart attacks. I also started her on medications to control her blood pressure and cholesterol.

Christine rejoined the Women's Healthy Heart Program to resume her exercise and diet program. But this time she made stress management her first priority, since it was anxiety, work obligations, and difficulty managing her time that had led her to drop out before. She now makes time each day for taking care of herself. The other women in the program support her and sometimes call her if she misses a class—to keep her accountable to her commitment.

Christine had been so caught up in her role as a caregiver that she ignored her early warning signs for a heart attack. Today she tells other women never to ignore themselves—that their life is important and that taking care of our personal health is something we all must do. With her new commitment and the support of other heart patients, Christine will become more and more healthy, resilient, and happy. I want you to take time every day to take care of yourself even before you develop the kinds of warning signs Christine had.

SOCIAL SUPPORT MAY INCREASE LONGEVITY

Some close relationships can actually give us stress. But preventing illness and living a long healthy life depend on your strengthening your bond with others. For anyone who has a chronic illness, social support is especially important. In study after study, the findings are the same: people with many social contacts—a spouse, a close-knit family, a network of friends, a religious or other group affiliation—live longer and are healthier. A full, rewarding social life can nourish the mind, emotions, and spirit. Good physical health depends as much on our social support as it does on a strong, well-functioning body.

Taking Action: Your Plan to Expand Your Social Network

A strong network of family, friends, and health care professionals is key to your optimal wellness. Even before you begin the Women's Healthy Heart Program in Part III, you can start *now* to increase your support by following these three steps:

STEP 1: EVALUATE YOUR CURRENT SOCIAL NETWORK

Personally and professionally, we all need support. Some important types of support include:

1. Emotional support, or someone you trust with your most intimate thoughts, anxieties, and fears, and who trusts you
2. Social support, or someone you enjoy being with, who helps you cope with disappointments, and who celebrates your joys
3. Informational support, or someone you can ask for advice on major decisions
4. Practical support, or someone who will help you out in a pinch (a neighbor or co-worker)

Who can you turn to for emotional, social, informational, and practical support? Try to identify these key people in your life, and work to nurture these much-needed relationships. If you are having trouble thinking of people in any one of these areas, please realize that this is an important task and you have to do it. Reach out to broaden your personal relationships.

STEP 2: IF YOU AVOID RELATIONSHIPS AND SUPPORT, IDENTIFY REASONS WHY

If you work hard all week and decide to be alone with your family on Friday nights, that is a healthy choice—you're tired, and you need time for rest and recovery. Yet if you stay home day and night, week after week, and pull out of all social activities, you really need to evaluate your behavior. Are you hiding from relationships? Are you afraid to talk about your illness with friends and family? Are you suffering from mild depression? If you have trouble figuring out why you've isolated yourself, you need to make an appointment with a counselor. This professional can help you determine the reasons you are avoiding social interaction and help you set personal goals to broaden your social network.

STEP 3: FOCUS ON BUILDING SUPPORTIVE RELATIONSHIPS

I think many times we women can get into the pattern of "doing nothing" socially and forget how invigorating it feels to be around other people. That's why I want you to start with one day a week, and make plans now to be with other people. Write a list with specific steps you can take this week to increase your social network. Keep at it. You may call one or two friends who are busy or out of town, but your third or fourth calls could result in a plan. Go with a friend to a movie or art show. Invite a neighbor over for tea or to see your garden or ask advice on decorating. Have your rabbi or pastor to lunch or dinner. Sign up for a computer class with a girlfriend. Join some mall walkers with a buddy. Phone for the catalog of events at the local Y, college, university, community, or senior center.

There are countless enjoyable ways in which you can reconnect to the world and work on your health as a whole person.

Behavioral Interventions

Along with increasing your social network, there are some other ways you can reestablish harmony within your body's physiological systems. Without question, the chemicals produced during moderate exercise can be extremely beneficial and improve the function of your immune system. The regular aerobic and strengthening exercises discussed in Chapter 9 are very effective in training your body to deal with stress under controlled circumstances. Volumes have been written about the health benefits of good nutrition, and we'll get into that too in Chapter 10.

Still, some of the most effective stress interventions, that cost very little money, are mind/body therapies. Learning relaxation response, deep abdominal breathing, progressive muscle relaxation, and visualization or guided imagery is enjoyable, and I'll give you instructions on them in Chapter 12. But you can find numerous classes and instructors—as well as video- and audiotape courses—all over the country. Other ancient disciplines, such as yoga, can also help you train your body to become less reactive to life's stressors. Studies show that when you can create a strong mental image using mind/body or relaxation techniques, you actually feel "removed" from stress and negative emotions.[15] This mindfulness, or focusing on the moment, can also help you move beyond destructive habits and center you on your health and inner healing.

Take time to learn the mind/body exercises so your stressful moments are not as intense or taxing, and so you develop a greater sense of control and decrease your chance of heart disease. There is a strong link between your heart and your mind. Chronic stress and anger can increase your risk of heart disease. Think about where you turn when life gets overwhelming and which relaxation techniques you are going to use to reduce your stress.

So you can start right away on the relaxation techniques in the Women's Healthy Heart Program, but I'd also like you to turn to Part II and check out your heart to make sure it's in great shape.

PART II

Examining Your Heart

6

Your Guide to the Symptoms and Diagnoses of Cardiovascular Disease

"**S**o if I stay at a healthy weight, eat right, and exercise daily, I can avoid heart problems. The prescription seems too easy!" Ellen, age forty-one, is an outgoing advertising sales representative who wanted a clear formula for good health all wrapped up in a neat little box and tied with a bow. The problem, as I explained to Ellen, is that heart health doesn't always work that way. Your formula for prevention and healing depends on your personal risk factors and on the type of heart disease you may have.

The healthy heart program discussed in Part III is geared to deter cardiovascular disease (especially blood vessel–coronary artery disease, including hypertension and stroke) as well as help you heal from it. But some diseases of the heart may not be affected by lifestyle measures. With these diseases, no matter how much you exercise, watch your weight, or spend time de-stressing, you will still need a doctor's help and possibly medication to keep you healthy. These heart diseases affect the heart's arteries, rhythm, valves, and muscle. You may need medications or even surgery to correct these heart problems. (In other cases, you may need to do little more than keep an eye on the problem.)

Some of these heart problems, such as mitral valve prolapse (MVP), mandate a conservative wait-and-see approach by your doctor, depending on the symptoms and the severity of the problem. Most people with MVP live an active, normal life. Other, more serious heart diseases, such as ventricular arrhythmias, can be fatal if treatment is not sought immediately. Treatment will involve medications or surgery, depending on the particular problem.

Finally, some of these problems can result *from* a heart attack, including mechanical, electrical, and some valve problems. With these diseases, there is no marked difference in how they manifest in men and women, but I'll comment on the similarities and differences for each one.

THINKING LIKE A DOCTOR

In this chapter, I want to demystify your heart health care by teaching you to think like a doctor and to understand more of the medical language we use. I believe that once you understand the "medical" thought process of assessing symptoms, examining a medical history, and considering treatment options, it will be easier for you to implement a prevention or treatment plan.

WHAT IS HEART DISEASE?

Before I take you through these diseases, let me first define these key terms.

- *Heart disease*—a general term that refers to diseases of the heart muscle, the arteries that supply the heart muscle (coronary arteries), the rhythm of the heart, and the valves.
- *Cardiovascular disease*—a general term that includes not only heart disease but also blood vessel diseases, such as stroke, high blood pressure, or peripheral vascular disease.

A Powerful Pump

Before we discuss particular diseases, let's look at how a healthy heart works. Visualize your heart as a pump. Although it's no bigger than your fist, weighing between 7 and 15 ounces, this pump is an amazingly powerful organ—it keeps you alive. Located in the middle of your chest, slightly to the left, it is the origin of all the major blood vessels that connect and branch off to deliver blood throughout your body (see Figure 6.1).

Your heart is divided into four chambers: the right atrium, the right ventricle, the left atrium, and the left ventricle. The atria (upper chambers) receive the blood, while the ventricles (lower chambers) pump the blood. In a healthy heart, blood is prevented from flowing from one side to the other by the septum, a thin wall of muscle that divides your heart in the middle. The right-sided chambers accept blood that is returning from the other parts of the body and send it to the lungs to be oxygenated. The left ventricle delivers blood to the aorta, where it goes to the vital organs.

The heart has four valves—the tricuspid, mitral, pulmonic, and aortic. They are composed of small flaps of tissue (leaflets) that open and close, depending upon the changes in pressure in the atria, ventricles, or vessels behind and in front of them. The valves ensure that blood flows one way when the heart is contracting or relaxing.

The mitral and tricuspid valves sit between the two atria and the two ventricles (see Figure 6.2). These valves regulate blood flow from the atria to the ventricles, by opening when your heart fills with blood and then closing as the heart contracts. The pulmonary and aortic valves guard the openings from the ventricles to the aortic and pulmonary arteries.

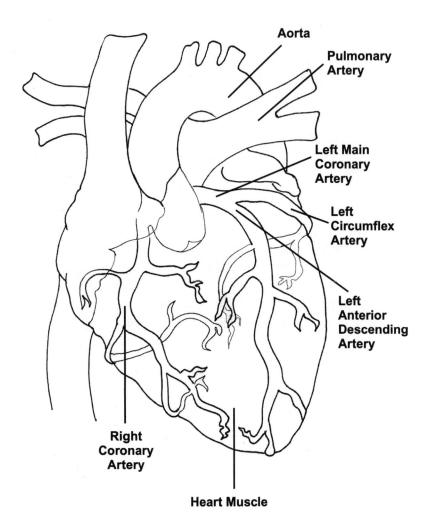

Aorta

Pulmonary Artery

Left Main Coronary Artery

Left Circumflex Artery

Left Anterior Descending Artery

Right Coronary Artery

Heart Muscle

Figure 6.1
A Closer Look at Your Heart

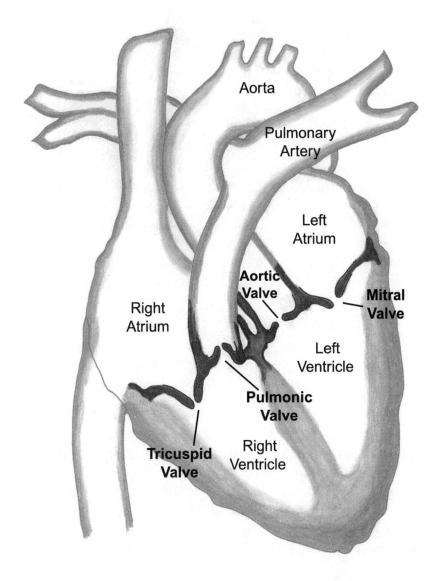

Aorta

Pulmonary
Artery

Left
Atrium

**Aortic
Valve**

**Mitral
Valve**

Right
Atrium

Left
Ventricle

**Pulmonic
Valve**

**Tricuspid
Valve**

Right
Ventricle

**Figure 6.2
The Heart's Valves**

Arteries Carry Blood Throughout the Body

Oxygen-starved blood enters the right side of your heart and is pumped through the pulmonary artery before traveling to your lungs to become enriched with oxygen. In your lungs, the blood exchanges carbon dioxide for oxygen. The blood then goes back to the left side of your heart, where it is pumped outward through the aorta to the arteries in your body.

The Electrical System Charges Your Heart

Your heart pumps blood to the lungs and body organs and tissues through an organized sequence of contractions of its four chambers, which are jump-started by the heart's electrical system—specialized tissues that produce minicharges of electricity that directly trigger cardiac contractions.

Every contraction of the heart is preceded by an electrical impulse that tells it to expand and contract, and each cell in your heart works together to keep the beating heart synchronized. Under normal conditions, the heartbeat is a synchronized action and repeats itself about 60 to 100 times a minute.

Heart Rhythm Problems

Thirty-two-year-old Anna came to see me because of a slow resting pulse rate. A slim, athletic runner, Anna was in training for the New York Marathon. While many athletes have a slow resting heart rate, Anna's heart rate was unusually low, at 38 beats per minute.

During the exam, Anna told me about having heart palpitations and a history of mitral valve prolapse. During the examination, I checked her neck and noticed that her thyroid was enlarged. I then did an ECG, which showed a regular but slow heart rhythm. Anna had a complete workup, including a blood test to detect any thyroid problems, and we discovered that she had hypothyroidism, an underactive thyroid grand. This common disease of the thyroid can potentially be serious to the heart, resulting in reduced heart function.

Anna realized that her voice had become deeper, and she was fatigued, both effects of the hypothyroidism. After starting on thyroid medication, her heart rate returned to 55 to 60 beats per minute, which is within the normal range (about 60 to 100 beats per minute). She was able to continue training and finished the New York Marathon in her best time ever.

Arrhythmias

SIGNS AND SYMPTOMS

I know from personal experience how frightening and unnerving palpitations can feel. One night recently I sat up in bed with my heart racing. For a few seconds, it felt like my heart would not slow down. When I took my pulse, it was 120 beats per minute, considerably faster than my resting pulse. I took some deep breaths and tried to relax for a few minutes, and my pulse finally slowed down. I then realized that the decongestant I had taken for my stuffy nose had revved up my heart rhythm.

My patient Genevieve, age thirty-eight, an attorney in New York, constantly fights court deadlines, along with extensive travel. Recently she complained of also fighting chronic sinus problems for several weeks, taking decongestants, yet her lifestyle did not slow down. She was on the go and living off a diet filled with coffee and a lot of chocolate.

When Genevieve experienced palpitations, she went to see her internist. He sent her for a Holter monitor test (see page 182), which revealed frequent premature ventricular contractions (PVCs), or early heartbeats that originate from the lower chamber of the heart. When she was referred to me, I explained to Genevieve that the most likely cause of the frequent PVCs was the combination of decongestants, chocolate, and stress. I recommended that she cut back on the coffee and chocolate and, once the chronic sinusitis improved, eliminate the decongestants. When her symptoms diminished, the Holter monitor test was repeated. This time the results showed resolution of the arrhythmia.

Jenny, a fifty-eight-year-old freelance journalist, came to see me for an evaluation of palpitations that occurred almost daily. She said that initially the episodes of a racing heartbeat had lasted for less than a minute, but that now they were lasting up to forty-five minutes, making her feel light-headed and breathless.

Accompanied by her husband, Jenny and I spoke about the problem and her personal medical history. Then she went to the examining room, but before I could follow her, her husband asked to speak to me alone. He said that Jenny had been under tremendous stress and needed some Valium. This medication, he told me, would solve the problem. But he was wrong—Valium is *not* a treatment for heart rhythms, so please don't fall into this misconception.

After the examination, I spoke with Jenny and her husband and told them that I thought she was having an arrhythmia. I recommended an echocardiogram and the Holter monitor as methods of assessment. Unfortunately, her health maintenance organization did not approve these tests until ten days had passed.

Meanwhile, about a week after the initial examination, Jenny called me to say that she was experiencing the symptoms while getting her hair styled at a local hair salon. I told her to go to the emergency room. She did, and there she was diagnosed as having a supraventricular tachycardia, with a heart rate of 140 beats per minute. The ER doctors gave Jenny some medication (not Valium!) to slow her heartbeat. Jenny then had a procedure called *radiofrequency ablation* (see page 408) to eliminate the arrhythmia altogether.

Interestingly, after Jenny was discharged from the hospital, her HMO approved her Holter monitor exam. So much for managed care! Her husband's reaction was most surprising—he couldn't believe that Jenny's problem hadn't been anxiety.

The first thing I tell patients when they come to see me with palpitations is to sit down, take a deep breath, relax, and describe the sensation. Some patients tell of feeling that their heart skipped a beat or that it was fluttering in their chest. Others tell of having an irregular or very fast or slow heartbeat. More serious arrhythmias may cause you to have chest pains, feel dizzy, faint, or have a hard time catching your breath. A few flutters occasionally should not cause panic in a woman with a normal heart. The severity of an arrhythmia depends on the presence or absence of symptoms and your heart's health. If you have any concerns about your heart rhythm or symptoms, see your doctor.

WHAT IS ARRHYTHMIA?

An arrhythmia is a change or disturbance to your normal regular heart rhythm. This may mean that the heart rate is fast (tachycardia), slow (bradycardia), or irregular. Tachycardias originate either in the ventricles (ventricular tachycardia) or in the atria (supraventricular tachycardia). Many women I see come in because they are experiencing palpitations, skipped beats, pounding heartbeats, or a fluttering in the chest. These symptoms are often frightening but in most cases not serious. What is important when it comes to an arrhythmia is to understand why it happens in the first place.

Arrhythmias happen when the heart's natural pacemaker (called the *sinus node*) becomes accelerated by caffeine, chocolate, alcohol, tobacco, a decongestant, stress, or a medical condition such as thyroid disease. The heart's pacemaker may also slow down because of medical conditions such as hypothyroidism. In general, these arrhythmias resolve when the trigger (condition or substance) is removed.

Sometimes the heartbeat is altered because of an underlying abnormality to the heart muscle, as in a heart attack or with heart valve problems. High blood pressure or reduced heart function may also result in arrhythmia.

WHO'S AT RISK?

Arrhythmias may occur at any age, but they are commonly experienced at certain ages, which is how I've grouped them here. Keep in mind that the severity of an arrhythmia is determined by the symptoms and the underlying heart function.

AT ANY AGE

Sinus tachycardia. With tachycardia, you feel a rapid heart rate. It
  happens because the sinus node sends out electrical signals faster
  than normal. Sometimes this is appropriate, as in exercise or in
  response to infection or fear. Sinus tachycardia can happen at

any age as a result of caffeine, medications, or chocolate. Sometimes it is a clue to the presence of thyroid disease, lung disease, or reduced heart muscle function.

Sinus bradycardia. Sinus bradycardia is defined as a heart rate of less than 60 beats per minute. This slow heartbeat may be the normal pulse of a very fit person, or it may indicate a sluggish thyroid gland or be due to medications. A person with this condition may have no symptoms at all. If you are symptomatic and experience dizziness or feel faint, then you may need treatment.

UNDER AGE FORTY

Premature supraventricular contractions or premature atrial contractions. In these conditions, a beat, occurring in the atria (upper heart chambers), causes your heart to beat early—before the next regular heartbeat. They are more common as you get older, and if they occur occasionally without symptoms in a woman with normal heart function, they may not be serious. If they occur frequently and are associated with dizziness, light-headedness, or fainting, your doctor must check them out.

Supraventricular tachycardia and paroxysmal supraventricular tachycardia. This series of rapid, early beats in the atria speed up the heart rate. In paroxysmal supraventricula tachycardia, repeated periods of very fast heartbeats begin and end suddenly.

Wolff-Parkinson-White syndrome (WPW). In this condition, accessory pathways between the atria and the ventricles cause the electrical signal to bypass the normal route and arrive at the ventricles too soon and to be transmitted back into the atria. As the electrical signal ricochets between the atria and ventricles, very fast heart rates may develop. If you have WPW and experience rapid heartbeats, shortness of breath, and fainting, you should be evaluated immediately. The treatment of choice is radiofrequency ablation, which eliminates the accessory conductive tissue.

Premature ventricular contractions. In this condition, an electrical signal from the ventricles causes an early heartbeat that generally goes unnoticed. The heart then seems to pause until the next beat of the ventricle occurs in a regular fashion. The strong beat that is felt is the normal beat after the pause.

AGES FORTY TO FIFTY

Premature ventricular contractions

Premature supraventricular contractions or premature atrial contractions

Supraventricular tachycardia

AGES FIFTY AND UP

Sick sinus syndrome. With this arrhythmia, you experience a group of abnormal heartbeats that are thought to be caused by a malfunction of the sinus node, the heart's "natural" pacemaker. Although the syndrome is slowly progressive, you may stay asymptomatic and need no treatment. In some cases, a pacemaker is used to assist cardiac function.

Atrial fibrillation. In this arrhythmia, electrical signals in the atria are fired rapidly and irregularly, resulting in a completely irregular heart rate. Atrial fibrillation more commonly occurs in older women who have a history of high blood pressure, coronary artery disease, congestive heart failure, or thyroid disease. Unfortunately, women have a worse outcome after treatment than men. We don't understand why. Although less common, it may occur in younger women, particularly those who have *Wolff-Parkinson-White syndrome* or are heavy alcohol drinkers. (For more on atrial fibrillation, see page 366.)

Ventricular tachycardia. In this condition, the heart beats fast due to electrical signals arising from the ventricles (rather than from the atria). This arrhythmia is most common in women with heart disease. It may occur in the first few hours of a heart attack or several days afterward. The treatment depends on a woman's symptoms and the amount of heart muscle damage she has had from her heart attack. (For more on ventricular tachycardia, see page 367.)

Ventricular fibrillation. In this condition, electrical signals in the ventricles are fired in a very fast and uncontrolled manner, causing the heart to quiver rather than beat and pump blood. This arrhythmia is associated with sudden death, requiring quick action with an electrical shock to recover a normal heartbeat. It is most common in women who have heart disease.

THE DOCTOR'S QUESTIONS

Your doctor's questions will focus on the actual symptoms and potential underlying cause of your arrhythmias. Questions may include:

1. How frequently do you have the palpitations? Daily? Weekly? Monthly?
2. Are you dizzy or light-headed?
3. Did you faint when you had the palpitations?
4. Do the symptoms occur with exertion?
5. Do you have heart disease?
6. Have you had a heart attack?
7. Do you have a history of heart murmur?
8. Are you taking over-the-counter cold medications? If so, what are the ingredients?
9. How much caffeine and chocolate do you ingest?
10. Are you under stress?

TESTS YOU MAY NEED

An ECG is the first test used to get a baseline evaluation of your heart rhythm. If it is done at the time of the arrhythmia, your doctor can see the arrhythmia and determine where it occurs: in the atria (meaning it is atrial or supraventricular, "above the ventricles") or in the ventricles (meaning it is ventricular). Ventricular arrhythmias are more serious, especially if caused by heart disease.

If the ECG does not give the answer, a Holter monitor may be used, a twenty-four-hour recording of the heart rhythm. Because arrhythmias do not always show up on a daily basis, I prefer the event recorder to the Holter monitor. This diagnostic test records the arrhythmia for a longer time, which increases the ability to make a proper diagnosis. In fact, a host of studies confirm that event recorders are more beneficial than Holter monitors in diagnosing arrhythmias.[1]

An echocardiogram may be done to evaluate your heart muscle or valve function as a potential cause of the arrhythmia. Finally, your doctor may do a stress test to see if your arrhythmia is provoked by exercise.

OTHER POSSIBLE DIAGNOSES

Sometimes the symptoms of arrhythmias are similar to the symptoms of heart attack or stroke. For that reason, a thorough and accurate diagnosis is most important.

YOUR ACTION PLAN

Depending on the nature and cause of your arrhythmia, treatment may be as simple as eliminating an offending food, such as caffeine or alcohol, or stopping a certain medication that is triggering the irregular beat. In more serious cases, a medication or invasive procedure may be used to control or eliminate the arrhythmia.

When your heart rate is extremely high, the heart muscle becomes overworked and inefficient in pumping blood. This problem can result in fainting, shortness of breath, or even heart failure. Your doctor may prescribe a medication (see pages 365–367) to prevent rapid heartbeats and overwork of the heart muscle.

Other treatments may include cardioversion, an electrical shock to the heart to regulate the rhythm. This treatment is used for ventricular tachycardia, ventricular fibrillation, and atrial fibrillation. Sometimes medications are used to convert atrial fibrillation to regular rhythm and then maintain regular rhythm. In addition, blood thinners are used to prevent stroke in atrial fibrillation. For those people who have life-threatening ventricular arrhythmias, such as ventricular fibrillation or ventricular tachycardia, implanted defibrillators are used. This treatment detects abnormal rhythms and sends an electric shock when they occur.

In women who have very slow heart rates associated with symptoms of shortness of breath, weakness, or fainting, pacemakers are used to maintain a normal heartbeat. A pacemaker is implanted under the skin and sends signals to your heart, should your heartbeat become so slow that it is ineffective for pumping and the electrical signals do not work correctly.

Radiofrequency ablation is a procedure that may be considered for supraventricular tachycardia or Wolff-Parkinson-White syndrome. This procedure (discussed in Chapter 16) may be used to eliminate the heart tissue causing the arrhythmia.

Blood Vessel Diseases

Blood vessel diseases, including hypertension and stroke, are very common. These diseases are also highly preventable and treatable using the lifestyle measures outlined in Part III, along with medications if needed.

High Blood Pressure, or Hypertension

When Monique was referred to me by her primary care physician, she was frightened when I said she needed immediate treatment for her high blood pressure. While this thirty-six-year-old African American woman was a little overweight, she was very active, working full time as a law school professor while raising two small children. She even went to the gym twice a week with several colleagues to use the weight machines. Still, at 170/100, her blood pressure was rising near the danger zone, which mandated treatment.

After taking Monique's family history, I learned that both her mother and grandmother had had heart attacks before age sixty and that her older sister, age forty-four, had a history of diabetes, angina, and hypertension. Not only do African American women get hypertension at younger ages, they have an increased risk of getting stage 3 hypertension (greater than 180/110).

Monique realized the seriousness of the problem and wanted to avoid having an early heart attack, like her mother and grandmother. After beginning blood pressure medication and a daily exercise program, along with a healthy low-fat diet, Monique's blood pressure had dropped within normal limits (130/85) by the time she returned in three months.

SIGNS AND SYMPTOMS

While some people with high blood pressure have symptoms such as headache, dizziness, shortness of breath, nausea (vomiting), or the warning signs of stroke (see page 142), in most cases there are no symptoms at all. In fact, Monique did not know her blood pressure was high until she saw her primary care physician for treatment of bronchitis. This silent killer does its damage in complete silence.

High blood pressure prematurely ages blood vessels, making them stiff and inflexible, which results in higher pressure in the vessels. Hypertension stimulates atherosclerosis, increasing the risk of heart attack, stroke, and kidney disease from the buildup of plaque in the arteries that carry blood to the heart muscle, brain, and kidney.

WHAT IS HYPERTENSION?
High blood pressure is a blood pressure reading of 140/90 or higher. It is categorized as either *primary* (essential) or *secondary*. Primary hypertension has no underlying cause. More than 20 percent of those with hypertension have secondary hypertension, which may be caused by medications (such as cold preparations) or other medical conditions (such as kidney disease, obesity, or endocrine conditions).

Normal blood pressure	less than 130/85
Optimal blood pressure for heart health	120/80

WHO'S AT RISK?
High blood pressure is common among women at midlife and affects more than half of women over the age of forty-five in the United States. Women of this age commonly have the following risk factors:

- Obesity
- Diabetes
- Sedentary lifestyle
- Stress
- Alcohol excess
- High dietary intake of salt

The risk for hypertension increases as you get older, and African American and Hispanic women have an increased risk. African American women living in the United States have the highest prevalence of high blood pressure in the world, a fact that they must take very seriously. Not only does high blood pressure develop at an earlier age in African Americans (in their mid-thirties), they also have a higher prevalence and a greater rate of stage 3 hypertension (blood pressure higher than 180/110). Compared with whites, African Americans are 1.8 times more likely to have a fatal stroke, 1.5 times more likely to have heart disease death, and 4.2 times more likely to have hypertension-related kidney disease.

Except for age and race, the risk factors are all within your control, meaning you can choose to make lifestyle changes to stop the damage of hypertension before it is serious. If left untreated, high blood pressure greatly increases your risk for heart attack, stroke, kidney disease, and heart failure.

THE DOCTOR'S QUESTIONS

Your doctor will start the diagnostic process by taking your medical history, asking such questions as:

1. Do you have a history of high blood pressure?
2. How long have you had high blood pressure?
3. Do you have a family history of high blood pressure?
4. Do you have headaches, dizziness, or shortness of breath?
5. Do you have a history of stroke?
6. Have you started on any new medications?
7. Do you have a history of diabetes, heart attack, elevated cholesterol, smoking, weight gain, or swollen legs or ankles?
8. Are you physically active?
9. What are your stressors?

TESTS YOU MAY NEED

Of all the types of heart disease, high blood pressure is the easiest to diagnose, using a simple blood pressure check (see page 177–179). If your blood pressure has been elevated for a while, your doctor may order tests to see if it has caused problems to other major organs. They include blood tests to check your electrolytes and two tests of kidney function: blood urea nitrogen (BUN) and creatinine. A urinalysis is also done to evaluate the presence of protein, which is seen in kidney damage due to high blood pressure and diabetes. Because the heart muscle can thicken in response to the high blood pressure, an echocardiogram may be taken to check for heart function and heart wall thickness. When blood pressure goes untreated, the heart can no longer compensate and muscle function diminishes, resulting in heart failure.

Additional testing, such as a magnetic resonance angiography (see page 196) or a sonogram of the kidneys, may be done to evaluate for other causes of hypertension.

OTHER POSSIBLE DIAGNOSES

Although most women with high blood pressure have *essential* hypertension (high blood pressure with no known cause), some conditions may cause high blood pressure, including:

- Kidney disease
- Oral contraceptive use
- Gestation (blood pressure may improve after pregnancy)

A thorough medical evaluation is important to get to the cause, if any, of your hypertension. Then the condition can be effectively treated so you do not have complications later on.

YOUR ACTION PLAN

The first goal of treating hypertension is to avoid it; don't get to the point where you have symptoms. While some lifestyle changes, such as losing weight, regular exercise, following a low-salt diet, stopping cigarette smoking, and reducing stress can help to reduce blood pressure, medications may be needed. Some commonly used medications to treat hypertension include diuretics, ACE inhibitors, and beta-blockers (see Chapter 14). Get your blood pressure checked regularly.

Control of mild and moderate hypertension (see page 178) with lifestyle changes or medication lowers the risk of coronary heart disease and stroke. Long-term control of hypertension may lower overall coronary disease by 25 percent and stoke by nearly 40 percent.

If you have severe hypertension or a hypertensive emergency, which happens when you have a severe elevation of blood pressure along with headache, vomiting, visual impairment, or other symptoms of a stroke, you will need to be hospitalized for treatment. At that time, your doctor will evaluate to see if you had a stroke and will treat your hypertension with medications under close monitoring.

Stroke

Sixty-eight-year-old Louise knew something was wrong when she suddenly felt dizzy and had to sit down quickly for fear of falling. She was watching her grandchildren swim in her club's pool when everything started spinning. Luckily, some friends sat with her while her grandson called 911. Medical help came within minutes. Louise was diagnosed and spent several days in the hospital for tests. She went to a rehabilitation center for three weeks to work on some muscle weakness on her left side and now continues to lead a very active life.

Preventing a stroke from ever happening in the first place should be your overriding goal. If you've had one stroke, it's more important than ever to take charge of key risk factors to prevent a second. You can easily start to control your blood pressure, put a stop to smoking cigarettes, cut back or stop alcohol use, and start walking. Research confirms that women who walk regularly three or more times each week had a reduced risk of heart attack and stroke.

SIGNS AND SYMPTOMS

As with a heart attack, certain signs or feelings may alert you or a loved one that a stroke is happening. Some of these include a sudden numbness or weakness of the face, arm, or leg, usually localized to one side of the body. For example, your left hand, arm, and side of your face may feel tingling or numb, while your right side feels normal. You may have difficulty speaking (aphasia) or understanding what is being said, or you could feel totally confused. Other symptoms of stroke include:

- Sudden difficulty in seeing out of one or both eyes
- Sudden difficulty in walking, loss of balance, lack of coordination
- Sudden dizziness

- Sudden severe headache with no known cause
- Problems with memory and emotions
- Difficulty swallowing (dysphagia)

WHAT IS STROKE?

Stroke, a common form of cardiovascular disease, is blood vessel disease in the brain. It may be caused by a plaque rupture in an atherosclerotic artery to the brain, or by hemorrhage of a brain blood vessel, or by obstruction of a brain blood vessel by a clot.

Some physicians refer to stroke as a brain attack (as opposed to a heart attack). An obstruction in the brain can affect you in myriad ways, depending on the type of stroke, the area of the brain affected, and the extent of the brain injury. The attack or injury can affect your senses, motor activity, and ability to understand speech.

Almost 80 percent of all strokes are *ischemic*, which means that they happen with the rupture of plaque, much as a heart attack is triggered. A clot obstructs blood flow to an area of brain, resulting in damage to brain tissue. With an *embolic stroke*, a piece of clot (embolism) forms in a blood vessel away from the brain or in a heart chamber. This clot breaks off, travels through the bloodstream, and lodges into a blood vessel in the brain. Atrial fibrillation, an irregular rhythm that originates in the heart's upper chambers and impairs the normal emptying of blood from the atria to the ventricles (see page 135), may cause this type of stroke.

An *aneurysm* is a pouch filled with blood in a weakened area in the arterial wall. In a *hemorrhagic stroke*, an aneurysm bursts in the brain and the blood leaks around the brain tissue, impeding and damaging it. This results in an inability to think, speak, or move, depending on where the stroke occurred. Hypertension can worsen an aneurysm, or even cause one to burst.

WHO'S AT RISK?

The common risk factors for stroke include:

- High blood pressure
- Smoking

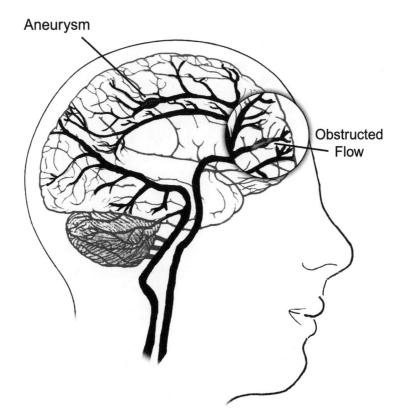

Aneurysm

Obstructed
Flow

Figure 6.3
Arteries of the Brain

- Elevated cholesterol
- Diabetes
- Sedentary lifestyle
- Family history
- Atrial fibrillation

THE DOCTOR'S QUESTIONS

Your doctor will ask questions about symptoms you may feel, your personal risk factors for stroke, and any medical condition that may predispose you to having a stroke. In many cases, family members will be answering these questions for you. Some possible questions include:

1. What risk factors do you have for stroke?
2. Have you experienced any dizziness? Headache? Inability to speak? Weakness in arms or legs?
3. Did you faint?
4. Do you have palpitations or a history of irregular heartbeat?
5. When did your symptoms start? How long did they last?

TESTS YOU MAY NEED

Your doctor will run tests to evaluate how much damage occurred during the stroke, as well as risk factors or conditions that predisposed you to a stroke. One test used to detect stroke damage is the CT scan, which can localize areas of brain infarction and identify hemorrhage. A carotid Doppler (see page 195) is used to take an ultrasound of the carotid arteries (the arteries on the right and left sides of your neck that lead to the brain). The carotid Doppler will help your doctor identify areas of narrowing where plaque rupture may have occurred. Magnetic resonance angiography (MRA) may be ordered; this test uses powerful magnets to provide images of the blood vessels of the brain and the carotid arteries (see page 195).

If your doctor finds you had an embolic stroke, an ECG may be used to evaluate whether you have atrial fibrillation. An echocardiogram is used to evaluate the presence of clots in the heart chambers or assess communication between the right and left sides of your heart. If the atrial fibrillation comes and goes (called *paroxysmal atrial fibrilliation*), a Holter monitor or event recorder is used to evaluate the heart rhythm.

OTHER POSSIBLE DIAGNOSES

Your doctor may find that you had a *transient ischemic attack* (TIA), which is a small stroke or ministroke. In some cases, a TIA precedes a stroke. In fact, of the people who have had one or more TIAs, more than a third will later go on to have a stroke.

A TIA is therefore a warning sign or predictor of stroke. It may have the same symptoms as a stroke, but they last only a few minutes or a few hours, then the symptoms resolve. If you have a TIA, do not ignore it—get help immediately.

With a TIA, your doctor will evaluate your arteries using a carotid Doppler or three-dimensional carotid MRA. If you are symptomatic and have carotid obstruction greater than 60 percent, you may be referred for surgery called *carotid endarterectomy*, during which plaque is surgically removed from the carotid artery. New techniques, such as carotid stents, are also used. One of the risks of surgery, however, is that more plaque could be knocked loose and cause a stroke. This risk is reduced if you have the surgery in a hospital where this procedure is frequently performed.

YOUR ACTION PLAN

Because the cause of stroke may vary, the treatment will be just as varied. That's why an accurate diagnosis is crucial to determine if you did have a stroke and what actual damage it created. *If you presently have stroke symptoms, your action plan should be to seek immediate medical attention.* If the stroke is caused by a blood clot, your doctor will immediately administer a clot-busting drug (tissue plasminogen activator, or TPA) to restore blood flow. In order for TPA to be effective, you must be treated within three hours of the start of symptoms. TPA is not used for hemorrhagic stroke. Other medications may include cholesterol-lowering drugs, aspirin or other blood thinners, and blood pressure medications. One study has shown that women are less likely to get blood-thinning medications after stroke when compared to men.[2]

If atrial fibrillation is diagnosed, a blood thinner, such as heparin or Coumadin, is routinely used. Other drugs to restore regular heart rhythm (see pages 365–367) may also be prescribed.

With stroke as with any chronic illness, family support and caregiver counseling are extremely important to your health and your family's health. If your doctor has recommended stroke rehabilitation, take advantage of it. A trained medical therapist can help you relearn how to use parts of your body that were weakened by the stroke. You will also learn how to manage your lifestyle to avoid any more problems.

Valvular Heart Disease

Valvular heart disease occurs when the heart valve does not close completely, resulting in backward leakage of blood (regurgitation), or when the valve is narrowed, so blood flow is impeded (stenosis), or both. Upon listening to your heart, your doctor may first hear the condition as a murmur. Heart murmurs are sounds, heard from the stethoscope, that are different from the normal closing sounds of the left- and right-side heart valves.

Although Jessica, age twenty-eight, experienced heart palpitations almost daily for five months, she was afraid to get them checked out. When she reached the point that she thought she could be having a heart attack, this young mother of eighteen-month-old twins came to see me.

Faulty Valves Make Your Heart Work Overtime

Normal heart valves are smooth and thin. But when valves become scarred and thick from infections or aging, they may be unable to open and close properly. Then your heart is forced to work harder to pump blood throughout the body. Over time, this can weaken your heart and cause symptoms such as leg swelling and shortness of breath.

During the examination, Jessica described the palpitations as short bouts of her heart racing. She felt them most when she was lying in bed perfectly still. Listening to her heart, I identified the murmur of mitral valve prolapse (MVP; see below). Her ECG showed a normal heart rhythm, but the event recorder showed rare premature atrial contractions. An echocardiogram of her heart confirmed the diagnosis of mitral valve prolapse, with minimal back flow or regurgitation of blood.

I explained to Jessica that the racing pulse she experienced is often associated with mitral valve prolapse. This congenital condition was not new and had been present her entire life. After the consultation Jessica was relieved that she wasn't having a heart attack. Her prescription was to lessen her symptoms with aerobic exercise, a healthy diet, and other preventive lifestyle choices.

In my practice, I consult with many women who have mitral valve prolapse. Before they understand their condition, they often become anxious when they experience these palpitations and are convinced that they have a serious heart disease. Yet once they understand the facts about MVP, they are able to move forward with active, normal lives.

Mitral Valve Prolapse

SIGNS AND SYMPTOMS

In most cases, no symptoms will alert you to the fact that you have mitral valve prolapse. Some women experience chest discomfort, fatigue, anxiety, difficulty in breathing, and palpitations or abnormal heartbeats. Your doctor may first hear the murmur during a checkup, as the abnormal motion of the valve causes a clicking sound.

Keep in mind that symptoms alone do not clinch the diagnosis of mitral valve prolapse. Above all, don't assume that you have MVP based solely on reading this section! Each symptom should be evaluated individually. For example, palpitations may be caused by an arrhythmia, while chest discomfort and shortness of breath, as you know, can be early warning signs of a heart attack. The only sure way to secure an accurate diagnosis is to have specific tests done.

WHAT IS MITRAL VALVE PROLAPSE?

Mitral valve prolapse, a disease of one of the heart valves, is often an inherited problem. Like all heart valves, the mitral valve is a one-way passage. In normal circumstances, the mitral valve closes to prevent blood from flowing backward into the left atrium (the upper left heart chamber) while the heart is ejecting blood out of the aortic valve. In MVP, one of the leaflets of the valve billows backward into the left atrium, allowing some blood to flow back, or regurgitate into the left atrium. This regurgitation happens at a time when the blood is supposed to be moving forward. In MVP, the mitral valve leaflets are thickened, a result of the proliferation or overgrowth of tissue.

For the majority of women, this congenital condition (existing since birth) is benign and is associated with a normal life expectancy. The more serious complications of mitral valve prolapse—arrhythmia, heart failure, and stroke—are seen in some situations with severe mitral regurgitation and thickening of the heart valve. Men over fifty are more likely to have complications of MVP.

WHO'S AT RISK?

After the original description of mitral valve prolapse was published more than three decades ago, it was thought to be the most common form of valvular heart disease—and even more common in women. Experts believed that MVP was found in 5 to 10 percent of the population, with women outnumbering men by two to one. A few years ago, however, this statistic was questioned by the Framingham Heart Study,[3] which found the prevalence of mitral valve prolapse to be only 2.4 percent—not the documented 5 to 10 percent. Why the discrepancy? One reason is that the earlier research had studied only people who already had symptomatic disease. Another explanation is that at the time the data was collected, our techniques to image the valve were not as accurate as they are today. Interestingly, men over fifty with MVP are more likely to have complications than women.

THE DOCTOR'S QUESTIONS

1. Do you have a history of a heart murmur?
2. Do you have a family history of MVP?
3. Do you experience palpitations?
4. Do you have chest discomfort or shortness of breath?

TESTS YOU MAY NEED

During a thorough physical examination, your doctor will listen for a heart murmur. If mitral valve prolapse is suspected, your doctor may order an echocardiogram. These tests check heart and valve function and evaluate the amount of blood regurgitation. Determining the degree of thickening of the valve and the amount of regurgitation allows your doctor to know how serious the condition is and if any further steps need to be taken.

The echocardiogram clinches the diagnosis. Other tests that may be used to evaluate associated symptoms include an ECG, a Holter monitor, and a stress test.

OTHER POSSIBLE DIAGNOSES

If you are experiencing chest pain, an exercise echocardiogram may be used to evaluate the possible causes. If you have shortness of breath or fatigue on exertion, it may indicate a moderate to severe leakage of the heart valve. The exercise echocardiogram will be able to distinguish between valvular heart disease and coronary artery disease.

Amelia, age thirty-one, came to see me when she became breathless while walking up a flight of stairs and could no longer vacuum her house. This young mother of three told of having a rapid heartbeat almost daily. When I examined her, I found that her heart murmur was caused by a severe leakage of the valve. An echocardiogram confirmed the leakage. Her heart muscle function was normal (a good sign). Amelia had surgery to repair the mitral valve prolapse, and she now walks and vacuums and has no trouble running after her three small children.

YOUR ACTION PLAN

Treatments for MVP vary depending on how much the valve leaks and on the associated symptoms. If you have documented MVP (that is, it is seen on the echocardiogram), antibiotic therapy may be required whenever you undergo certain medical procedures, such as dental work (including cleanings), colonoscopy, or some gynecological procedures. This therapy, called *antibiotic prophylaxis*, will help prevent endocarditis, or infection of the valve. If you have mitral valve prolapse with severe mitral regurgitation or shortness of breath, your doctor may do further testing to see if you need valve repair or replacement.

Palpitations and Mitral Valve Prolapse

Arrhythmias caused by mitral valve prolapse vary according to type and frequency; some increase with exercise, and some are associated with symptoms such as lightheadedness or fainting. In my experience, arrhythmias sometimes occur less frequently with regular aerobic exercise, perhaps because the exercise reduces the norepinephrine circulating in the body, resulting in a lower pulse rate and lower blood pressure. The evaluation of palpitations in the presence of mitral valve prolapse is similar to those outlined on page 136.

Mitral Stenosis

Fifty-nine-year-old Susan first noticed shortness of breath when she was riding her bike to the park with her two grandsons. At first she thought the cause was that she was out of shape, being ten pounds overweight and working as a legal secretary for the past decade. But one night when she started having palpitations while watching television with her husband, she knew something more serious was going on.

One of Susan's friends in my Women's Heart Program suggested that she see me, and Susan immediately made an appointment.

While we were talking about her health history, Susan said that she had had rheumatic fever as a young child. Then during the physical examination, I detected a heart murmur, an indication that she might have heart problems. I ordered an echocardiogram, and the results confirmed that an abnormal valve, or mitral stenosis, was restricting blood flow in the heart. Rheumatic fever is one cause of this heart disease.

SIGNS AND SYMPTOMS
Symptoms of mitral stenosis include shortness of breath, fatigue, palpitations, irregular heartbeat, and swelling of the ankles or legs.

WHAT IS MITRAL STENOSIS?
Mitral stenosis is a narrow mitral valve that restricts blood flow from the left atrium to the left ventricle. It is an uncommon valve abnormality because the usual cause is rheumatic fever, which is not regularly seen.

WHO'S AT RISK?
Women who are at greatest risk of mitral stenosis are those who have a history of rheumatic fever.

THE DOCTOR'S QUESTIONS
At the consultation, your doctor may ask you the following questions to get an accurate diagnosis:

1. Are you experiencing unusual fatigue on exertion?
2. Do you have any shortness of breath?
3. Do you have a history of rheumatic fever?
4. Do you have a history of palpitations?
5. Do you have a history of a heart murmur?

TESTS YOU MAY NEED
During the physical examination, your doctor will listen for a heart murmur. An echocardiogram will be used to further determine the extent of the valve damage. Other tests commonly used include an ECG, a Holter monitor, and an event recorder.

OTHER POSSIBLE DIAGNOSES

Anyone who has heart valve problems such as mitral valve prolapse, mitral stenosis, aortic stenosis, or certain congenital defects is at increased risk for endocarditis. Endocarditis is an infection of the heart valves. Symptoms of endocarditis include fever, chills, and sweating. To diagnose the condition, your doctor will perform an echocardiogram to confirm the heart murmur, and draw blood to culture for infection. The culture will let your doctor see the growth of bacteria and inflammatory cells on the valve (known as vegetation). In some cases of endocarditis, a transesophageal echocardiogram (see page 186) is performed, to give your doctor a better view of the small growths on the heart valves.

YOUR ACTION PLAN

Treatment for mitral stenosis varies, depending on the severity of the problem and symptoms. If you have mitral stenosis, your doctor will prescribe antibiotic prophylaxis (see page 151) to use when you undergo certain medical procedures. You may be given medications to slow your heart rate and return you to normal rhythm (see Chapter 14). Blood thinners are used to prevent stroke. In cases of moderate to severe mitral stenosis with symptoms, you may require mitral valve replacement.

Aortic Stenosis

Mona's story is one I've shared with many of my patients. Not only does it detail the serious nature of a particular valvular disease, especially with older women; it also shows how a proper diagnosis and medical treatment can resolve a problem and give women back their quality of life.

Mona, a sixty-five-year-old grandmother, was referred to me by her ophthalmologist after she had lost her vision in her right eye because of cholesterol obstructing the blood vessel to that eye. Mona saw a cardiologist two years before she saw the ophthalmologist or he referred her to me. She did not tell the ophthalmologist that she had previously seen a cardiologist for a heart valve problem. After asking her question upon question, I eventually found out that for the last two to three weeks, Mona had experienced left arm discomfort while walking up the subway stairs. The symptoms were relieved when she rested, and they never occurred while she was walking on the sidewalk or while watching television. She had had a hysterectomy fifteen years earlier and was on Premarin. While Mona had smoked for approximately thirty years, she had quit three years earlier. From her personal history, it appeared that Mona had had an early warning sign of a heart attack.

Mona had a definite heart murmur that indicated that she had the valve problem called aortic stenosis (AS). She had a bruise above her right eye, and when I asked her about the injury, Mona said she had tripped. I specifically asked if she had fainted (a common symptom in severe aortic stenosis), but she said no.

To make an accurate diagnosis, the first step was to confirm whether Mona had severe aortic stenosis, coronary artery disease, or both. The usual procedure of diagnosing coronary artery disease with a stress test was too dangerous. Severe aortic stenosis contraindicates a stress test, as exercise could result in sudden death. Instead, we started with an echocardiogram, which is the best test for looking at the heart valves. Mona's echocardiogram showed that her aortic valve was so calcified that it barely opened, and her ECG indicated that her heart muscle was thickened. With asymptomatic AS, regular follow-up and monitoring by the physician, along with echocardiography, are standard treatment. But severe aortic stenosis like Mona's requires prompt treatment. In fact, if her valve were not replaced within five years of the onset of her symptoms, she would most likely die. (If she had been fainting, the chances were great that she would be dead within three years if the valve were not replaced.)

Mona's personal history and the test results made it clear that she had to be admitted to the hospital to have her valve replaced. She underwent an angiogram, which showed normal coronary arteries, so the only operation she needed was an aortic valve replacement. In less than one week after her valve replacement, Mona was discharged from the hospital, and in just three weeks, she was back to her normal daily activities.

SIGNS AND SYMPTOMS

Because obstruction of the aortic valve impedes blood flow out of the left ventricle, women with severe aortic stenosis may experience angina, chest discomfort, fatigue, shortness of breath, heart failure, or fainting (*syncope* is the medical word for fainting).

WHAT IS AORTIC STENOSIS?

Aortic stenosis is a condition that happens when the aortic valve is thickened and narrowed, leading to the development of abnormally high pressure in the left ventricle. The left ventricular wall becomes thickened as well. When the aortic valve becomes diseased over time, the leaflets thicken and the valve becomes calcified. When this happens, the body's organs (including the brain) receive an insufficient supply of oxygen-rich blood, because the narrowed valve is keeping it from getting out of the heart to these vital organs.

In the United States, calcified valvular disease is the most common cause of AS. More than 25 percent of adults over the age of sixty-five have calcified valves, with a significant obstruction occurring in 1 to 2 percent of these.

WHO'S AT RISK?

While rheumatic fever used to be a common cause of aortic stenosis, today the most common cause is age-associated degeneration and calcification of the aortic valve. This usually leads to symptoms in the seventies and eighties.

THE DOCTOR'S QUESTIONS

Your doctor will ask questions such as the following during the examination:

1. Do you have chest discomfort?
2. Do you have shortness of breath?
3. Have you ever fainted?
4. Do you have a history of a heart murmur?

TESTS YOU MAY NEED

Your doctor will do an echocardiogram to check the function of the aortic valve and heart muscle. The results of this test may lead to an angiogram, depending on the severity of the disease, to evaluate for coexisting coronary artery disease.

OTHER POSSIBLE DIAGNOSES

Coronary artery disease is another possible diagnosis: its symptoms mimic those of aortic stenosis, and it can coexist with aortic stenosis.

YOUR ACTION PLAN

Valve replacement is the treatment for aortic stenosis. This operation has a 95 percent success rate in patients with normal heart function and no coronary artery disease. In mild or moderate AS with no symptoms, antibiotic prophylaxis is given prior to certain procedures (see page 151), and periodic follow-up with the doctor is recommended. Serial echocardiograms may be done, as indicated. If you have no symptoms at the diagnosis but later develop symptoms, your condition may be worsening. See your doctor for an evaluation.

Aortic Regurgitation

SIGNS AND SYMPTOMS

With moderate to severe aortic regurgitation, you may feel shortness of breath or fatigue upon exertion, or you may have heart failure.

WHAT IS AORTIC REGURGITATION?

Aortic regurgitation is a leaky aortic valve, where the blood flows backward into the left ventricle and is then pumped out. Sometimes it occurs with an enlargement of the aortic root (the place where the aortic valve is attached) because of chronic hypertension or connective tissue diseases such as Marfan's syndrome.

WHO'S AT RISK?

You may be at risk for aortic regurgitation if you have had rheumatic fever, a congenital bicuspid aortic valve, endocarditis, aortic stenosis, or hypertension.

THE DOCTOR'S QUESTIONS

During the examination, your doctor will ask questions to see if you've experienced:

- Shortness of breath
- Fatigue
- Chest discomfort
- Difficulty sleeping flat on your back
- Swelling in your ankles or legs
- High blood pressure or diabetes
- History of heart murmur
- Palpitations or rapid or irregular heartbeats
- Fainting

TESTS YOU MAY NEED

If you have no symptoms and the disease is mild to moderate, your doctor will do echocardiography and follow-up periodically. Sometimes an exercise echocardiogram is performed to see if the aortic regurgitation worsens with exercise.

OTHER POSSIBLE DIAGNOSES

Other possible diagnoses include heart failure due to other causes (see page 160).

YOUR ACTION PLAN

If you have severe aortic regurgitation and yet are still asymptomatic, an ACE inhibitor may be prescribed to delay the onset of symptoms. With severe symptoms, a valve replacement may be necessary to resolve the problem. Asymptomatic aortic regurgitation is followed with regular doctor's visits and periodic echocardiograms.

Heart Disease from Diet Drugs

Priscilla came to see me after her gynecologist found that her blood pressure was extremely high, at 165/100. This thirty-one-year-old graduate student was about forty pounds overweight, and her doctor had put her on Meridia (sibutramine), a new diet pill, to help her reduce.

Upon hearing about the drug Priscilla was taking, I explained to her that extreme hypertension is one of its side effects in some women, particularly those who are prone to blood pressure problems. While she had never experienced high blood pressure, she realized the seriousness of this disease.

I took Priscilla off the diet drug and explained the Women's Healthy Heart Program (see Part III). I showed her how to calculate how many calories she needed to take in each day to lose weight and how, by exercising more than half an hour each day, she could speed up her weight loss. But for the time being, Priscilla needed to get her hypertension controlled, so I prescribed a beta-blocker and a diuretic (explained in Chapter 14).

In three months, Priscilla came back for a follow-up visit. She had lost fourteen pounds using the dietary suggestions in Chapter 10, and she was walking almost an hour each day. She was still taking her hypertension medications, and her blood pressure had dropped back into a normal range for her age.

SIGNS AND SYMPTOMS
You may feel shortness of breath and fatigue, depending on the severity of the valve damage. On physical examination, your doctor may hear a heart murmur.

WHAT DIET DRUGS CAUSE HEART DISEASE?
The connection between popular diet drugs and heart disease became much publicized in the late 1990s. In particular, the problematic combination of the diet drugs fenfluramine and phentermine (fen/phen), originally described in 1997 in the *New England Journal of Medicine*, increased serotonin, a hormone that reduces appetite.[4] Yet it is believed that the increased levels of serotonin damaged the mitral and aortic valves, resulting in mitral and aortic regurgitation. Some of the dieters who used fen/phen required valve replacement.

POPULAR WEIGHT LOSS DRUGS AND YOUR HEART

- Fen/phen, the drug combo of fenfluramine and phentermine, is no longer available. The severity of heart disease from fen/phen appears to be related to the duration of time it was used. Many who stopped the drug combo reported an improvement in their symptoms.

- Herbal fen/phen, available at most health food stores, is touted as a "natural" weight loss compound. Be cautious about anything that is said to be natural (see Chapter 11). Herbal fen/phen has the potential to be life-threatening because it contains ephedrine, which may cause arrhythmias and hypertension in those susceptible to these problems. (It does not cause the same type of valvular heart disease as fen/phen.)

- Meridia (sibutramine) is an appetite suppressant intended for those who are obese, with a body mass index greater than or equal to 30, or who have a BMI of 27 and also have diabetes or increased cholesterol. Cholesterol levels improve with the weight loss associated with Meridia. Meridia is said to help you eat less at each meal. If you have untreated high blood pressure, arrhythmia, heart failure, stroke, or coronary artery disease, avoid this drug. It may also greatly increase blood pressure in some who have this tendency.

- Orlistat is another weight loss medication that decreases fat absorption. It does have short-term effectiveness, and its use is not associated with heart or vascular disease. Still, because it decreases fat absorption in the intestines, it is associated with gastrointestinal upset. If you use it, you should have counseling for lifestyle modification—cutting calories and increasing exercise and activity.

WHO'S AT RISK?

If you took the popular diet combination fenfluramine and phentermine (fen/phen), you may be at risk for this heart problem.

THE DOCTOR'S QUESTIONS

1. Did you take this medication?
2. For how long were you taking the medication?

3. Are you now experiencing shortness of breath or fatigue?
4. Do you have palpitations?
5. Have you experienced rapid heartbeat?
6. Do you have any swelling in the ankles or legs?

OTHER POSSIBLE DIAGNOSES

Another type of vascular disease, pulmonary hypertension, was also associated with diet drugs. In this condition, blood vessels in the lung become constricted, resulting in an inability to oxygenate blood properly and subsequent lung damage. Pulmonary hypertension is a rare disease, occurring in one in half a million women over the age of thirty. In women on fen/phen, the incidence of pulmonary hypertension was three times higher.

TESTS YOU MAY NEED

If you have taken fen/phen, see your doctor. An echocardiogram will be done to evaluate any potential damage to your heart valves. If your valve has abnormalities, then before you undergo any invasive procedure, such as dental work, an antibiotic will be prescribed to prevent endocarditis (see page 151).

YOUR ACTION PLAN

Get your heart checked out. If the valves have abnormalities, you may be prescribed antibiotic prophylaxis. Some recent studies show great encouragement in this type of heart disease, as in some women the heart valves improve over time.[5]

Heart Muscle Diseases

Heart Failure

After Eloise, age seventy-one, had been ill for five days with no improvement, she finally called her doctor. She described the flulike symptoms of fatigue, congestion, and chest tightness. But when she told her doctor that she could not sleep lying down because she became extremely breathless and her heart started pounding, she was told to call 911 immediately. Knowing that Eloise had hypertension and was a diabetic, her doctor realized that she could have far more serious problems than the flu.

After being admitted to the hospital and going through a battery of tests, Eloise was diagnosed with systolic heart failure. She was given medications to lower her blood pressure and reduce the fluid buildup in her body. Within a few days, she had stabilized and was released to go home.

SIGNS AND SYMPTOMS

With *systolic heart failure*, heart muscle function is reduced. You may have fatigue on exertion and swelling of the ankles and legs. Fluid may accumulate in your lungs, which causes shortness of breath. You may find it difficult to sleep completely flat because of breathlessness.

The symptoms of *diastolic heart failure* include shortness of breath, chest tightness, and wheezing, which occur in the presence of normal heart function. You may have difficulty breathing when lying flat and may even need to sleep sitting up in a chair. This type of heart failure may be due to coronary artery ischemia, heart attack, diabetes, hypertension, or hypertrophic cardiomyopathy, a condition where the heart muscle is severely thickened.

WHAT IS HEART FAILURE?

As a result of living longer, more and more women may be faced with heart failure, especially those who survive a heart attack. There are two types of heart failure. Systolic heart failure results when reduced heart muscle function makes your heart unable to pump enough blood to your body's organs and tissues. With diastolic heart failure, your heart contracts normally, but when it is relaxed, the pressure inside your heart is higher than it should be. This elevated pressure is transmitted back to the lungs and results in shortness of breath.

WHO'S AT RISK?

Heart failure is the leading hospital discharge diagnosis in women over sixty-five years of age with a six-year mortality rate of 65 percent. High blood pressure is the leading cause of heart failure in the United States. The next leading cause is coronary artery disease.

THE DOCTOR'S QUESTIONS

To make an accurate diagnosis of heart failure, your doctor will ask questions like these:

1. Do you have shortness of breath?
2. Have you experienced fatigue?
3. Can you sleep lying flat on your back? Does this cause breathing discomfort?
4. Do you have swelling in your ankles or legs?
5. Do you have high blood pressure? Diabetes?
6. Have you had a heart attack?
7. Do you have valvular heart disease?
8. Do you have a history of heart murmur?
9. Do you have thyroid disease?
10. Do you have palpitations or rapid or irregular heartbeats?
11. Have you fainted recently?

TESTS YOU MAY NEED

In addition to the findings of the physical examination and the answers to your doctor's questions, further tests will help determine the diagnosis. An echocardiogram will be used to evaluate heart function or valve abnormalities; it can also distinguish between diastolic and systolic heart failure. An ECG may also be used if there are rhythm problems. If your doctor needs further assessment, you may be tested with a Holter monitor or an event recorder.

Other possible tests include a chest X ray and blood tests to check for electrolytes, glucose, and kidney and thyroid function.

OTHER POSSIBLE DIAGNOSES

Heart failure is the result of long-standing and untreated hypertension, untreated valvular heart disease, viral infections to the heart muscle, hypothyroidism, incessant tachycardia, or heart attacks.

YOUR ACTION PLAN
Once your doctor has diagnosed you with heart failure, different medications can be used, depending on the kind of heart failure you have. The best medications for systolic heart failure are the ACE inhibitors, as studies confirm they improve survival.[6] A diuretic may be used to relieve the shortness of breath and reduce the fluid overload. Nitrates are given if the underlying cause is ischemia (shortage of the blood supply to the heart muscle). Other forms of treatment can include:

- Digoxin, to increase the contractility of the heart (used in systolic but not in diastolic heart failure)
- A blood thinner, to reduce stroke if there are clots in the left ventricle or with atrial fibrillation
- A beta-blocker, to reduce levels of circulating adrenaline that are released (in systolic heart failure) or to relax the heart muscle (in diastolic heart failure)
- Exercise, once acute symptoms are resolved

Peripartum Cardiomyopathy

SIGNS AND SYMPTOMS
Signs and symptoms of peripartum cardiomyopathy include shortness of breath and edema.

WHAT IS PERIPARTUM CARDIOMYOPATHY?
Peripartum cardiomyopathy is a form of heart disease that causes heart failure during the last trimester of pregnancy.

WHO'S AT RISK?
Peripartum cardiomyopathy is not common, occurring in one out of every ten thousand pregnancies. But the risk is greater in women over thirty who have had previous pregnancies and in African American women.[7] Women who are pregnant with twins or multiples also have an increased risk.

THE DOCTOR'S QUESTIONS

Your doctor will ask the following:

1. Are you experiencing unusual shortness of breath?
2. Are you fatigued?
3. Are you having heart palpitations?
4. Do you have leg swelling?

TESTS YOU MAY NEED

An echocardiogram is ordered to make this diagnosis.

OTHER POSSIBLE DIAGNOSES

If the problem is not peripartum cardiomyopathy, it might be heart failure due to other conditions discussed in this chapter.

YOUR ACTION PLAN

Treatment includes medications to reduce fluid and regulate the heart rhythm. Within six months after delivery, 50 to 60 percent of women experience a complete recovery. But even if the problem is resolved, there is an increased risk of a recurrence with subsequent pregnancies.

While the various types of heart disease discussed in this chapter are very complex in nature, most are effectively treated with lifestyle changes, medication, or even surgery if necessary. While this book cannot replace a proper and accurate medical diagnosis, it does explain the various ways heart disease manifests itself in the body—the signs and symptoms—as well as how it is diagnosed, treated, and prevented. But it's important to remember that each woman is different. Once your doctor determines what type of heart problem, if any, you have, he or she can prescribe an effective medical and lifestyle plan that can resolve your symptoms and prevent further problems.

7

The Women's Healthy Heart Checkup

Over the last two hundred years, we have come a long way in our diagnosis and treatment of heart disease in women, but the majority of medical breakthroughs have been in the last thirty years. It was long considered highly improper for a male doctor to put his ear to the chest of a woman patient, so until a young French physician named René-Théophile-Hyacinthe Laënnec invented the stethoscope in 1819, women probably never received accurate heart exams. Dr. Laënnec rolled up twenty-four pieces of paper into a cylinder shape, then put one end to a patient's chest and the other to his ear. He realized that not only was he able to hear the woman's heartbeat, but the heartbeat was louder and clearer than when heard with an ear to the chest.

I realized just how far we had come from the time of Laënnec the day my patient Sharon's husband said, "So which test will you use first? I want to hurry up and get to the bottom of Sharon's problem."

Sharon, age forty-seven, sat quietly in my office while her husband, the CEO of a large computer software corporation, did not hesitate to offer his advice on testing her for heart disease. Six months earlier Sharon had had a complete evaluation of her heart after having been told, during hospitalization for appendicitis, that she had a leaky heart valve. Before she had a chance to answer my questions and update me on her recent health history, her husband had determined that she definitely needed an ultrafast CT scan, an X ray that looks at the amount of calcium in the arteries. (Calcium tends to be found in larger amounts in older plaques and can signal diseased arteries.)

As I told Sharon and her husband, there is no one test that diagnoses all heart problems. Open discussion between patient and doctor gives clues about tests that will be most helpful in making the correct diagnosis.

Guidelines for Choosing the Best Doctor

Your doctor is your advocate and will tell you what your symptoms mean. He or she may run tests, diagnose you, prescribe proper treatment, and be a dependable source of information for how to deal with the worries and anxieties that accompany any illness.

Get Recommendations from Friends

Your aim is to find a qualified health care professional with whom you feel comfortable sharing your concerns about your health. Some women ask their friends for recommendations, but do check the physician's credentials. You can also call a local hospital for referrals. The combination of insurance and managed care constraints can make it difficult to find the best doctor for you; check the list of doctors who will accept your insurance provider.

Understand Your Personal Preferences

One of the most important steps to take when selecting a doctor is to know yourself, including your personal likes and dislikes. Do you feel more comfortable with a woman or a man? Should your physician be the same age as you, or older, or younger? Do you have a preference about educational background? These questions are important to consider when making your decision.

Another important criterion should be that the doctor's location is convenient for you to reach when coming from home or your place of work.

Narrow the Search

As you go through the process of choosing a physician, try to find answers to the following questions about each candidate.

- Is the doctor board certified or board eligible in cardiology? (Has he or she passed the standard exam in cardiovascular disease given by the American Board of Internal Medicine?)
- Is the doctor involved in any academic pursuits, such as teaching, writing, or research? A doctor who is may be more up to date on the latest developments in the field.
- Where does the doctor have hospital privileges, and where are these hospitals located? Some doctors may not admit patients to certain hospitals, an important consideration for those with chronic health problems.
- Does the doctor accept your particular type of health insurance, or is the doctor a member of the medical panel associated with your HMO?
- What is the demeanor of the doctor's office staff? Are the office hours convenient, considering your work and personal responsibilities? Do they have after-hours coverage, in case of an emergency?

Remember, board certification and diplomas are not the only criteria for making a good selection. You want to be able to trust your health care professional with your life.

Choosing a Cardiologist

Because of managed care, you may wonder whether or not your doctor (a generalist or an internist) is referring you quickly enough to a cardiologist. Many people who see a primary care doctor for heart disease worry a great deal about whether they are getting the right treatment. Some convincing studies suggest that people who see cardiologists for their heart disease are more aggressively treated for elevated cholesterol and are counseled about exercise and diet more than those who see a generalist.[1]

As a rule, if your symptoms are not quickly reversed or managed with medication and lifestyle changes, you should talk with a cardiologist. Especially if you have coexisting illnesses—hypertension, diabetes, insulin resistance, or high cholesterol—that can complicate the management of your heart problem and you are experiencing increasing anxiety or sick days, you should consult with a heart specialist.

REFERRAL TO A CARDIOLOGIST IS BENEFICIAL FOR:

- Women who have had a heart attack, coronary artery bypass surgery, or angioplasty/stent
- Women with symptoms that require further cardiac testing to confirm the diagnosis
- Women with a family history of heart attack, stroke, or sudden death
- Women with high cholesterol or blood pressure
- Women who require a cardiac procedure such as angiography or cardiac surgery
- Women who need an evaluation of arrhythmia
- Women who need an evaluation of heart murmur

A cardiologist specializes in understanding the structure and function of the heart and the cardiovascular system and their specific diseases. There are several kinds of cardiologists, so knowing your cardiologist's area of expertise is important. Different types of cardiologists may work together in a group or heart and vascular institute like the one at Lenox Hill Hospital.

TYPES OF CARDIOLOGISTS

Today most cardiologists are superspecialized because of the groundbreaking techniques and treatments that are available for cardiovascular diseases. Some specific subspecialties include:

NONINVASIVE AND CLINICAL CARDIOLOGISTS. These doctors, of which I am one, focus on the diagnosis, treatment, and prevention of cardiovascular diseases, heart attack, heart failure, hypertension, and high cholesterol. Clinical cardiologists perform diagnostic tests, such as stress testing, echocardiography, exercise echocardiography, and exercise nuclear studies.

INTERVENTIONAL CARDIOLOGISTS. These cardiologists perform coronary angiography and interventional procedures, such as coronary artery angioplasty. They open up clogged coronary arteries with balloons and place stents, and some open up carotid arteries with significant plaque.

ELECTROPHYSIOLOGISTS. These doctors are specially trained in the treatment of arrhythmias. They are trained to put in pacemakers and perform electrophysiology studies, which evaluate the rhythm system of your heart.

THE CARDIOLOGIST AS PATIENT ADVOCATE

It is important to have a noninvasive or clinical cardiologist as your patient advocate. Winona, a thirty-seven-year-old college professor, is a good example of why. This young professional woman had a stent placed in her artery after a heart attack. At her last visit with her interventional cardiologist, he told her, "The artery is open, and you're fine."

But Winona didn't feel fine. During the consultation, she told him that she lived in constant anxiety that the chest discomfort would return again. She wanted to exercise but was paralyzed with fear. Sadly, she felt she could not discuss this with the doctor who had performed her procedure, especially after he had given her a "clean bill of health."

The interventional cardiologist was correct in his assessment— the stent *was* open, and Winona was doing well. But she didn't *feel* that well, and that was a warning sign. She knew that there was more to heart disease than just fixing the plumbing. While her plumbing was in working order, Winona now needed an advocate—a noninvasive or clinical cardiologist whom she could see regularly to assess her heart's health, address risk factors, and help her to move beyond fear into healing and health.

As Winona realized, the cardiologist who placed the stent was vital to her for performing this precarious invasive procedure. Yet now she needed a doctor who was objective and who could monitor her prevention program and make decisions about further treatment or procedures, should symptoms reoccur.

Be Your Own Health Advocate

Even though your doctor is your advocate, you must also become your own health advocate today, especially if you're in a managed care program: the doctor you have today may not be in your program next month. Make sure you keep your own file of medical records. In order to get copies for you *and* your cardiologist, you may need to call the different medical offices or hospitals where you had tests or treatments. Get them before you go in for your appointment with your cardiologist. If an office or hospital asks you why you want a copy of your records, all you need to answer is that you want your own copy. I am astonished at how many women come to see me, seeking a second opinion, without any medical records, not even important test results or evaluations. When I ask them why they didn't bring them, they all say, "I didn't want to offend my doctor." But getting a second opinion is your right as a person! If your doctor gets upset, that's not your problem. Your biggest concern is you—and your health is a priority.

The information you will need to bring to consult a doctor will include the following:

- Reports of ECG and cholesterol tests
- Echocardiogram, Holter monitor, and angiogram reports, if done
- Medical records from any hospitalization

- Records of any past surgeries
- List of current medications, previous medications, and any known allergies to medication or contrast (the dye injected into the arteries during an angiogram)
- List of supplements you are taking

Ask Questions

I met Sarah, age forty-one, after one of my lectures at the 92nd Street Y in Manhattan. Her doctor had scheduled her for a thallium stress test, she said, but the thought of having an intravenous line inserted, even for a short period of time, frightened her. Sarah asked if there were other options for tests she could take. I recommended that she ask her doctor about getting an exercise echocardiogram. Sarah walked away with a sense of relief that she could try something else to diagnose her condition.

If you don't ask, you may not learn about alternatives! At the end of your consultation, ask any questions you may have regarding your health, medications, or lifestyle changes. If your cardiologist recommends a test, medication, or procedure, ask about its benefits, risks, and side effects. Let your doctor know about any fears you may have, and see if there are other healthy alternatives that you may choose.

As a cardiologist today, I am both a partner and a coach to my patients. I am a a cardiac specialist with the tests I order or medications I prescribe, and I am a fitness and nutritional coach with the exercise and diet plan I outline for my patients.

Write Down Your Concerns and Get Answers

Before your appointment with any doctor, write down a list of questions concerning your condition. Bring them, with a pen and a pad of paper, to the appointment. Openly talk about these concerns with your doctor. Write down the responses, so you can refer to them later. If your doctor feels you need special treatment for a condition but it is not covered in your managed care plan, write down your doctor's view. Then call your plan to discuss how you may get that treatment covered.

Sometimes you can appeal to a managed care or insurance company to get special treatment covered. Before you call, write down your questions, and as you ask them, write down the answers you receive. Continue up the chain of authority until you are satisfied that you have spoken with someone who understands your policy.

Get a Second Opinion

While your doctor is the trained professional who fully understands the heart, no one knows your particular body better than you do. Do not be satisfied with the statement "I'm the doctor, and I know best." If you do not feel comfortable with the diagnosis, or if you do not understand what its ramifications are, ask your doctor if more testing is necessary. Or seek a second medical opinion until you feel that your concerns are adequately addressed.

Recently Gloria came to see me for a second opinion on her unremitting chest pain. Gloria had previously been diagnosed with heart disease and had undergone an angioplasty and stent about a year before. Yet even after this procedure, she had daily chest pain. Gloria also smoked and got no exercise, yet she was never referred to a cardiac rehabilitation program. In fact, her doctor told her, simply, "Exercise," without giving her specific instructions. When Gloria had asked him for help with smoking cessation, he looked at her and said, "It's going to be difficult. You just need to suck it up and deal with it."

Can anyone blame Gloria for seeking a second opinion? She realized it was her body and her heart, and that she owed it to herself and her loved ones to find the best answers for treatment and prevention.

To your second evaluation, bring a copy of all your medical records, including all tests and results. Also write down your detailed questions and specific concerns, and bring this list with you to the consultation. Be sure to disclose any unusual symptoms and feelings so that this doctor can better interpret the results of the physical examination and the laboratory testing.

REASONS FOR A SECOND OPINION

- You are unable to communicate with your doctor.
- You need a doctor with specific expertise in one area.
- You need another point of view regarding a surgical or procedural option.
- You do not feel better on current therapy.

Your Checkup Appointment

I ask my patients to write down a list of their concerns ahead of time and bring the list with them for the visit. Many times patients forget to tell me about problems they had in the past or about medications they have taken. Yet to make an accurate diagnosis, I have to know all I can. Before your visit, write down:

- Your health concerns
- Symptoms you've noticed
- Past illnesses and medications
- Your family history of heart disease or other illnesses
- Medications you are taking now; medications you've taken in the past
- Your lifestyle habits (diet, exercise, smoking)
- Causes of stress in your life
- Questions you have about your heart

Some medications or herbs may increase blood pressure or heart rate, so be sure to place all your medications and nutritional supplements in a bag and bring them to your healthy heart checkup. Your doctor will let you know which ones are safe—and which may not be used safely.

The Visual Check

Even if you do not feel any signs or symptoms, your doctor may get an idea of your cardiovascular health by looking and listening.

- *Heart rate and rhythm.* Your doctor can feel your pulse to check your heart rate and rhythm. By checking the pulses in your neck, groin, and feet, then using a stethoscope to check the arteries in the neck for irregular, weak, or abnormal sounds, your doctor may find an obstruction to blood flow.
- *Heart sounds.* Using a stethoscope, your doctor will listen to your heartbeat and check for a murmur, which could indicate abnormal heart valve function.
- *Swelling.* The doctor will examine your legs and ankles for swelling. The medical term for swelling is *edema*, which means an abnormally large amount of fluid between your body's cells. This swelling may occur as a result of heart failure, or kidney or liver disease, or an obstruction in the vein that carries blood to the heart. If your doctor presses your leg or ankle and the skin does not spring back quickly, edema is present.
- *Breath sounds.* With a stethoscope, your doctor will listen to your heart and lungs. Crackling sounds may indicate fluid in the air sacs of the lungs, a possible sign of heart failure.
- *Body color.* Your doctor will notice if you are pale, a possible indicator of anemia or weak blood flow. If you have bluish skin tones (called *cyanosis*), or bluish fingertips or lips, your heart may not be meeting your body's oxygen needs.
- *Eyes.* Your doctor may use a special instrument, called an *ophthalmoscope*, to check the blood vessels in the back of your eyes. The condition of these vessels may indicate the condition of the other blood vessels in your body.

During the examination, your doctor will talk to you about any past or present symptoms or health problems (as explained in Chapter 7). If your doctor doesn't ask the "right" questions, then openly volunteer any helpful information as this may save your life. To avoid serious problems now and later in life, you have to educate yourself about your heart.

Understanding the Healthy Heart Tests

In the rest of this chapter, I want to go over the tests that are normally done on healthy women, as well as some specific tests for diagnosing heart problems. I will explain how and why each test is used—the procedure, what you will feel, the precautions, and the pros and cons. This will help you start to think like a doctor, as you interpret the test results in relation to your physical symptoms. By interpreting test results as fully as possible, your doctors can give you the best diagnosis and the most effective treatment if you need it.

During a consultation, your doctor will look for specific medical problems, such as elevated blood pressure, a rise in blood sugar or cholesterol, or even a heart murmur. These problems can be treated early, before they do damage to your heart. Your doctor may then discuss important changes you can make in your lifestyle, measures that may benefit your heart and overall health.

Because each of my patients is different, to evaluate for heart or blood vessel disease I do not have a certain order of tests. The testing one person undergoes may be significantly different from someone else's, depending on the symptoms and the findings I make during the physical examination. Just because your mother or sister had a specific test does not mean that you will also need that test. Again, I have to stress that there is no one specific test to diagnose heart disease.

Age-Appropriate Tests

Tests may vary according to age. For example, while I recommend that all women have a baseline cholesterol screening at age twenty, I usually wait until the patient is forty for an ECG, unless she is having specific signs and symptoms that warrant this test sooner.

Using the "Tests for Healthy Women" chart, you can identify the specific tests that are suggested for your age group. If any heart problems are identified after the checkup, your doctor can move forward with further testing. A personalized treatment regimen will help to resolve the problem and decrease or reverse your risk of heart disease.

TESTS FOR HEALTHY WOMEN

	Under 40	40 to 50	over 50
Blood pressure	•	•	•
Lipid profile	•	•	•
Blood chemistry	•	•	•
Urine analysis		•	•
ECG		•	•
Stress test			•*

* Under certain circumstances, stress testing is done for asymptomatic women over fifty who are sedentary prior to starting a vigorous exercise program.

Note: Stress testing is not a screening test for heart disease. This means that it is not routinely ordered for women without symptoms of coronary artery disease. There are two situations in which a stress test may be ordered for asymptomatic women: One is for sedentary women without symptoms who are planning to start a vigorous exercise program and the other is for women with multiple risk factors for coronary artery disease.

Testing Your Cholesterol

A simple blood test can tell you whether you have enough good cholesterol or too much bad cholesterol. With this test your doctor will measure your lipid chemistry—the total cholesterol, including the HDL ("good") cholesterol, the LDL ("bad") cholesterol, and triglycerides. This test is called a *fasting lipid profile*. The test should be done after an overnight fast.

CLASSIFICATION OF LDL, TOTAL, AND HDL CHOLESTEROL (MG/DL)*

LDL cholesterol

Equal to or less than 100	Optimal
100–129	Near or above optimal
130–159	Borderline high
160–189	High
Equal to or more than 190	Very high

Total cholesterol

<200	Desirable
200–239	Borderline high
>240	High

HDL cholesterol

<45	Low
≥60	High; reduces risk of heart disease

*This test is for women of all ages.

TRIGLYCERIDE SCREENING FOR WOMEN

Less than 200 mg/dL	Acceptable
Less than or equal to 150 mg/dL	Optimal

Testing Your Blood Pressure

The blood pressure in your arteries is measured by a quick, painless test using a medical instrument called a sphygmomanometer, in millimeters of mercury (abbreviated as mm Hg). Your blood pressure is given as one number over another, representing systolic over diastolic pressure. Normal readings range from 90/60 to 130/85. You are considered to have high blood pressure if either number is regularly beyond this range.

THE 120/80 RANGE IS OPTIMAL

Doctors now believe the optimal blood pressure for women is around 120/80. This is especially important in women with diabetes: diabetes combined with high blood pressure puts enough stress on the kidneys to risk heart attack. Researchers have now shown that as blood pressure rises above 120/80, cardiovascular disease may gradually increase.[2] For a discussion of high blood pressure, or hypertension, see pages 138–142.

LIFESTYLE MEASURES MAY LOWER BLOOD PRESSURE

If your blood pressure is 140/90 and you do not have diabetes or heart disease, I would recommend that you try a three-month lifestyle program (increasing exercise, modifying your diet, losing weight, and de-stressing) to see if you can reduce your blood pressure. If these lifestyle measures do not work, or if your blood pressure was 160/100 or greater, your doctor will probably want to start you on blood pressure medications (see Chapter 14). If your blood pressure is categorized as stage 3 (see the "Screening of Hypertension" chart) hospitalization is often the safest prescription. This will allow your doctor to run the necessary tests and administer medication to bring the pressure down quickly.

IS LOW BLOOD PRESSURE SERIOUS?

When a woman has low blood pressure, I evaluate that number in the context of that individual. For example, if she has a blood pressure reading of 90/60 and has no symptoms, such as fatigue or dizziness, and can do all her activities, then this low reading is not a cause for concern. But if she feels tired or dizzy, then I like to do further testing to evaluate the exact cause of the low reading.

CAUSES OF SYMPTOMATIC LOW BLOOD PRESSURE

- Dehydration
- Anemia
- Abnormal heart rhythm

During your healthy heart checkup, your doctor may have picked up on warning signs that need further investigation. So other tests commonly used to evaluate the cardiovascular system may be in store for you. As you read about these tests, use the diagram in Figure 7.1 to see which part of your heart is being tested.

WHAT DO THE NUMBERS MEAN?

Category	Systolic (upper number)	Diastolic (lower number)	Follow-up
Optimal	less than 120	less than 80	Routine check
Normal	121–129	81–84	Recheck in 2 years
High normal	130–139 or	85–89	Recheck in 1 year
Hypertension			
Stage 1	140–159 or	90–99	Confirm in 2 months
Stage 2	160–179 or	100–109	Evaluate in 1 month
Stage 3	180–209 or	110 +	Evaluate in 1 week

Source: "The Sixth Report of the Joint National Committee on Prevention, Detection, Evaluation, and Treatment of High Blood Pressure," *Archives of Internal Medicine* 157 (1997): 2413–2446; "AHA/ACC Scientific Statement: Consensus Panel Statement Guide to Preventive Cardiology for Women," *Circulation* 99 (1999): 2480–2484.

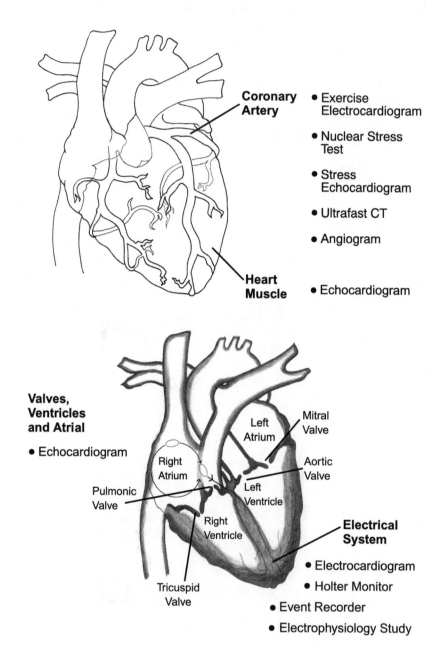

Coronary Artery
- Exercise Electrocardiogram
- Nuclear Stress Test
- Stress Echocardiogram
- Ultrafast CT
- Angiogram

Heart Muscle
- Echocardiogram

Valves, Ventricles and Atrial
- Echocardiogram

Right Atrium

Pulmonic Valve

Left Atrium

Mitral Valve

Aortic Valve

Left Ventricle

Right Ventricle

Tricuspid Valve

Electrical System
- Electrocardiogram
- Holter Monitor
- Event Recorder
- Electrophysiology Study

Figure 7.1
Testing for Heart Disease

Checking Your Heart Rhythm

Tests to Evaluate Heart Rhythm

Electrocardiogram
Holter Monitor
Event Recorder
Electrophysiology

The electrical system of the heart usually gives a smooth, regular rhythm. You might compare it to the electrical system of your car engine, which precisely distributes electrical impulses so that the engine runs smoothly. If your heart rhythm is irregular, the irregular pumping action of the heart may cause a drop in the blood flow from the heart. This can cause shortness of breath (especially with activity), light-headedness, dizziness or fainting, and loss of consciousness.

Electrical problems can cause the heart rhythm to sputter, to race, to be irregular, or in some cases to be extremely slow. These rhythm problems can result in palpitations, which are skipped beats or abnormal sensations of the beat felt in the chest. While not every woman feels these palpitations, they can be annoying or extremely disabling and anxiety-producing.

Electrocardiogram

The electrocardiogram (ECG) is one of the first tests I order for rhythm disturbances, suspected heart disease, and possible heart attack. This test gives a graphic record of the heart's electrical impulses and is commonly used to see if the heart is damaged. The ECG can detect heart attacks, ischemia, or decreased blood flow to your heart muscle, and record the heart rate and rhythm.

Because the ECG is most beneficial if you are actually having heart symptoms, the results may be normal if you have no symptoms, even if you do have a heart problem. That's why the physical examination and discussion with your doctor are crucial for an accurate diagnosis. If the ECG is abnormal or if your chest discomfort suggests coronary heart disease, further tests may be needed.

THE PROCEDURE: The ECG is usually done in your doctor's office by the nurse or technician and takes only five minutes. During the test, you will lie comfortably on your back while small sticky pads called *electrodes* (or *leads*) are attached to specific points on your neck, chest, arms, and legs. These electrodes record the path of electrical impulses through your heart muscle on graph paper. Your doctor will read this recording to see if there are abnormalities.

WHAT YOU MAY FEEL: You will feel sticky pads applied to your chest, arms, and legs; they make better contact between the leads and the points on your body. Avoid using body lotions or oily bath soaps prior to the test, or the sticky pads will slide across your skin.

PRECAUTIONS: There are no precautions with the ECG.

THE UPSIDE: The ECG is a quick, noninvasive procedure that in some cases can alert your doctor to the presence of arrhythmia, heart attack, or ischemia.

THE DOWNSIDE: The ECG is sometimes uninformative. Your doctor may find your ECG normal, even if you have a heart problem. In fact, many women who have had heart attacks have normal ECGs. In women with coronary artery disease, the ECG is often normal during rest (but may be abnormal during symptoms).

Holter Monitor

The Holter monitor is a twenty-four-hour ECG recording of the heart's rhythm. Its purpose is to evaluate changes in heart rhythm over a twenty-four-hour period. It is used to evaluate palpitations or skipped heartbeats.

THE PROCEDURE: With the Holter monitor, tiny electrodes are applied to your chest, and the wires are attached to a small tape recorder. While wearing the monitor, you can make notes in a diary when symptoms happen so that later the symptoms can be compared to the heart rhythm at the time. For example, if you feel weak or dizzy at two P.M., you write it down in your diary. At dinnertime, you may feel flushed and light-headed. Again, you write down these symptoms. Your doctor will compare your notes with the readings on the Holter monitor.

Some monitors have a button on the side that can be used to precisely identify the time an abnormal rhythm happens.

WHAT YOU MAY FEEL: You will feel the sticky pads of the tiny electrodes as they are applied to your chest.

PRECAUTIONS: There are no precautions with the Holter monitor.

THE UPSIDE: By analyzing the twenty-four-hour recording, the abnormal rhythms can be identified.

THE DOWNSIDE: The abnormal rhythm must happen during the twenty-four-hour period that you are wearing the monitor to be correctly discovered and diagnosed. If the abnormal rhythm does not occur during that time, your doctor will order further testing to make an accurate diagnosis.

Event Recorder

I find the event recorder especially helpful for women who have infrequent episodes of abnormal rhythm or intermittent palpitations, or whose symptoms are difficult to identify, because it can give an ECG recording at the time of the symptoms.

THE PROCEDURE: The event recorder is a small tape-recording device about the size of a beeper. One commonly used recorder is directly applied to the chest at the time the symptom is occurring.

Then the telephone receiver is placed over the recorder. The recorder transmits a short ECG recording via the telephone line to a central recording station. These results are then directed to your doctor.

Another device, known as a continuous loop recorder, requires the daily attachment of electrodes. This device can be programmed to do an ongoing monitoring of the heart, but to record only when you are having symptoms, by pressing a button on the recorder. This device is particularly beneficial in women whose palpitations are short term.

Event recorders and continuous loop recorders are usually ordered for a thirty-day period. It is important that during this time you do all your normal daily activities, so that there can be an accurate evaluation of your heart rhythm. Write down your symptoms in a diary, so that they can be correlated with the heart rhythm.

WHAT YOU MAY FEEL: The event recorder requires the placement of the recorder over your chest; there is no discomfort. In some instances, the electrodes are directly applied to the chest.

PRECAUTIONS: There are no precautions with the event recorder.

THE UPSIDE: The recording is made at the time the symptom is occurring.

THE DOWNSIDE: For very short arrhythmias this type of event recorder may not record your arrhythmia fast enough.

Checking Heart Muscle Function Noninvasively

Tests for Heart Muscle Function

Echocardiogram (resting echocardiogram)

Echocardiogram (Resting Echocardiogram)

The most common test to evaluate heart muscle function is the echocardiogram, or ultrasound of the heart. A resting echocardiogram is specifically used to evaluate the functioning of the heart muscle and the valves.

WHEN IS AN AN ECHOCARDIOGRAM INDICATED?

I order an echocardiogram for women who have heart murmurs, an abnormal baseline ECG, and hypertension to see if there is any heart muscle damage or abnormal valve function. I might use this test to check the extent of heart muscle damage after a heart attack, to evaluate the cause of heart failure, or to diagnose valvular heart disease.

WHAT IS AN ULTRASOUND PROBE?

Many women are familiar with ultrasound probes from pregnancy, when they saw ultrasound images of their baby. An ultrasound probe is like a miniature radar machine that produces images of the heart using sound waves. The recorded waves show the shape, texture, and movement of the valves on the resulting echocardiogram. They also measure the size of the heart and its chambers and can detect any excessive fluid in the membrane that surrounds the heart.

THE PROCEDURE: The resting echocardiogram is done by a technician in your doctor's office or in an outpatient testing lab. A specially trained cardiologist then interprets it. You will remove your clothing above the waist, including your bra, and lie on a table on your left side. Gel is applied to your chest, then an ultrasound probe that resembles a microphone is applied. The technician places the probe over different areas on your chest, using slight pressure. The transducer emits high-frequency sound waves that create visual images of your heart and indicate the blood flow to different parts of your heart.

WHAT YOU MAY FEEL: You will feel the gel on your skin, then light pressure as the transducer rubs along your chest.

PRECAUTIONS: There are no precautions with the echocardiogram.

THE UPSIDE: This echocardiogram is noninvasive, fast, and easy to administer. It gives information about the heart muscle and valves and is an excellent way to assess valve problems and structural abnormalities in people with arrhythmias. When an ECG reveals no changes or only subtle changes, it can also detect heart muscle damage. It assesses heart function, a very important determinant of survival after a heart attack, without any radiation.

THE DOWNSIDE: The accuracy of the test depends on the skill of the technician and the physician interpreting the test. In people with lung disease such as emphysema, it is difficult to get good studies.

THE TRANSESOPHAGEAL ECHOCARDIOGRAM MAY BE THE BEST TEST WHEN:

- Assessing for valvular heart disease
- Checking the function of artificial heart valves
- Looking for blood clots in the heart chambers
- Seeking the cause of an unexplained stroke, such as a clot in a heart chamber
- Evaluating for clots in the left atrium, prior to a cardioversion (a direct current shock) for atrial fibrillation

---

Transesophageal Echocardiogram

A transesophageal echocardiogram may be used to give your doctor a better view of your heart valves. This test is commonly used to evaluate regurgitations of the mitral valve (see page 148) and to give a more accurate assessment of the regurgitation. In some cases, your doctor may order it to diagnose vegetations (outgrowths on the membranes lining the heart valves) in endocarditis, mitral valve disease, clots in the left atrium, or problems in communication between the right and left sides of the heart, or to evaluate the function of artificial heart valves.

THE PROCEDURE: With the transesophageal echocardiogram, you are given sedation and a local anesthetic to your throat. A tube with a tiny ultrasound transducer at its tip is inserted into the esophagus. Because the mitral valve is one of the posterior structures of the heart, it is better imaged from the esophagus, which is behind your heart.

THE DOWNSIDE: The greatest downside is that it is uncomfortable to swallow the tube. The local anesthetic will numb your throat and prevent gagging. The test should be avoided if you have difficulty swallowing or a history of ulcers or bleeding from the esophagus or stomach.

Checking for Coronary Artery Disease Noninvasively

Tests for Coronary Artery Disease

Exercise Electrocardiogram (stress electrocardiogram)
Nuclear Exercise Electrocardiogram (thallium stress test)
Exercise Echocardiogram (stress echocardiogram)
Pharmacological Stress Tests
Ultrafast CT (electron beam CT)

Exercise Electrocardiogram (Stress Electrocardiogram)

The most common use of the exercise ECG is to diagnose coronary artery disease (CAD). It increases the work of the heart so that your doctor can see if you experience the same symptoms you may have previously described. The earliest signs of coronary heart disease are often present only under exertion. Your doctor will watch for differences between the exercise and resting electrocardiogram. The exercise ECG may also be used for fitness assessment, or to evaluate blood pressure during exercise, or to evaluate exercise-induced arrhythmias.

THE PROCEDURE: Before the stress test, your doctor will take your personal medical history to make sure you are not having a heart attack (a contraindication to any stress test). Once you have been screened for the test, a nurse or technician will attach ECG leads to your chest and a blood pressure cuff to your arm. Then you walk or run on an exercise treadmill or pedal an exercise bicycle. As you do, an electrocardiogram is taken and your blood pressure is continuously monitored. The test increases in intensity every few minutes until you are tired or have symptoms, or until the ECG becomes abnormal.

During the test, your doctor will watch for the response of your heart rate and blood pressure, both of which will normally increase. Your heart is monitored for irregular heartbeats, since the presence of arrhythmias may be a clue to more serious coronary artery disease.

To make the diagnosis, your doctor will look for certain changes in the ECG that may indicate reduced blood flow to your heart muscle. These changes can help predict whether CAD is present. While the test can help detect CAD in men about 90 percent of the time, in women it is only half as accurate. About half the time, women have abnormal ECG test results but have normal coronary arteries. Such a test is called a *false positive test*. *False negative tests* may be a problem for some women because they do not achieve a high enough heart rate to accurately diagnose CAD: either they may stop before they reach an adequate heart rate, or their medications keep the heart rate from increasing high enough. If your ECG is negative, yet you still have signs and symptoms of heart disease, your doctor will order further diagnostic testing.

WHAT YOU MAY FEEL: If you are a sedentary person, you may feel tired and stiff and have muscle aches after the exercise ECG, as if you had walked a few city blocks. If you have angina, this test may provoke chest pain, shortness of breath, or throat tightness.

PRECAUTIONS: This test should not be performed if you are having a heart attack or have uncontrolled hypertension, unstable angina, acute heart failure, an active heart infection, or aortic stenosis. If you are able to take the test, do not eat for four hours beforehand. Be sure to ask your doctor whether you should take your normal daily medications—do not assume that you should not take them. Sometimes medications, such as digoxin, give a false reading to the test. To avoid errors, be sure to let your doctor know about all medications, vitamins, or supplements you have taken. During the test, if you experience palpitations or chest pain, tell the doctor, and the test will be immediately stopped. If you have any signs of cardiac problems, such as an abnormal electrocardiogram, fall in blood pressure, unsteady gait, light-headedness, or cold or clammy skin, the test will be stopped immediately and the necessary treatment will be administered. Emergency equipment must be present at the location where the test is administered.

THE UPSIDE: The test is generally safe and easy to administer, and it can give a quick assessment of your heart's function during exercise.

THE DOWNSIDE: As many as 50 percent of exercise stress tests give false positive readings in women. There is a small risk of a heart attack, particularly in people whose symptoms have become unstable. To prevent a heart attack, the physician takes a medical history and evaluates your ECG, before you step on the treadmill.

WHAT THE RESULTS MEAN: If a woman's test is negative and she has achieved an adequate heart rate, then the outcome is considered good, and she is not considered to have heart disease. But it's important to be sure she reached a diagnostic heart rate (85 percent of age-predicted maximum heart rate) before the test is confirmed negative. In some cases, a woman may have a false negative test if she didn't reach an adequate heart rate. The nuclear exercise stress test or exercise echocardiogram is a better and more accurate test in most cases.

For any woman, a positive test result should be followed up with additional testing, such as a nuclear exercise ECG, an exercise echocardiogram, or a coronary angiogram (see Chapter 16). CAD may be diagnosed on an exercise ECG test if the test result is positive. An angiogram is usually the next step. A positive result should not be assumed to be a false positive, which occurs when the results of a test are positive yet there is no conclusive evidence to confirm it. The exercise ECG should not be the first test for a woman who has baseline ECG changes, because it may result in a false positive. An exercise echocardiogram would be preferable.

Nuclear Exercise Electrocardiogram (Thallium Stress Test)

In a nuclear exercise electrocardiogram, a tiny amount of radioisotope (not a dye) is injected into a vein at peak exercise. This radioisotope goes into the heart muscle and helps to picture the blood flow pattern in the heart muscle. A scanning camera records the pattern. If part of the heart muscle is damaged, it does not take up the radioactive isotope. If the scan shows *reduced* uptake during exercise that normalizes with rest, that indicates an obstructed artery without heart damage. In areas where the isotope is able to flow (perfuse), the artery is unobstructed. This test can give useful information about the pumping action of the ventricles and vital information about the blood supply to the heart muscle.

THE PROCEDURE: Before the test begins, a small IV line is started so that the isotope can be injected into your vein. Then you exercise on a treadmill. At the completion of the exercise, you lie down on a table under a scanning camera. A technician, under the supervision of a nuclear cardiologist, takes images of your heart. You then wait a few hours so that you can be reimaged in a resting state. The doctor will analyze the resting and stress images and make a comparison between the two.

WHAT YOU MAY FEEL: You may have symptoms of increased physical exertion.

PRECAUTIONS: The precautions for this test are the same as for all stress tests.

THE UPSIDE: The nuclear stress test increases the ability to detect coronary heart disease to about 90 percent, higher than the 50 percent detection rate of the exercise ECG. If the nuclear stress test is normal, your chances of significant heart disease are usually quite low. The referring doctor will usually have the test results at the end of the day or the next day.

THE DOWNSIDE: Occasionally the imaging is not accurate in large-breasted women, giving false positive results.

WHAT THE RESULTS MEAN: The nuclear stress test may produce one of several results.

1. Normal blood flow (perfusion) at rest and exercise. This is a normal result—the isotope was able to flow unobstructed.
2. Areas of reduced perfusion at exercise and rest. This result is consistent with previous heart damage.
3. Reduced perfusion at exercise; normal perfusion at rest. This result denotes an ischemic-reduced blood supply to the heart muscle, indicating a coronary artery is blocked. If this result occurs in multiple areas, then more than one coronary artery is blocked. In that case, the test may be followed up with an angiogram.

Did you know that women with positive stress tests are less likely to be sent for coronary angiography than are men?[3]

Exercise Echocardiogram (Stress Echocardiogram)

A variation of stress testing is exercise echocardiography, which, like the stress ECG, is done during exercise. Using ultrasound as the imaging technique, your doctor will look for exercise-related or -induced wall motion abnormalities that indicate the presence of coronary artery disease. Because coronary artery anatomy is fairly standard, doctors can pinpoint the abnormal wall segment and the exact blocked artery as the wall segment improves with rest. Many doctors find the exercise echocardiogram to be the best stress test for diagnosing heart disease, particularly in women.

THE PROCEDURE: A resting echocardiogram is performed first; then you have two options:

1. You exercise on a treadmill. When you reach the maximum heartbeat, you are quickly guided to a table, where an exercise echocardiogram is taken.
2. You take the test on a special table to which a bicycle is attached. The bicycle is also connected to the echocardiogram. You pedal the bicycle while lying down on the table, and the echocardiogram (heart imaging) is taken throughout the test.

WHAT YOU MAY FEEL: The test may bring on your symptoms. For example, you may develop fatigue, shortness of breath, and even arrhythmia.

PRECAUTIONS: The precautions for this test are the same as for all stress tests.

THE UPSIDE: The test uses no radiation and lets your doctor evaluate symptoms for CAD and valvular heart disease at the same time. The test is quick, taking only about forty-five minutes. The results are available immediately. Studies have suggested that this may be the best initial stress test for women, given the limitations of the exercise ECG.[4] This particular test is also beneficial as it lets your doctor determine whether your symptoms are due to valvular or arterial disease.

THE DOWNSIDE: This test is not valuable if the images that come out of it are not good, or if you cannot exercise enough during the test to get measurements. Often it is difficult to image women who have lung disease, such as chronic bronchitis or emphysema.

WHAT THE RESULTS MEAN: This is an excellent test for distinguishing symptoms of shortness of breath from coronary artery disease, heart failure, or valvular heart disease. It is more accurate for women than the stress ECG. The echocardiogram shows areas of the heart that have reduced motion with exercise, implying a narrowed artery. It can diagnose the area of the affected heart muscle; then an angiogram is used to determine the exact point or extent of blockage in the artery.

Pharmacological Stress Tests

If you cannot do enough walking, running, or pedaling to allow the exercise test, a medication called *dipyridamole* can do the work for you. This medication is injected, followed by thallium, as in the nuclear stress test. Dipyridamole causes the coronary arteries to dilate, or expand. While normal arteries can dilate, obstructed arteries cannot. This alternative works well for women who have arthritis, back pain, lung disease, or other problems that prevent exercise. The test is contraindicated for those with asthma.

If you have asthma and need a pharmacological stress test, another medication, *dobutamine,* is the drug of choice. This drug mimics exercise by increasing blood pressure and heart rate. Both medications are useful for women with arthritis, peripheral vascular disease, or orthopedic conditions that limit their ability to walk. Dobutamine may also be used in conjunction with the nuclear stress test or stress ECG.

It is extremely important to be off caffeine and decaffeinated beverages prior to the dipyridimole test, as they counteract the effects of the medication.

Some common side effects of dipyridimole include headache, dizziness, and palpitations. These symptoms can be reversed with aminophylline, a drug that is commonly used for asthma. Side effects of dobutamine include palpitations, atrial and ventricular arrhythmias, and nausea.

Ultrafast CT (Electron Beam CT)

There are still more tests doctors use to diagnose the presence of heart disease. While these tests have benefits, they are neither standard nor widely used.

WHAT DOES THE ULTRAFAST CT LOOK FOR?

Ultrafast computerized tomography or electron beam CT is one of the newer techniques used to test for atherosclerotic heart disease. It is very fast (it takes only twenty minutes) and relatively safe, with low doses of radiation and no needles or injection of dye.

Ultrafast CT looks for the presence of calcium, a marker for the presence of coronary artery plaque. Though calcified plaques are stable and hence less likely to rupture, their presence may signify the presence of noncalcified or vulnerable plaques. The greater the amount of calcium, the greater the likelihood that coronary artery disease is present. Some studies show that high calcium correlates to a greater likelihood that a heart attack may occur in two to five years.[5] The ultrafast CT may prove to be most beneficial for those on cholesterol-lowering medications, in order to follow the regression of the calcification, indicating less plaque.

ARE THERE SPECIAL PRECAUTIONS?

The test is not recommended for asymptomatic people or for those under the age of forty who have no risk factors. This test is not a substitute for stress testing or angiography and is not necessary in women who have had a heart attack, bypass surgery, or PTCA/stent (see page 396) or who have been diagnosed with CAD. This test may not eliminate the need for further testing. Unlike an angiogram, it does not give us the percent of stenosis (narrowing) of a particular artery, and it does not tell us whether symptoms are due to an obstructed artery.

WHO WOULD BENEFIT MOST?

While this test may have some benefit as a follow-up test for cholesterol-lowering therapies and for high-risk but asymptomatic women, its role is still emerging; it has not been shown to be better than the evaluation of risk factors to predict heart disease. The test may prove to be most beneficial for those on cholesterol-lowering medications, in order to follow regression of the calcification. If you have a low calcium score, it does not mean you have no risk. A low calcium score is not a license to give up exercise, eat fatty foods, or start smoking again.

Checking for Blood Vessel Problems

Tests for Blood Vessel Problems

Carotid Doppler
Magnetic Resonance Imaging
Magnetic Resonance Angiography

Carotid Doppler

A carotid Doppler test is an ultrasound of the arteries in the neck that appear to be narrowing because of plaque accumulation. This narrowing puts you at a higher risk for a stroke.

Magnetic Resonance Imaging

While magnetic resonance imaging (MRI) is not one of the initial tests your doctor will use, it may be used to target some forms of heart disease. MRI uses powerful magnets instead of radiation to generate a computerized image of the heart and blood vessels. Currently it is used to image the aorta and carotid arteries and to evaluate congenital heart disease.

Magnetic Resonance Angiography

Magnetic resonance angiography (MRA) uses powerful magnets to visualize blood vessels, giving the percentage of obstruction. It is not used for the routine diagnosis of coronary artery disease and is being evaluated in medical and research centers for this purpose.

Where Do You Go from Here?

Testing can be very confusing. I can tell by the looks on my patients' faces that they are frightened about the possible test results and that not knowing how many tests or procedures they'll need weighs heavily on their minds.

After you undergo stress testing, your doctor will assess the following points before methodically deciding whether to begin treatment or if you need further testing and procedures for diagnosis.

- *Your symptoms before and during the test.*
- *Duration of exercise.* Studies show that if the exercise lasts thirteen or more minutes in people with positive tests, the prognosis over the next year is as good as for people without coronary artery disease.[6]
- *Recovery heart rate.* This is a marker for improved survival. One study reported in the *New England Journal of Medicine* showed that if you have CAD and your heart rate decreases twenty beats within the first minute postexercise, your survival is better even with CAD.[7]
- *Number of segments involved.* The more segments affected on the nuclear exercise ECG or stress echocardiogram, the more disease or arteries involved.

As I've mentioned, after an abnormal stress test, women are given less follow-up testing than men. Past studies show that women are less likely than men to be referred for further testing.[8] We can change this outcome if more doctors become aware that women's greatest health threat is heart disease, and if women learn to speak up when they have signs and symptoms of heart disease, and seek immediate treatment.

If a test is positive, this result may call for further testing, which can be done in your doctor's office. If the nuclear stress test is positive, your doctor may recommend a coronary angiogram (see page 393).

It's your heart—never lose sight of that! It is your right to know the findings of all tests, so I want you to insist on understanding the results. If your doctor dismisses your concerns, do not hesitate to dismiss your doctor.

Keep in mind that as with any illness, taking control and reversing heart disease starts with an accurate diagnosis and a thorough understanding of all the risk factors. Using one or more of the tests described in this chapter, your doctor will determine the state of your heart health. If there are problems, your doctor has the resources to decide how to best treat your specific problem. Although heart disease can sometimes be complex to treat and call for lifestyle changes, effective medications, and surgical procedures, the results of treatment can be good if treatment is begun early on. If the tests find that you have no heart problems, make it your goal to keep your heart healthy by following the program outlined in Part III.

PART III

The Women's Healthy Heart Program

8

Your Commitment

Of all my patients, Linda, age forty-seven, was the one who resisted change the most. Even after she had a heart attack, she denied that she needed to eat or live differently.

I first met Linda in the coronary care unit during her recovery. While reviewing her chart, I noticed that she had several serious risk factors for heart disease. Not only was she greatly overweight, but she smoked a pack of cigarettes every day, had high blood pressure, and had just been diagnosed with type 2 diabetes. Linda also had a family history of early heart disease: her mother had died suddenly from a heart attack at only forty-six. Linda was at high risk for yet another heart attack if she did not make some immediate lifestyle changes.

She and I talked at length about her health habits, including:

- *Diet.* Linda was a "night eater." She ate little during the day except for colas and crackers, and then when she got home, she ate a huge fatty meal and sugary snacks until bedtime.
- *Exercise.* Linda had been physically active in the past, playing sports in high school and college, but she rarely exercised now.

As a full-time computer programmer, she sat most of the day and then watched TV in the evening.

- *Smoking.* Linda had smoked since high school. Several years before her heart attack, she tried to quit but gained almost thirty pounds. In the past year, she had even increased her daily smoking by half a pack.
- *Stress.* This was a big problem for Linda. She had recently gone through a divorce and was frequently tense because of having "more month than money," as she put it. Her financial stress caused her to eat and smoke even more.

After I got to know Linda, I realized that the chance of her changing any of her harmful behaviors was slim, simply because she felt that her excuses for continuing them were valid. For example, she said she could not exercise because she had no time. When I suggested easy ways that she could fit exercise into her day, she immediately gave me reasons why they wouldn't work. I suggested that she get a treadmill at home; she replied that she had one, but it was broken, and she could not afford to get it fixed. I recommended that she join the Y near her apartment. She said that wouldn't work because she didn't like to work out with people she didn't know.

About her unhealthy eating habits, Linda's excuses went on forever: she had no time to eat during the day; food made her sick in the morning; food allergies kept her from eating fruits and vegetables; and so on.

Perhaps Linda's biggest episode of denial came when we discussed her family history. When I explained that this too was a risk factor for heart attack, her response was revealing: "My mother was so different from me. She was uneducated about heart disease. Not only was she obese, but she ate high-fat foods, smoked cigarettes, and was sedentary. My mother just had no clue about healthy living."

Linda was in total denial of her own personal risk: she herself fit her mother's profile. Still, knowing about your risks and doing something about them are two different things—and two different states of mind and body. It would take a lot of motivation and eye-opening education for Linda to see her grave situation—and she is not alone.

Many women who have suffered major heart attacks or undergone heart surgery still do not acknowledge that heart disease is a reality in their lives.

A Mountain of Excuses

Tragically, too many of the women whom I treat seek help only *after* they have had a heart attack or when they've harbored symptoms for many days and weeks. Some, like Linda, are in total denial of their risk. The majority of women whom I see take care of their families before taking care of themselves. When they tell me, "I'll never get a heart attack," or, "I'll take care of it later," they are reflecting these priorities.

Do any of the following excuses sound familiar?

- "I'll start an exercise program after my daughter gets her braces off next month."
- "I'm so busy this week with work and the kids. If I still have this pain, I'll call the doctor next week."
- "My blood pressure is off the chart, but I'm going to wait and see the doctor after the holidays."
- "Yes, I know I smoke, but only to ease my stress. Justin goes off to college soon, and I won't feel as much stress. I'll quit then."
- "My diet can wait until after my daughter's bridal shower."
- "If this is related to heart disease, I'd rather not know. My husband could never raise these kids without me."
- "I can't get sick right now. My kids are young, and my family could never get along without me, so I keep moving."
- "I don't think this is a heart problem. I probably just pulled a muscle in my chest while carrying those boxes a few weeks ago."
- "I really can't stress my husband now about my own health concerns. He was just diagnosed with congestive heart disease and is very depressed."
- "My doctor told me I had to start exercising, but I don't have time for one more commitment right now."

- "My chest pain can wait until after my husband is discharged from the hospital."

The list goes on. Often by the time a diagnosis of heart disease is made and proper treatment has begun, the heart muscle has been seriously or even irreparably damaged.

One of my greatest desires as a cardiologist is to figure out why it is so difficult to prevent heart disease in women—and why some women ignore or deny the signs and symptoms of heart attack even when they are having one. I've had patients who fear dying young from heart disease—as their mothers and fathers did—but won't take care of themselves, stop smoking, or try to lose weight. I've had women in the midst of a heart attack with terrible pain or pressure say to me, "Do you think I'll be well enough to host my dinner party tomorrow night?" I've had patients tell me they don't have heart disease even *after* they've had bypass surgery or angioplasty with a stent to keep the blocked artery open. I've even had some patients pretend not to have symptoms of breathlessness, dizziness, or atypical pain for fear I'd mention the words *heart disease*.

It breaks my heart to see women I care about throwing away their health, losing precious time with their loved ones and friends, cutting their lives short with a problem they could have prevented. Please make sure you understand the full extent of your risks, and please face the facts! Don't hide your head in the sand. Don't try to deny the reality of your risk or your need to take steps to prevent heart disease or to heal your condition. I assure you, you can make changes and help yourself feel better and stay well.

I know change can be frightening, so I want to talk to you some more about how to perceive your disease.

Facing Reality

The Health Belief Model

As you make your commitment to change the bad habits that increase your risk for heart disease, I want you to understand something called the *health belief model*. I hope that it will help you understand better your own attitude toward your body and health. The health belief model was developed by psychologists to explain how and why people stick to a diet or exercise program, or take medications as prescribed. First, they comply if they perceive that they are at risk for a particular disease. Second, they comply if they believe that the disease is serious enough to prevent or treat and that the prescribed prevention, treatment, or intervention will be effective. Third, they comply if they believe that the personal costs of intervention will not inconvenience them or be dangerous.

How does the health belief model relate to women and heart disease? If the Women's Healthy Heart Program is to be effective, a woman must first accept the fact that she is at risk for heart disease. This acceptance is the biggest wall I run into in treating my patients: most women simply do not perceive themselves to be at risk. Because they do not feel vulnerable, they do not seek an effective diagnosis, or take prevention measures, or undergo life-saving treatment. After all, it's hard to make the commitment to prevent heart disease if you feel you are actually at greater risk for breast cancer. So they avoid making crucial lifestyle changes that could save, lengthen, and improve the quality of their lives.

Perhaps they don't face the truth because they fear how their lives will have to change. But even if fear is at the root of their denials, it's the denial of the risk of heart disease that keeps them unhealthy.

It's true that any change is frightening. But isn't losing your life or putting your loved ones through pain and grief far more frightening than facing the reality of health issues? If I could make the commitment for you, I would. But making the commitment to prevent heart disease is up to you.

Women in Denial

All women—yes, even you and I—have some risk for heart disease, depending on particular risk factors. To think differently is to ignore a reality. Yet a revealing study done on a highly educated group of women, all graduates of Stanford University, shows the popular mis-

conception about women and heart disease. The Stanford study surveyed 600 women about their attitudes on hormone replacement
therapy (HRT) and the prevention of heart disease. The investigators conducted this study because at that time, in 1995, they felt that
not enough menopausal women took HRT to prevent heart disease.
(Now it's clear that HRT is not advisable for heart disease prevention at menopause.)

The study found that the majority of the women (73 percent)
thought they had less than 1 percent risk of developing heart disease
by age seventy. By contrast, more than half (52 percent) perceived
that that their risk of developing breast cancer by age seventy
was greater than 10 percent. Interestingly, 35 percent of the women
said that the risk of breast cancer influenced their decision not to
take HRT.[1]

Another, similar survey was taken by the American Heart Association on 1,000 women, between twenty-five and forty-five. In this
study, only 8 percent of the women thought they were at risk for
heart attack, and only 1 percent felt at risk for stroke.[2]

A few years ago, after poring over all the research, I was stunned
by these women's misperception that heart disease was not a serious
health threat. Wondering if this misperception was true in women
who already had heart disease, I did my own study of patients enrolled in the Women's Heart Program, some of whom had already
had heart attacks. I asked each of these women, ages fifty to seventy,
to describe on a 1 to 10 scale what her perceived risk of heart disease
had been before she was admitted to the hospital.

- Choosing 1 meant that the woman had felt sick enough to go
  to the hospital but had not believed that she was having a heart
  attack.
- Choosing 5 meant that she knew a heart attack was a possibility.
- Choosing 10 meant that she knew a heart attack was a strong
  possibility.

I then sorted my patients' feedback into two groups: low perception and high perception. Low perception meant the women had felt
their personal chances of having a heart attack were minimal; high

perception meant they had been aware of the symptoms and knew they were heart-related. I was shocked when I found that *61 percent of my own patients who had already-diagnosed heart disease had a low perception of their risk!* Only 39 percent had had a high perception of their reality prior to admission and acknowledged that they were overweight or sedentary. In other words, most had denied that they had heart disease!

The most striking thing about this small study is the high number of women *with coronary artery disease* who, on the day they went to the hospital, mistakenly thought they were at *low risk* for heart disease! The women in the low perception group were more likely to believe that breast cancer was a woman's greatest health threat and were less likely to acknowledge that they were sedentary or overweight. In fact, the women in both groups (high and low) were equally overweight, but the women in the low perception group were less fit and active than their high perception counterparts. The women in the high perception group were more in tune with their risk factors.

This brings us back to the health belief model and how the low perception of risk is associated with a low perception (or even denial) of risk factors like obesity and a sedentary lifestyle. For these women, their own beliefs were an important barrier to getting healthier and preventing further heart damage.

Women's perceptions of heart disease risk are in striking contrast to those of men. We doctors know that *most* men believe they *are* at risk for heart disease and are more likely to adopt lifestyle habits to prevent it. In fact, in years past, most heart awareness campaigns on hypertension, cholesterol, and warning signs of heart attack have been directed at men. Only in recent years has an attempt been made to alert women to their risk of heart disease—and we are still only in the beginning stages of this vital life-saving campaign. Since our teenage years, Americans have been indoctrinated to believe that heart disease is for men and breast cancer is for women.

Kelly, age forty-four, never missed her annual gynecological exam. This mother of two teenagers was an officer in the Junior League and president of a local cancer organization. Because her mother had been diagnosed with breast cancer at a young age, Kelly was passionate about this cause and spent hours educating women about the importance of monthly breast self-exams and routine mammograms. Several years ago at her annual physical, Kelly's doctor mentioned that her blood pressure was unusually high and that her weight and cholesterol had also increased dramatically over the previous year. Unsure about the significance of these risk factors, Kelly's doctor referred her to me to discuss possible treatment to prevent heart disease.

Even though Kelly was emphatic that she detested medication, I convinced her to start taking a drug to lower her dangerously high blood pressure and to reduce her risk of a heart attack or stroke. We then discussed her diet, which consisted mostly of processed or fast foods because of her busy lifestyle. I suggested that she try the Mediterranean-style diet (see Chapter 10), which uses whole grains, fruits, nuts, and vegetables, among other foods, and eliminates foods high in saturated fat. I then sensed some resistance from her about making these heart-healthy changes.

But the real block to improving Kelly's health was exercise. When I explained to her that exercise was crucial to reduce her blood pressure, lose weight, and increase her protective or HDL cholesterol, her response was "I hate to sweat." Kelly was used to being busy but sedentary, but now she had to own up to the fact that she was developing heart disease—and that it was up to her to make changes to prevent it from becoming a controlling factor in her life. We had to start somewhere, and after I pushed some more, she finally agreed to start exercising and to regularly take medication to control her hypertension. She started on the Women's Healthy Heart Program, and in a few short weeks she felt so much better that she became passionate about her heart's health. Since then, as a result of simple changes in her diet and daily exercise, Kelly has lost about twelve pounds, her blood pressure is in the normal range, she has reduced her dose of medication, and her cholesterol levels are healthier. This young mother sees her fight against heart disease as a new mission in her life, and she now volunteers with the American Heart Association to teach other women about this killer disease.

Making the Commitment to Change

Quite honestly, it is rare that I meet a woman who openly acknowledges that she is at risk for heart attack and who takes proactive steps to decrease that risk. In fact, most women who have heart attacks are shocked. They ask, "How did this happen to me? Was it my genes, my hormones, or my lifestyle?"

In most cases, it was all three, since heart disease is a multifaceted disease. More than half of all cases of heart disease result from lifestyle factors—lack of exercise, overweight, high blood pressure, smoking—but 25 percent may be related to family history and reduced estrogen levels at menopause, which are associated with higher levels of cholesterol and reduced flexibility of the arteries.

So what does this mean to you? Whatever your risk factors may be, the most tried and true way for you to prevent heart disease—and the least intrusive—is to take control and change your health habits permanently. This involves making many lifestyle changes, including increasing your exercise, modifying your diet, stopping cigarette smoking, and taking time each day to de-stress. The key to preventing heart attack is to acknowledge that these changes *will* put you back in control, and control, or self-efficacy, is essential for wellness. Commit yourself to making the following lifestyle changes:

- Move around more. Follow "Your Exercise Prescription" in Chapter 9.
- Modify your diet. Follow "Your Healthy Heart Eating Plan" in Chapter 10.
- Find out what supplements really work, and what supplements do not. Following the advice in Chapter 11, adjust the supplements you take to decrease your risk of heart disease.
- De-stress and unwind throughout your day by following "Your Stress Reduction Program" in Chapter 12.
- Stop smoking—today! See Chapter 13 for "Your Stop Smoking Program."

Are You Ready to Change?

"Wait a minute. You're asking me to make many changes. I know myself well, and if change involves a great deal of effort, I'll probably quit the plan before I even start." Fifty-five-year-old Patricia was quite honest when we discussed the Women's Healthy Heart Program and the proactive ways she could decrease her risk of heart disease.

I will tell you what I told her: Before you begin to make the changes necessary to protect your heart, it's important to assess your own readiness. If you are still in denial about your risk of heart disease, then the chances are low that you will stick with any wellness program. But if you face reality and commit yourself to making a wellness program a regular part of your lifestyle—your daily routine— then the chances are great that you will maintain the program. If you start out gradually, making small changes instead of dramatic ones, you are more likely to stick with this program for the rest of your life.

To give you an idea of how real a difference readiness can make, let me tell you about my experience with swimming. I had never been a swimmer and had failed many times at swimming lessons. Yet my husband, Robert, loves to swim. Many times I'd wanted to join him in the pool, but I'd always been afraid of the deeper water.

About five years ago, I mentioned my fear of swimming to my friend Dave, director of the May Center for Health, Fitness, and Sport at the 92nd Street Y. A week later my telephone rang, and a woman named Leslie told me she was the pool director at the 92nd Street Y. I was scheduled for my first swimming lesson, she said, the following Thursday at 7:30 P.M. Before I could protest, she hung up the telephone!

The next week, somewhat hesitantly, I went to the swimming lesson. I got in the water, and while the instructor showed me how to breathe under water and move my arms and feet to stay afloat, I faced my fear. I must admit that halfway through the lesson, the instructor paused to remind me to remove my hand from the side of the pool! Now I'm finally getting better at swimming—but only because I made that commitment to overcome my fear of the water.

We all fear making some kind of change, but if you can think of making these changes for your health as developing a new kind of skill—as swimming was for me—then the chances are great that you will succeed in meeting your goals.

The Five Stages of Change

Knowing that any change is difficult, especially as we grow older and more set in our habits, I want to help you figure out how best to change your lifestyle. Dr. Joseph Prochaska at Brown University developed five key stages by which people make permanent lifestyle changes.[3] Review each one, then decide which one you are in now. Going through each one honestly will help you get into your health program and then stay in it.

Stage 1: Pre-contemplation (Denial)

Remember my patient Linda? She had experienced a heart attack and was risking another, yet she was in total denial that heart disease was a problem for her. Linda typifies a woman in the pre-contemplation or denial stage of heart disease. In this stage, you do not really consider that you have a problem that may affect or end your life. For instance, if your friend invites you to go to a cholesterol screening with her, you will not think it important to go.

Sadly, for those who have several risk factors for heart attack, denial could delay good medical treatment and cut years off your life.

Stage 2: Contemplation (Considering Making Change)

The fact that you are reading this book shows that you are at least in the contemplation stage of making changes. In this stage you are ready to accept information. Some common statements my patients have made when contemplating these changes include:

- "Maybe I should watch my cholesterol and my weight. How can I learn how to do it?"
- "You know, I've noticed that I'm really out of breath when I

walk the dog. Maybe an exercise program would help me get back in shape."
- "Wow. I didn't know that steak had so much saturated fat in it. I've been thinking of cutting down on red meat or giving it up altogether."
- "You're going to Weight Watchers? I've been wanting to join to lose the ten pounds I gained last year."
- "I resent paying the high price of cigarettes now. This may be my new incentive to quit smoking."

When my patients actually acknowledge that they should be making lifestyle changes, I know there is some hope. When you consider or acknowledge that you may, in fact, have a problem, you are one step closer to actually seeing results!

Stage 3: Preparation (Making the Commitment to Change)

When you reach Stage 3, you are really taking initiative to do something about making the changes. Whether it involves calling Weight Watchers, moving past the meat department at the grocery store to get to the fruits and vegetables, or vowing not to buy cigarettes after work, you have taken a specific step to get ready for change.

Preparing for change involves making a definite plan and setting a date for making the change. I like to refer to this stage as finally putting your feet on the treadmill—then turning it on!

Stage 4: Action (Taking Steps for Change)

In Stage 4, you put real action behind your words and begin to change your lifestyle habits. Some actions may include:

- Walking fifteen minutes after dinner each night.
- Starting a new eating plan and adding more fresh fruits and vegetables.
- Going to a SmokEnders meeting and stopping smoking.

- Taking time each day to meditate or de-stress.
- Avoiding the butcher shop and going to the fish market instead.
- Going to the aerobics class at the Y three times a week.
- Meeting friends to walk around the track at your local high school.
- Writing down what you eat in a diet journal, to show how many calories you had.
- Switching to 1 percent fat milk instead of 2 percent.
- Taking the stairs to your office instead of the elevator.

The exciting part of taking action is that you will see results. As you change your lifestyle to decrease your risk of heart disease, you will start to look forward to these new activities and enjoy the benefits they yield.

Stage 5: Maintenance (Change Becomes Part of Your Routine)

When the heart-healthy changes you make have become as regular a part of your daily routine as brushing your teeth or washing your hair, you have reached Stage 5. If you maintain your new healthy habits for several months, you will stick with them for good, working only to resist any possibility of relapse.

Maintaining the Commitment

Relapses Do Happen

"I really was changing my lifestyle and had even reached Stage 5 with my exercise program," Charlotte told me. "I was so proud that I'd lost twenty-two pounds and that my doctor reduced my high blood pressure medicine. But look at me now." At forty-six, Charlotte had regained the weight she had lost the year before and was frustrated by her relapse from exercise.

"I was walking every evening after work without fail. Then last winter I got the flu. Somehow being in bed for ten days and feeling fatigued for weeks after that put me in my old lazy mode again. I regained the weight, and now I can hardly manage to get the kids off to school, much less walk each day. I'm a total failure."

I quickly let Charlotte know that she was *not* a failure. It's quite normal to have a slip-up or relapse after you make a lifestyle change. Even Olympic athletes tell of having an off season, where they just can't get motivated to press on with their workouts. When this happens to you, you must review the reasons you made the change in the first place and set new short- and long-term goals.

Set Realistic Goals

In anything we do, having a goal is vital for success. Without a specific goal, you have no way to measure your growth. In making a lifestyle change, setting a goal will help turn your initial enthusiasm into reality. In overcoming a relapse, you can set goals for organizing your time, in order to get back into your heart-healthy habits. And you can get some help from your family and friends to do so.

As you recover from a slip-up, make sure the new goals you set are specific. Give yourself a time limit, to allow for evaluation. And write down your goals so you can visualize the commitment, such as:

1. I will walk one mile, three times a week, for one month.
2. I will substitute sugarless gum and candy for cigarettes for two weeks.
3. I will measure my food this week and stay under 1,400 calories per day.

Be sure the goals you set are realistic so that you can actually achieve them. Your goals will also be a good baseline from which you can improve. Review your goals frequently, and make changes accordingly.

Some of my patients set goals that are too high. Paula, a fifty-one-year-old accountant, came to see me after suffering with angina for several months. She was frightened by the shortness of breath and pain and sought advice on how to relieve the problem. I explained the Women's Healthy Heart Program, and Paula was extremely enthusiastic about adding exercise and a healthier diet to her health habits. In fact, she left my office saying, "Don't worry, Dr. Goldberg. Next time you see me, I'll be a new woman—twenty pounds lighter and physically fit."

Well, the next time I saw Paula was the following week, and she was *neither* twenty pounds lighter *nor* more physically fit. In fact, she could hardly sit in the chair by my desk because of the pain in her lower back. In her enthusiasm to take charge of her health, she had started her "own" vigorous exercise regimen: she woke up early to swim at the local gym, then walked during her lunch hour, and two days each week she came to the Women's Heart Program at Lenox Hill Hospital.

Now all that exercise would have been wonderful if Paula's body had been ready to tackle it. But it wasn't. Paula was so gung-ho, she took the adage "no pain, no gain" to heart and found out the hard way that, especially when you haven't exercised in a while, this adage is not true.

Please, as you make plans to start the Women's Healthy Heart Program, establish goals with your doctor that are *reasonable* for your age and physical condition.

Suggested Goals

1. *I'll check with my doctor before I start any exercise program.*
2. *I'll start slowly to create a lifetime of good health habits.*
3. *I'll schedule exercise and de-stressing time every day.*
4. *I won't give up when setbacks occur.*
5. *I'll eat smaller portions at each meal.*
6. *I'll listen to my body and back off when it seems stressed or tired.*

Be Prepared for Motivational Lapses

If you think you can succeed with this healthy heart plan, then you can. If you feel that this plan is setting you up for another failure in your journey to lose weight, exercise, or stop smoking, it probably will, *but* you do *not* have to think in this negative way.

To reach your ultimate healthy heart goals and maintain them, perseverance is the key. As you begin the program, try to stay focused on your goals even when obstacles or stumbling blocks occur. Do this in the following ways:

- Believe in yourself and your particular health goals.
- Take time out for yourself to ensure you meet these goals.
- Take responsibility for your own health—only you can make necessary lifestyle changes.
- Practice the visualization exercise described in Chapter 12, and see yourself feeling good and healthy. Imagine yourself fully immersed in the Women's Healthy Heart Program. Use this visualization as a motivator to get back into action. Visualization without action won't help you!
- See making healthy change as the opportunity of a lifetime. You can finally make a difference in your well-being—and your future health.

Focus on the Benefits

As you proceed with the Women's Healthy Heart Program, keep reminding yourself of the many benefits you'll receive. Not only will you feel better, but you'll look better, your clothes will fit again, and you may even make new friends, especially if you participate in a group weight-loss, aerobics, or spinning class. One patient, Andrea, age forty-nine, achieved her goal of losing sixty pounds in a popular weight-loss program. Her past eating habits, she said, had been stealing every part of her life, from her health to her looks to her energy to her relationships. She's now at a normal weight and also has normal blood pressure and cholesterol levels. By losing the weight, she was able to reclaim her joy of living—and her heart's health.

Focus on the Reality

I hate to use fear as a motivating factor, but in some situations knowing the facts—that heart disease is a reality in your own life—can have a positive effect. Many patients are more willing to change serious risk factors for heart disease, I've found, when they perceive the impact on their health and well-being.

As fifty-six-year-old Nancy said, "When I came to grips with the fact that I was a walking time bomb, being a smoker with out-of-control hypertension and high LDL cholesterol, I knew I had no choice but to obey the doctor's orders. The facts were obvious, and the prescribed therapy—losing weight, changing my diet and exercise habits, and stopping smoking—was not costly. I had everything to gain and nothing to lose."

Focus on Yourself

For once in your life, you have permission—in fact, you have doctor's orders—to focus on yourself—to really love *you*!

I want you to read the next five chapters carefully and to approach each lifestyle change deliberately and slowly. Realize that sometimes you will not feel like exercising. Some days you may eat a fudge brownie (or two!) or finish the rest of your child's ice cream cone. But then you'll know to cut out sweets for the rest of the week. You may stop smoking for three weeks, then break down and have a few cigarettes while dining with friends. That's not failure. That's human! Just remind yourself that you did quit, and get back on the wagon again.

You may be thinking, "I will exercise when summer is over," or, "I've never been successful in maintaining an exercise or healthy eating program." That may be, but now you know that you need to do this, for yourself and your loved ones, in order to stay healthy or get healthier and prolong and improve your life. Remember, you are not going to make these heart-saving changes all at once. You can make the changes slowly—over the next three months, six months, even a year or a lifetime. But you do need to get started. As you read the next five chapters, you will learn that making healthy heart changes is not difficult. I'm going to teach you some easy, convenient ways to stop unhealthy lifestyle habits—such as inactivity, poor diet, and cigarette smoking—and in doing so reduce your risk for heart attack.

Keep in mind that following the healthy heart prevention steps is a process, not an end. You did not gain those thirty pounds in one week. Nor did you get high blood pressure or high LDL cholesterol and triglycerides suddenly.

To change long-standing behaviors over time, you will need to recommit to your health and to yourself every day. But with an open and willing spirit, you can start right now to do something positive and healthy for yourself—and your heart.

9

Your Exercise Prescription

If you're like many of my patients, you probably cringe when you think of making time to exercise each day. Maybe you're faced with a time crunch because you must balance too many work commitments with a demanding family life. Or perhaps you're juggling caregiving for aging parents while working full time and volunteering in the community. Whatever is keeping you too busy to exercise, I have answers for you in this chapter.

If you have coronary artery disease or symptoms that may be due to heart disease, or if you are over fifty and are at high risk for heart disease, then you should have a medical evaluation before starting an exercise program. If you have high blood pressure, get your blood pressure evaluated, and make sure it's regulated with medications if necessary. (If you've had a heart attack, a good place to start your exercise program is in a monitored cardiac rehabilitation program, as I explain in Chapter 15.)

Aerobic Exercise Is the Foundation

I believe that aerobic exercise and physical activity are the foundations of any heart disease prevention program. Physically moving around reduces many risk factors all at the same time. For example, when you exercise regularly, not only will you lose weight but you can reduce your blood pressure and even decrease your chance of getting diabetes. How's that for time efficiency?

Regular aerobic exercise benefits your heart in many ways. For one thing, it reduces the amount of adrenaline circulating in your body. This relaxes the blood vessels, resulting in a slower pulse rate and lower blood pressure. It also helps to raise your HDL ("good") cholesterol and lower your LDL ("bad") cholesterol and triglycerides. In fact, studies show that just three hours of walking each week (about half an hour each day) can reduce a woman's risk of heart attack by 35 percent.

Heart-Boosting Benefits of Exercise

Improves insulin sensitivity
Improves HDL ("good") cholesterol
Improves endurance
Improves resting systolic blood pressure
Increases resting metabolic rate
Reduces LDL ("bad") cholesterol
Reduces percentage of body fat

Resistance Training Strengthens Your Body

For years it was thought that resistance training (or strength training) was harmful for the heart because of increases in blood pressure. Now we *know* that resistance training is actually *good* for your heart. The best healthy heart exercise program includes both aerobic exercise and resistance training. Resistance training helps improve heart health by reducing blood pressure, changing fat into muscle, and increasing your metabolic rate. While aerobic exercise is low resistance and rhythmic and uses multiple muscle groups simultaneously, resistance training uses tension and resistance on individual muscle groups. Recent studies have revealed that half of all women over age sixty-five cannot lift a ten-pound weight with one arm.[1] That means they're not fit at a very basic level, and their hearts are probably not as strong as they should be. But resistance training for three to six months can improve muscular strength and endurance by 25 to 100 percent, depending on the workout and the woman's initial level of strength.[2] To me, this fact confirms the need for all women—no matter what their age—to work at building muscle mass, along with their regular aerobic exercise.

Medical research has shown that resistance training is important in the prevention of sarcopenia, the age-related loss of muscle mass that is associated with reduced muscle strength and reduced aerobic power. If you have sarcopenia, you may feel like you have less energy to do your daily activities. Being sedentary, not exercising, and menopause all accelerate the process of sarcopenia. But you can prevent sarcopenia with resistance training. You may even reverse it with consistent exercise.

Benefits of Resistance Training

- Increased muscle tone and definition
- Increased muscle size
- Increased strength
- Decreased percentage of body fat
- Improved endurance during aerobic activity

Benefits of Exercise

Exercise Boosts Positive Feelings and Improves Mood

Studies show that exercise helps restore the body's neurochemical balance and triggers a positive emotional state. Exercise reduces anxiety and stress; when you move around more, and are working hard physically, it's difficult to worry about daily problems. All that's on your mind is getting through the routine—*not* the problems you face each day.

Exercise has been shown to improve mood in women with depression. It also releases endorphins, which are brain chemicals that are natural mood elevators.

When I leave an exercise class, I can definitely feel the difference from when I arrived. My muscles feel less tense, and I stand straighter. My outlook on life is more positive, and my energy level is greater.

Exercise Boosts Bone Strength

Exercise is a prescription for your overall health, but it also definitely strengthens your bones. Revealing studies report that weight-bearing exercises (exercises where you are standing on your feet)—walking, aerobic dance, climbing stairs, racquet sports, and resistance training— are all crucial to increasing bone mass. While swimming is a super aerobic activity and good for the cardiovascular system, it is not weight bearing.

Generally bone mass peaks between ages twenty-five and thirty for women; then the tide turns. At some point, usually around thirty-five, women begin to lose bone, sometimes at a rate of 1 percent per year. During the five to ten years after menopause (usually forty-five to fifty-five), the rate increases to about 4 percent per year.

Weight-bearing exercise stimulates the cells that make new bone. By doing more weight-bearing exercise, we encourage our bodies to form more bone and can delay or actually reverse osteoporosis, which results in painful or debilitating fractures. By adding resistance training, you improve your muscle strength and flexibility and reduce the likelihood of falling as you get older. When you consider that one-third of all women who live to age ninety will break a hip because of osteoporosis, daily exercise is a small price to pay to keep bones strong and fracture-free!

BONE BOOSTER

Two studies involving more than eight hundred older adults found that those who walked the equivalent of twenty to thirty minutes per day had much denser bones than did inactive adults.[3] Numerous studies have reached similar conclusions; in premenopausal, post-menopausal, and elderly women, weight-bearing exercise, such as walking, can stimulate bone mass to stay strong.[4]

Exercise Decreases Risk of Cancer

As exercise strengthens your heart and bones, it also reduces your risk of cancer. Studies have shown that regular physical activity can reduce a woman's risk of colon and breast cancer.[5] The breast cancer benefit is especially seen in premenopausal women, under the age of forty-five.

No Matter What Your Age, Move Around More to Protect Your Heart

"I'm not a young athlete anymore," Dot said, "so don't expect me to start running." This forty-five-year-old woman had been a star athlete in college, running cross-country. But after working a sedentary job for almost twenty years, her most aerobic activity consisted of twisting around in her typing chair to open the bottom drawer on her desk. As a result, she had gained more than sixty pounds over a period of two decades. Last year, after Dot suffered a heart attack, she finally decided to take control of her heart's health with weight loss, diet, and exercise.

Many women do slow down with age, but that's no excuse to avoid physical exercise. In fact, as I tell my patients, you can't store up the benefits of exercise from your college days. You have to be continually active and do some sort of exercise throughout your life. By the same token, if you haven't exercised since college, don't be overly hard on yourself, and don't expect to have the same fitness level you had at eighteen. Get into an exercise regimen gradually so that you don't hurt yourself, make yourself too sore, or burn out.

Ruth, age fifty-two, has been a patient of mine for more than two years. Because of hypertension, she takes a low dose of blood pressure medication. As I was writing her first prescription for the medication, I told her that there was a chance she could get off the medication if she started a regular exercise program. She admitted that while she did have a treadmill at home, its current use was as a place to hang clothes. So I then wrote her an exercise prescription.

Evidently Ruth never took the clothes off the treadmill to start exercising, because she recently came to see me with symptoms of chest discomfort. At this visit, her lack of movement was clearly beginning to take its toll. Now thirty pounds heavier, she was extremely short of breath even after very limited activity, such as making her bed or walking to get her mail. I immediately scheduled her for a stress test, and although it did not show any signs of heart disease, it showed a lot about how unfit she was. Ruth was able to exercise only for four minutes, and during that brief period of time her heart rate soared to 160 beats per minute. While her blood pressure had started at 130/80, it skyrocketed to 200/100. These numbers convinced Ruth that she had to start doing regular exercise. I wrote her a new prescription and suggested that she sign up for the Women's Heart Program. Thankfully, her response was immediate: "How soon can I start?"

Get Physical

"What's left for me? I hate pumping iron just about as much as I hate walking at the mall. I'd ride my bike, but the last time I checked, the tires were flat. Is there any hope for me to get back in shape?" If you are like my patient Judith, forty-nine, and absolutely dread even the word *exercise*—much less actually doing it—the good news is that I have a loose definition of exercise. If some physical activity gets your heart pumping and burns calories, chances are that it can be classified as exercise.

When I write my patients a prescription for an individualized fitness program, the word *exercise* is often a barrier to their getting started. To many women, the word brings images of buff Olympic athletes and lean prima ballerinas. Don't let these images throw you! The key to dispelling your old negative impressions of exercise is to think of it as just another physical activity that you do in the course of your day. Activity that accumulates throughout your day counts, and it can include anything from doing housework chores and gardening to taking the stairs instead of using an elevator to riding bikes with your children or grandchildren. Your goal is to accumulate at least thirty minutes a day.

My mother has worked out her entire life—without ever stepping into a gym. She always incorporated the activities of daily living in her fitness regimen without even knowing it. Because she is a meticulous housekeeper, she is always busily scrubbing the floors, vacuuming, mopping, sweeping, or washing windows. My mother does not drive, so she walks almost everywhere she needs to go. She even walks to the market and carries her own heavy bags of groceries back home. She is proof to me that you can incorporate moderate activity into your life and reap the rewards of staying healthy.

Overcoming Common Barriers
to Exercise

No matter how you perceive exercise, you must move beyond any resistance you have to it and into an acceptance of activity as a way of life—for the rest of your life. See if you identify with any of these five common mental barriers that women have toward exercise.

BARRIER 1. MISPERCEIVING THE WORD *EXERCISE*.

I want you to think of exercise as any physical activity, including walking your dog each evening or mowing your lawn. It can mean taking an aerobics class with a group of women, or doing aerobics in the privacy of your own home with a good videotape. It can include normal daily routines such as vacuuming your floors, mopping the kitchen, planting flowers in your garden, carrying your groceries, taking a brisk walk during your lunch hour, or playing in the park with your children or grandchildren.

BARRIER 2: BEING TOO BUSY FOR EXERCISE.

Many of my patients complain that their busy schedules allow them no time for regular daily exercise. That's when I share my personal exercise history. When I was younger, I did not participate in competitive sports, and like many doctors-in-training, my biggest workout fifteen years ago was climbing the stairs of the hospital. Then one day my husband, Robert, and I received a flyer about a new gym opening up in Park Slope, near where we had lived. Robert was thrilled and wanted to check it out immediately. Upon touring the gym, we found it had all the amenities he wanted, including a big swimming pool. I agreed to join but was hesitant, since I had never considered myself an athlete and thought I wasn't "good enough." But I gradually came to love the exhilaration of physical motion. Today Robert teases me that although initially I was hesitant about joining the gym, now I'm never home because I'm always there in my free time.

My individualized exercise program combines my daily-life activity and my regular workout regimen at the gym, and yours can too. For example, I am an avid walker, and I walk to many of my activities. Because I now live in the heart of Manhattan, I can easily walk to my office early each morning, to the hospital to see patients, and to a nearby grocery store to pick up fresh produce before going home at night. For me, walking is my greatest ally in the prevention of heart disease. The additional time I spend in the gym during the week adds to my daily walking program and also gives me much-needed time to de-stress.

Here's a daily capsule of my regular physical activity, which is for a moderate fitness level. My small segments of aerobic exercise and daily activity add up to more than thirty minutes per day, the minimum daily requirement for heart health.

1. Walk to work (ten minutes round trip)
2. Walk to the hospital (twenty minutes round trip)
3. Take the stairs at work (fifteen minutes daily)
4. Weight training (a twice-weekly one-hour session with trainer to focus on upper and lower body and abs)
5. Spinning or aerobics class (three days each week, forty-five to fifty minutes per session)

The goals of my individualized exercise program include building endurance and boosting muscle strength and toning. Because I enjoy walking and resistance training, I get the double benefit of a weight-bearing exercise and a bone booster. Also, the time I spend at the gym brings me together with a strong social network of other women who enjoy exercise as well.

Now please think about your own routine: When are you already moving around? Where could you add more activity to get to thirty to forty-five minutes a day of movement?

BARRIER 3: THINKING THAT AEROBICS IS THE ONLY FORM OF EXERCISE.
In reality, aerobic exercise is simply any type of movement involving low resistance and repetition and that uses your large muscles. Aerobic exercise can be as simple as using your leg muscles to walk your dog or climb the stairs at work.

My patient Millie, age fifty, went to health spas all the time for stretching and meditation classes. But she hated to do any activity that made her heart beat faster. While she was very laid back, she was overweight and needed aerobic exercise to get back in shape. We discussed this several times, but at each visit Millie's blood pressure had increased. Finally it was near a danger zone, and I felt we had to get her into an individualized exercise program. I gave her my pep talk, and she quietly listened. When I was finished, she offered the common excuses, saying, "Well, I'm not going to an aerobics class. I hate to sweat, and I won't be able to keep up with the younger women. Besides, I'd look horrible in those skintight leotards."

I explained to Millie that she didn't have to go to an aerobics class—she could simply pick up her walking pace. Then she actually joined the gym and started to work out on the treadmill and exercise bicycle. Today, along with her daily exercise routine, she also attends a resistance training class twice a week. Her blood pressure has gone down, and she's lost weight.

BARRIER 4: FEELING THAT YOU MUST LOOK GREAT TO EXERCISE.

Another barrier many women have is the belief that they must look great to participate in an exercise program. My patients' excuses include "I need to lose weight *before* I go to the gym" and "I don't have the right kind of exercise clothes." I explain that they can't get into shape *before* they get into shape. Dieting to lose weight before you exercise is a common practice, but it's not successful over a long period of time. The weight you lose by dieting alone will usually creep back again—and you'll gain extra weight on top of that. Comprehensive studies confirm that you will lose more weight and keep it off if you combine exercise and diet.[6]

BARRIER 5: HAVING DIFFICULTY GETTING STARTED BECAUSE OF LACK OF INSTRUCTIONS.

My friend Mary is the most health-conscious woman I know. She has a very healthy diet, eating a variety of fresh vegetables, fruits, and grains, and she maintains a healthy weight. As administrator of cardiology in my hospital, her constant walking and stair-climbing time totals more than thirty minutes per day.

One day Mary told me she wanted information on the heart- and bone-boosting benefits of resistance training. She asked if she could try the exercise bands that we use in the women's program. I brought the brightly colored bands to Mary's office, where she hung them on a hook behind her door. The bands looked impressive hanging in her office, but when I saw that they were still in the same spot a few weeks later, I asked her why she hadn't used them. Mary replied, "You forgot to bring me the instructions. I have no idea what to do with the bands."

Needing instructions is a common barrier to beginning an exercise program. Once I gave Mary the instruction booklet and demonstrated how to hold and pull the bands to provide resistance, she started enjoying her new "portable" resistance workout and is still using the bands today.

How to Exercise

Sometimes it is hard to know where to begin, how long to exercise, and how hard to train. I wouldn't tell you or a patient "just exercise," any more than I would say simply "just take a pill." When I prescribe medication, I give an exact prescription that specifies the type of medication, the frequency it should be taken, and the number of days over which it's to be taken. The same goes for exercise—you need directions. You need to know how often to exercise, how hard, what kind to do, and for how long.

Frequency

Frequency means how many times a week you work out. Ideally, the frequency is half an hour or more per day for aerobic activity, along with resistance training two to three times per week. If you cannot commit to a thirty-minute block of a set workout, then you can break it up into shorter durations, such as three ten-minute intervals. If you find that difficult to do, cut back to three days per week until you build stamina and strength.

As you increase the frequency of your exercise program, monitor how you feel. You might want to keep a little purse-size notebook or journal, or make notes on your calendar about when you exercise and jot down how you feel afterward. After a few weeks, the workout may be easier to do.

Intensity

Intensity means how hard you are working during your activity. I recommend moderate intensity for aerobic activities because studies have shown that moderate intensity in exercise for women is enough to promote heart health if done regularly.[7] If you're already active, this intensity will be easy to attain. But if it's been a while since you were physically active, start with lower-intensity activities and build up to moderate ones. Remember that the regularity of exercise is what's most important for your heart's health.

Women frequently ask me how they can know if they're exercising too much or not enough. You can tell you've reached the right intensity if your heart is beating faster and you're breathing a little more quickly but you can still speak. *That* is a good level for optimal benefits.

To know exactly what intensity is best for you, use the following tips:

TIP 1: MEASURE INTENSITY BY HOW YOU PERCEIVE IT.

One way to measure intensity during a workout is to rate your exertion according to the Borg or Modified Borg Perceived Exertion Scale. This scale helps you translate the feeling of a specific physical effort into a number. The goal is to connect your mind and body to the work you are doing. I've adapted the Modified Borg scale to help you really "feel" varying demands of physical effort.

MODIFIED EXERTION SCALE

1. Rest (sitting in a chair)
2. Very light (just warming up)
3. Moderate (starting to enter the work zone)

4. Somewhat strong
5. Strong
6. Moderately strong (you're working hard and are able to talk about it)
7. Very strong
8. Outside your fitness zone
9. Exhaustion
10. Beyond exhaustion

On this scale, a perceived exertion of 5 to 7 is in the target zone. You should feel as if you are working but still be able to talk.

TIP 2: KEEP TRACK OF YOUR HEART RATE.
Your exercise or training heart rate is a percentage of the maximal heart rate achieved on the stress test (usually 70 to 85 percent of the maximal heart rate). This number is calculated from the target heart rate zone equation (see the box following), which varies depending on your age, your fitness level, and whether or not you are taking medications that slow down the pulse.

To compute your heart rate zone, subtract your age from 220 and multiply this number by 70 percent. This gives you the low number of the heart rate zone. Now subtract your age from 220 and multiply this number by 85 percent to get your high number. It is important to keep your heart rate between these two numbers while exercising for maximum cardiovascular benefits.

If you've had a stress test, your doctor can give you your target heart rate from the test results. The target heart rate from your stress test is 65 to 85 percent of the maximal heart rate you attained on the stress test. This is the heart rate zone (or training zone) you should be exercising in after you do your warm-up, and it is one way you can measure your exercise intensity.

TARGET HEART RATE ZONE FOR AGE FORTY

Low zone: 220−40 = 180 × .70 = 126
High zone: 220−40 = 180 × .85 = 153
Target heart rate range: 126 to 153

Checking your pulse periodically through the workout helps you to monitor the intensity. If your pulse is higher than the target heart rate range, you may be working too hard. Slow down until your pulse is in the proper range, and stay at that pace to avoid injury.

The real problem is not how to figure out your heart rate but how to measure it while you're exercising. Taking your pulse is easier said than done, because you have to take it while you're moving around. You may have seen women in an aerobics class slow down their exercise and hold their wrists as they concentrate more on taking their pulse than on keeping the rhythmic beat!

TIP 3: KEEP TRACK OF YOUR PULSE MANUALLY.
Although it's not always easy, you can keep track of your pulse by placing your finger (not your thumb) on the artery on the side of your windpipe (your carotid pulse) or on the thumb side of your wrist. Continue your movement in place; do not completely stop while you count your pulse rate for fifteen seconds. Multiply this number by four to get your total pulse for one minute. Speed up or slow down your exercise pace to keep your heart rate within the target range. Continue to check your pulse periodically to make sure you are not overdoing it (or going at a snail's pace either!).

HEART RATE FORMULA

15-second pulse rate × 4 = Total heart rate for one minute

TIP 4: USE A HEART RATE WATCH.
A good alternative to taking your pulse manually is to purchase a heart rate watch. These are commercially available. To use the

watch, you put the band that comes with it on your chest underneath your exercise clothes. This band transmits your heart rate to the special wristwatch you wear during exercise. To assess your heart rate during exercise, you merely look at the watch.

If you don't want to buy this special watch, you can use any watch with a second hand or a digital watch to keep track of the fifteen seconds.

MEDICATION CAN SLOW YOUR HEART RATE
In some cases (10 to 15 percent of the time), the Heart Rate Formula will not work. If you are on a medication that slows your heart rate, such as a beta-blocker or a calcium channel blocker, you could run all day and still not get your heart rate in the target range. If you are on a medication, consult your doctor for your target heart rate during exercise to be safe.

For the most effective way to measure the intensity of a workout, use a combination of the heart rate measurement methods along with my Modified Exertion Scale.

Type of Exercise

In choosing exercises for your individualized plan, remember that the one you choose should be one you enjoy doing. In most cases, the exercises and activities listed in the box are in the moderate-intensity category. But if you don't think you can start at that intensity, go with a lower-intensity activity and build upward. Consider the list as a general guideline.

SELECT YOUR FAVORITE ACTIVITIES

LOW INTENSITY
Ballroom dancing (light)
Bowling
Dusting (light)
Golf (with cart)
Water aerobics (slow tempo)
Yoga

MODERATE INTENSITY

Active play with children

Aerobics (low-impact, or arms at shoulder height and one foot on the
    floor)

Badminton

Ballroom dancing (fast)

Cycling (leisure)

Gardening

Golf (carrying clubs)

Mall walking (3.3 to 4 miles per hour)

Mopping floors

Stair climbing

Stationary cycling

Swimming (moderate)

Tae kwon do

Tennis (doubles)

Vacuuming

Walking, brisk

Washing windows

Water aerobics (moderate tempo)

HIGH INTENSITY

Aerobics (high-impact, or arms over head and jumping movements)

Basketball

Biking (hills)

Cardio kick-boxing

Dancing (fast)

Hiking

Jogging

Jumping rope

Karate

Rollerblading

Shoveling (fast)

Soccer

Spinning

Surfing
Swimming (fast)
Tennis (singles)
Water jogging

Duration

Whatever intensity you can handle—low, medium, or high—try to incorporate thirty minutes of it into your daily routine. Thirty minutes of moderate physical activity is a level that most healthy women can achieve, and it will promote heart health by lowering your heart rate and blood pressure. But if you need to lose weight, you'll have to aim for at least forty-five minutes of activity.

Whatever exercise you choose—running, biking, swimming, raking the leaves, or walking around your yard or the block—you'll be one step ahead of the game by starting to do it today.

Your Exercise Prescription

Now that you know some of the benefits of moving around more, along with common barriers women have toward exercise, it's important to individualize your program. In this section, I'm going to give you a specific Exercise Prescription (your Rx) to lose weight, lower your cholesterol, and build muscular strength. But first let me tell you about Lisa, age thirty-seven, whom I treated for hypertension last year. She went from detesting exercise to enjoying her daily workouts at home.

Lisa had become a little housebound after the birth of her twins, and while she did lose twenty-two pounds initially, she could not lose the remaining eighteen pounds of "baby fat" she had gained from the pregnancy. Even though she knew that exercise, along with her medication, could help her control high blood pressure and lose weight, she simply could not get motivated to start a regular program. In fact, each time I saw her, she had the same excuse: "Dr. Goldberg, don't worry! I'm still looking for the perfect exercise."

At one visit, I noticed that Lisa's weight and blood pressure had increased, and I finally told her, "If I could exercise for you, I would do it!" I think Lisa was a little shocked to hear how frustrated I was with her, and she said, "Dr. Goldberg, if you feel that strongly about it, I promise to start this week."

Searching for that perfect exercise is often just another excuse for not exercising. To help Lisa incorporate exercise into her daily routine, I explained that she was already moderately physically active—she just needed a regular workout program to help lose weight and strengthen her body. Losing weight and adding more exercise would help reduce her blood pressure too. That took some pressure off of Lisa, knowing that she was doing something good for her heart. After taking some notes about her daily activities, I drew the following chart for her:

LISA'S DAILY ACTIVITIES

Activity	Accumulated Time Per Day
Chasing the active twins (including bending, lifting, and carrying)	25 minutes
Walking dog in the evening	10 minutes
Household chores	25 minutes

Even though this was a good amount of light to moderate movement, Lisa needed more regular exercise and a resistance-training program to lose weight and lower her blood pressure.

Your Rx: Add Up Your Daily Activities

As you design your exercise program, I want you to incorporate moving around more and exercise into your daily routine. Using the following blank chart, write down the physical activities you normally do each day, along with the total amount of time. (Include any walking, running, lifting, pushing, pulling, bending, or stooping activities, and anything you do that increases your heart rate.)

MY DAILY ACTIVITIES

Activity	Accumulated Time Per Day
1.	
2.	
3.	
4.	
5.	

Your Rx: Set a Dedicated Workout Time

Once you've seen how active (or inactive) you are with regular daily activities, I now want you to establish a *set time for a workout or exercise at least three days a week*. The time can be in the morning before work or in the evening after dinner. Whenever you can block twenty to thirty minutes into your daily schedule for exercise, write it on your calendar, and don't let anyone interrupt your "heart-boosting time." In Lisa's case, she did get plenty of movement in her daily routine, but I convinced her that she also needed a dedicated time to work out—one that was set on her calendar and a priority in her life.

Your Rx: Find Activities You Enjoy

What activities do you enjoy? Using the box on pages 233–235, choose the exercises and activities you enjoy, and incorporate them in your workout plan.

Lisa used to enjoy going to a dance aerobics class and riding bikes, but with two small toddlers and no baby-sitter, these activities were now out of the question. I suggested she rent or purchase some exercise videos and try to follow a three-day-per-week regimen of regular exercise. The exercise videos would allow her to stay at home and care for her toddlers while doing a variety of movements and exercises at different levels of intensity.

I also encouraged her to buy some elastic exercise bands to use for resistance training. These bands help to strengthen the muscles we use every day. I gave her a few other ideas on how to build her "home-based gym," including a step bench (a plastic bench that comes with adjustable risers) and a fit ball, which is great for stretching your lower back and doing abdominal and leg work. (Her twins also loved stepping on the bench and rolling on the fit ball while Lisa held it!)

Lisa found a popular exercise video that included many dance movements performed to favorite songs. As she had promised, she followed the video three times a week and did the resistance bands on the opposite days (twice a week).

TYPES OF EXERCISE CLASSES

- **Low-impact aerobics**—uses arm and leg movements choreographed to music. At least one foot is on the ground at any given time. There are no jumping movements.
- **High-impact aerobics**—uses arm and leg movements choreographed to music. Includes jumping movements.
- **Body sculpting**—resistance (strength) training with free weights, resistance bands, and body bands.
- **Body conditioning**—combines features of low-impact aerobics and body sculpting; increases muscle strength with less chance of injury, as you put less stress on the musculoskeletal system than in high-impact aerobics.

HOW TO CHOOSE AN EXERCISE CLASS

1. Read the class description in the available brochure.
2. If you are starting to exercise or getting back from a long hiatus, choose a class that is geared to beginners.
3. Observe the class before you start, and pay attention to the class size. Look at the spacing between participants—you don't want someone's hand in your face while you're exercising.
4. Notice if there is a warm-up period before the moderate exercise portion: five to seven minutes of low-intensity aerobic exercise and stretching.

5. Watch the instructor. Is she facing the class and paying attention to participants who have trouble keeping up?
6. Does the instructor give alternatives for difficult-to-follow movements? (For example, if you have trouble coordinating the arm and leg movements, just do the leg movements. Or if you are getting tired, decrease the height of your arms.)
7. Does the instructor help to correct body alignment during the class?
8. Make sure that the moderate exercise or the training component of the class, which usually lasts thirty minutes, is followed by a cool-down period, mirroring the warm-up.
9. Are the instructors certified?
10. Does the music work for you?

Your Rx: Add Resistance Training

Along with setting a workout time, I want you to establish time for an individualized resistance-training program. It should include eight to ten exercises for the major muscle groups (arms, legs, shoulders, chest, back, hips, and trunk). The exercises should be performed two or three days a week with one or two sets, ten to fifteen repetitions per set. If you are using free weights or weight machines, increase the weight after you can comfortably perform fifteen repetitions.

Divide your resistance-training workout into low, moderate, and high sections, depending on the intensity of the activity and your experience with this exercise.

- **Low:** Using an elastic resistance band; using your own weight as resistance; lifting canned vegetables or fruit; lifting bags of groceries or a baby
- **Moderate:** Using a medium-intensity exercise band; using free weights, wrist and ankle weights, weight machines, or your body weight (in calisthenics or push-ups)
- **High:** Using heavier free weights (dumbbells or barbells) or weight machines

Like Lisa, you may want to get a colored elastic band from your local sporting goods store for your resistance workout. To start, do the following exercises eight to twelve times on each side of your body. In about two weeks, after you become used to the exercises, move to two sets of eight to twelve times each on each side of your body. You can do these exercises to get back into shape and protect your heart:

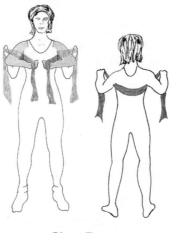

Chest Press

CHEST PRESS. In a standing position, grip the ends of the band in your right and left hands. Place the band around your back, running under the armpits. Holding both ends of the band, extend your arms out in front of your body, keeping your upper arms parallel to the floor and your hands about shoulder width apart. Pull the band taut, so there isn't any slack. Exhale as you bring your arms out in front of your body, matching the two ends together. Inhale as you release the tension, and let the bands go back to the starting position. Repeat this procedure eight to twelve times. Rest, and do another eight or twelve.

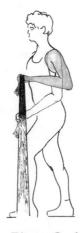

Biceps Curl

BICEPS CURL. Stand and place the band on the floor under your right foot and hold the other end with your right hand in a tight grip. Pressing your right elbow into the side of your body, bring your fist up toward your shoulder and then extend it back down to the side. Exhale as you curl your arm, then inhale as you return to your starting position; repeat eight to twelve times. Reverse sides to work your left bicep. Rest, and then do another set of eight to twelve repetitions.

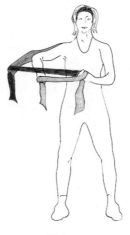

Triceps

TRICEPS. Stand with your legs about a shoulder width apart and your knees slightly bent. Take the elastic band, and wrap one end around each hand, keeping your hands approximately a shoulder width apart. Bring your right fist to the left shoulder to hold the band against your body. Holding the left forearm parallel to the floor, fully extend the right arm and then flex it back to the shoulder. Hold each movement, then lower and repeat eight to twelve times; reverse to the left side. Rest, and then do another set of eight to twelve.

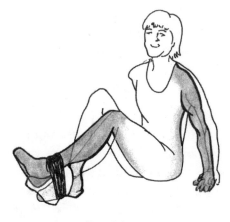

Quadriceps

QUADRICEPS. Sit on the floor, and tie each end of the band around your ankles. Then loop the elastic band under the arch of the right foot. Bend your knees so that your feet are flat on the floor, and then lean back on your hands or elbows. Extend and straighten your left leg, keeping your knees parallel. Hold for five seconds, then release. Remember to exhale as you extend your leg and inhale as you relax. This exercise should be repeated eight to twelve times on each side.

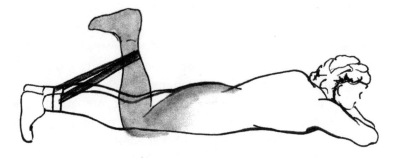

Hamstrings

HAMSTRINGS. Tie the band around your ankles. Lie facedown on the floor, resting your chin on your hands. One leg will be stationary, while the other leg is in motion. Exhale as you curl your right leg ninety degrees, then inhale as you lower your leg. Repeat this eight to ten times, then do the same with your left leg. Rest, and do another eight to ten repetitions with each leg.

Your Rx: Calculate Your Total Workout Time

You should aim to do your workout for at least thirty minutes, three times a week, but you can certainly do it every day. On the days when you're not doing your workout, do your resistance training, about fifteen minutes each time. Lisa tallied her total exercise time and found that it was forty-five minutes, three days a week, on nonconsecutive days, so her muscles had a chance to rest. On days when she was busy with her twins, she split the workout into separate segments. For example, if she didn't have enough time to do a total workout, she could work her upper body muscles one day and her lower body muscles the next. That way the muscles in each segment would be strengthened and then have a chance to rest.

Your Rx: Add Toning Exercises

After you have done your workout for four weeks, try these exercises to tone your muscles. While you are doing toning exercises, pay attention to your posture. I find that exercising in front of a mirror at the Y is helpful to make sure I'm following a proper form and that my posture is good and my arms and legs are coordinating their movements. If you work out at home, you can put a full-length mirror by your exercise spot to notice how you are standing and moving.

Lisa wanted to tighten her abdominal muscles after giving birth to twins, so I suggested the following six-minute abdominal workout that she could do at any time of the day, even while the twins were watching their favorite cartoon shows. Abdominal exercises are key to having good posture and avoiding back pain. With each abdominal exercise, do two sets of eight to twelve repetitions. Be sure to breathe properly: exhale as you work the muscle, and inhale as you relax it.

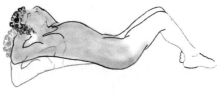

Crunch

CRUNCH. Lie on your back with your hands at the base of your neck, keeping your head and neck in line with your spine. Now contract your abdominal muscles, and exhale as you lift your shoulders. Your shoulders will rise a few inches, but your lower and middle back will still touch the floor. Hold for five seconds, then lower your shoulders, inhaling. Repeat eight to twelve times. (If you have low back problems, ask a physical therapist for specific instructions.)

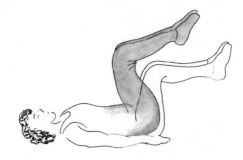

Curl

C U R L . Lie on your back with your knees bent and your feet flat on the floor. Exhale as you raise your hips and contract your abdominal muscles until your tailbone clears the floor. Hold for five seconds. Inhale as you release the curl. Repeat eight to twelve times.

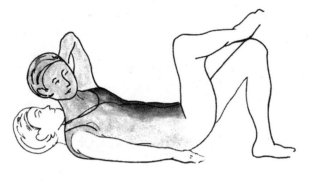

Twist

T W I S T . Lie on your back with your knees bent and your feet on the floor. Cross your right leg over your left thigh. Bring your right hand up and hold the base of your neck on that same side. Twist at the waist toward the left, and exhale while you bring your right shoulder toward your left knee. Remember to keep your elbow back. Inhale as you return to your start position. Repeat this movement eight to twelve times, then reverse and repeat on the other side.

Your Rx: Add Stretches for Flexibility

Flexibility, the ability to move your limbs through their full range of motion, is a key element of fitness, along with cardiovascular endurance and muscle strength. Flexibility varies from one woman to the next. You may be flexible enough to touch your toes yet have trouble doing crunches. Your best friend may be able to do crunches but unable to bend forward and touch her toes without stiffness. Flexibility helps to protect you from injury during exercise, and the best way to get this protection is through stretching before and after your workout.

A person's flexibility is determined by several factors, including:

- The intensity and types of physical activity performed
- Sex (women are more flexible than men)
- Age (flexibility decreases as you get older if you don't work at it)
- Temperature (warm muscles are more flexible than cold ones)

Numerous studies have shown that stretching makes muscles more elastic and increases the joints' range of motion. It may even enhance how long and hard you can exercise. Stretching is not just for joggers, ballet dancers, and athletes! Incorporate stretching into your overall fitness program before and after you walk, run, or do any physical activity.

The following six stretches will let you move more easily, avoid injury, and alleviate aches and pains. The entire stretching workout takes about four minutes total. Hold each stretch for twenty seconds, and be sure to work both sides of your body.

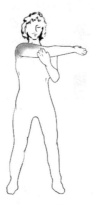

Shoulder Stretch

SHOULDER STRETCH. Stand with your feet a hip width apart, your knees relaxed, and both arms straight out in front of you. Extend your left arm and bring it across your chest. Your left shoulder should be pressed down away from your ear, and your left hand relaxed. Use your right hand to press your left elbow toward your chest and hold. You will feel the stretch in the upper right shoulder. Hold for twenty seconds, then do the same for the right arm and shoulder.

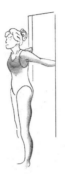

Upper Body Posture Stretch

UPPER BODY POSTURE STRETCH. Stand in front of a door with your arms outstretched at about a ninety-degree angle. Hold on to the doorframe with your hands at shoulder level, and stagger your stance, placing one foot forward. Brace yourself, then lean forward until you feel the stretch in the upper chest. Hold for twenty seconds.

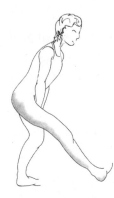

Hamstrings

HAMSTRINGS. While standing, bring your right leg forward with your foot flexed at the ankle. Your left leg should be bent while you lean forward with your hands on your left thigh. You should feel this stretch in the upper part of your right leg. Hold this position for twenty seconds and release; reverse to stretch the left hamstring.

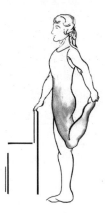

Quadriceps Stretch

QUADRICEPS STRETCH. Stand facing the back of a chair. Balance yourself by placing your right hand on top of the chair. With your left hand, pull your left heel up to your buttocks, bending the leg as you do this. Feel the stretch in your quadriceps, the muscle in the front of your upper leg. Hold for twenty seconds, then repeat with the right leg.

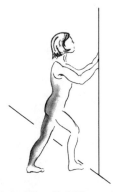

Standing Calf Stretch

STANDING CALF STRETCH. Stand about one foot from a wall. Put both hands on the wall, and move your right foot about three feet behind you. Shift your weight forward, keeping your feet parallel to each other and your right heel on the floor. Feel the stretch in your calf muscle. Hold for twenty seconds, then repeat with the left leg.

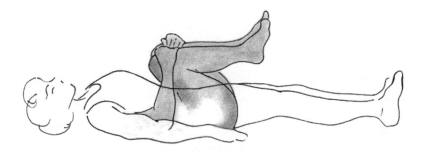

Low Back Stretch

LOW BACK STRETCH. Lie on your back, bring both knees to your chest together. Hold this position for twenty seconds and release.

Your Rx: Enjoy the Results!

These exercises will improve your balance, your posture, and the muscles you use in your everyday activities. After doing them for three months, Lisa started seeing results. She lost eleven pounds without cutting back on calories, and her blood pressure dropped back into the normal range for her age. Her stomach was flatter, her clothes fit better, and her muscles were tight instead of flabby. Lisa especially likes the fact that she does not have to leave her house to do the exercise program. She fits in her workouts using the exercise videotapes and the resistance band while her twins are napping. (Note: If you have home exercise equipment, such as a bicycle, a rowing machine, or a treadmill, you can change your resistance-training program from very low intensity, doing the movements without weight, to using low- to high-intensity resistance bands or dumbbells.)

You too can enjoy the results of getting to a normal weight and strengthening your muscles. Make a commitment to start an exercise program that's right for you, adapted to your daily life, and make it a priority.

Putting It All Together

Let's review your Exercise Prescription. As you progress with your individualized exercise program, check off each item in the following list:

- ♥ *Your Rx:* Add Up Your Daily Activities   _____
- ♥ *Your Rx:* Set a Dedicated Workout Time   _____
- ♥ *Your Rx:* Find Activities You Enjoy   _____
- ♥ *Your Rx:* Add Resistance Training   _____
- ♥ *Your Rx:* Calculate Your Total Workout Time   _____
- ♥ *Your Rx:* Add Toning Exercises   _____
- ♥ *Your Rx:* Add Stretches for Flexibility   _____
- ♥ *Your Rx:* Enjoy the Results!   _____

Measurable Healthy Heart Results from Exercise

Most of the women I treat are impatient to see results from the Exercise Prescription. In general, if you stick with it, you should notice improved endurance in just three or four weeks. If you find that you are not reaching your target heart rate or that it is lower than it was a month ago, that's a positive sign—it means you're experiencing the training response, with a lower heart rate and lower resting blood pressure. If this is the case, consider increasing the intensity of your workout, perhaps by increasing the speed or elevation on the treadmill, or by increasing the length of your workout from thirty to thirty-five or forty minutes.

Lower Systolic Blood Pressure

After exercising for about four weeks, you should notice that your systolic blood pressure is lower by eight to ten points. For some women, this difference may help them avoid hypertension medication altogether, which is desirable since every medication has some side effects. For others, the reduction in systolic blood pressure may help reduce the dosage of their medication. Always check with your doctor about altering dosages—do not do it on your own.

Higher HDL ("Good") Cholesterol Levels

It may take longer than six months to increase your levels of HDL ("good") cholesterol. Postmenopausal women may have to wait a full year. But with regular exercise, the average increase in HDL cholesterol is 10 percent. It continues to increase with continued exercise, so please don't give up.

Weight Loss and Lower LDL ("Bad") Cholesterol Levels

You may see moderate weight loss after three to six months of regular aerobic exercise. If you are also dieting, you may also see reduced LDL ("bad") cholesterol (by about 8 to 10 percent). But if the changes do not show up during your first months of exercise, don't give up or become frustrated. Over time small daily changes add up to a stronger, healthier heart. You may notice that you are less tired during the workday or have more energy to do your housework. These benefits will become noticeable and will eventually show up on the bathroom scale!

Lower Triglyceride Levels

Exercise, in combination with the Mediterranean-style diet presented in Chapter 10, and choosing foods low on the glycemic index are effective ways to reduce triglycerides and so to lower your risk of heart disease.

INCORPORATE MINIWORKOUTS INTO YOUR BUSY DAY

If you find that you cannot make a commitment of thirty continuous minutes for several days each week, then break up your exercise into "miniworkouts." Pulsed exercises are ten-minute workouts that can be done throughout the day and can provide aerobic fitness. Although the training response will occur more slowly, the result will be the same.

To keep from getting bored, vary the exercises and activities you do each day. Don't let the change of seasons prevent you from staying fit. If you enjoy walking in the park during the summer, consider joining an indoor aerobics class for the winter months, when you may not want to walk in ice and snow (unless you love it!). If you are passionate about beach volleyball, check out your local Y for the indoor volleyball schedule during cold months. Likewise, if you thrive on swimming in the lake, continue this water sport in an indoor pool.

If you do not like to exercise out of doors or with a group of people, rent or buy a few of the popular exercise videos and try them out in the privacy of your own home. There are instructional videos for all levels of fitness. You can get up ten minutes earlier in the morning before work or before your usual day starts, pop in the tape, and get moving—no matter how inclement the weather. When it comes to your heart's health, there are no excuses!

Four Tips to Exercise Safely

TIP 1: ALWAYS WARM UP BEFORE EXERCISING

Before you start exercising, you should warm up with five to ten minutes of walking, jogging, or a lower-intensity exercise. To increase flexibility, you should also stretch your limbs and move them through their full range of motion.

**SAFETY TIPS FOR ALL
TYPES OF EXERCISE**

- Always warm up before exercising.
- Finish exercising with a cool-down.
- Stay hydrated.
- Know your personal limitations.
- If the activity hurts, *stop*.
- If you feel dizziness or discomfort in your chest, arms, or throat, *stop*.
- Don't forget sunscreen if you are outside.
- Reduce your workout in hot and humid temperatures, or take it inside to an air-conditioned facility. If one is unavailable, take the day off.

Pay attention to the quality of your stretches. Don't think that you have to do ten or more to warm up. A few on each side should be enough. A few properly done stretching exercises will increase your flexibility safely and effectively.

One of the safest techniques for improving flexibility is the Static Stretch. To do it, you gradually stretch each body part as far as it will comfortably go, then hold it with a steady gentle force for fifteen to thirty seconds. You should also do the stretches on pages 246–249.

Never, ever jerk your body to lengthen a stretch. Don't ever bounce in place to stretch either, no matter who's told you that that's a good way to stretch. It isn't, and you can really hurt your joints and tendons by doing it.

If you are sedentary, you particularly need the relief from muscle tension and stiffness that stretching provides. When it is done the right way, stretching feels good. Improper or excessive stretching, however, actually increases the likelihood of injury.

As you stretch, if you feel any pain, *stop!* Discuss any pains you feel with your physician, or consult a physical therapist who can show you the proper way to stretch without creating injury.

TIP 2: STOP IF IT HURTS!

If you experience any shortness of breath, dizziness, nausea, or palpitations or chest pain during exercise, stop it immediately, and consult your physician before you try again.

TIP 3: STAY HYDRATED

Don't forget to stay well hydrated by drinking water before, during, and after you exercise. Dehydration reduces blood volume and causes less fluid to reach the brain, which keeps it from working efficiently and makes your body feel exhausted. Being even slightly dehydrated can reduce your concentration and slow your blood circulation. Drinking too little water during exercise negatively affects your coordination, endurance, and strength and may make you dizzy, nauseated, or crampy. Whether you are thirsty or not, drink water on a regular schedule instead of waiting until you are thirsty— which sometimes means you're already too dehydrated to exercise comfortably or effectively.

TIP 4: FINISH WITH A COOL-DOWN

A ten-to-fifteen-minute cool-down after your workout will allow your heart rate to decrease gradually and will help prevent muscle soreness. To cool down, walk at a slower pace, stretch, or ride a stationary bicycle.

Give It Time

With your Exercise Prescription, you will see short-term results of increased energy and well-being within days. It may take several weeks or months, however, before you see a significant reduction in weight, body fat, blood pressure, or cholesterol. But please keep at it! These heart-saving benefits will happen after a while. I've seen it time and again.

Start small, and build into a full exercise program that you look forward to doing every day. For example, if you start out walking and swimming, start with just ten minutes a day the first week. As you increase in strength and endurance, add five minutes the second week, then another five minutes the third week and so on until you get up to thirty minutes of exercise at least five times a week.

As you make plans to start your exercise program, establish goals with your doctors that are *reasonable* for your age and physical condition. If you are healthy, relatively fit, and have no signs of heart disease, work into a regular program of thirty minutes of aerobic or endurance exercise, five times a week, with resistance training three times a week. This would be ideal. But if you are out of shape and have several risk factors for heart disease, go slowly, listen to your body, and stop exercising immediately should you feel discomfort.

Watch for Burnout

After working out for several weeks, you may begin to feel sluggish and think that working harder might give you more energy. Don't be deceived. Working out *too* much or *over*training can sometimes cause malaise and sluggishness. If you have these symptoms, however, don't simply assume they come from overtraining. Heart disease and other medical conditions can have similar symptoms. Before you continue your exercise program, discuss any unusual feelings or symptoms with your doctor.

Starting today, you can reduce your risk of heart disease simply by moving around more. Instead of riding in your car or taking the subway, walk; carry packages or a briefcase; use the stairs instead of the elevator. Exercise and do physical activities you enjoy regularly. Add resistance training several times each week to boost your fitness and to help tone you up and trim you down.

If you stop exercising, you will lose the benefits you were building up. Exercise is not a short-term Band-Aid but a long-term commitment to which you must adhere to keep your cardiovascular system functioning at its peak. In other words, the aerobic activity you did yesterday does not count unless you do it again today, tomorrow, and for years to come.

Now as you start the Healthy Heart Eating Plan in Chapter 10, you are well on your way to increasing longevity and living heart healthy for your entire lifetime.

10

Your Healthy Heart Eating Plan

When I was a young girl, I was quite small for my age and a very picky eater. My mother occasionally fed me lamb chops for breakfast, simply because I wouldn't eat anything else.

Today I know better. Yet many women today who know what they should eat and what foods are not good for their hearts have yet to modify their diets. During a recent question-and-answer period at a community lecture I gave at Lenox Hill Hospital, for instance, a woman asked what I ate for breakfast. My usual first meal is whole-grain cereal, skim milk, and fresh fruit. Afterward we asked the audience members to write their evaluations of the lecture. On her evaluation, this woman wrote that it was excellent, but she said that I "should eat more for breakfast." She clearly had to get together her understanding of healthy eating and portion size before she could make the dietary changes to keep heart disease at bay!

Three decades ago it simply was not widely known how damaging the fat content of some foods (like lamb chops!) can be to heart health. Scientific studies as far back as the mid-twentieth century showed a correlation between a high-fat diet and heart disease,[1] but many doctors didn't warn their patients to eat fewer fatty foods. And many of the patients who were warned ignored the message. Even today patients who need to lose weight refuse to meet with our center's dietitian because, they tell me, "I know how to eat." Sure they may know, but they aren't *acting* on that knowledge. To stay healthy and get healthy, you have to eat healthy. Clearly, what you eat—and don't eat—makes a major difference in the prevention and treatment of heart disease and other chronic health problems.

You know that a healthy diet is important—that certain foods boost your immune system and help prevent illness or infection. And you know that red meats and other fatty foods can increase your risk of chronic illness. For example, the Nurses' Health Study (see page 86) showed that when the women ate 5 percent more saturated fat, their risk of heart disease increased by 17 percent.[2] And every further 5 percent increase resulted in another 17 percent increase! Other studies have confirmed that a diet high in trans fatty acids, a type of fat found in solid margarine and many processed baked foods, raises levels of LDL ("bad") cholesterol and reduces levels of HDL ("good") cholesterol.[3] To decrease your risk of heart attack, you want the *opposite* effect. Some heart-healthy monounsaturated fats (like olive oil) are actually beneficial, reducing the dangerous LDL cholesterol without lessening the beneficial HDL cholesterol.

Even if you already know basics about healthy nutrition, this third step in the Women's Healthy Heart Program may give you the incentive you need to make life-saving changes and implement a heart-healthy diet. Studies show that even women with diagnosed heart disease improve their health by eating certain foods that are good for their heart. For example, the Lyon Diet Heart Study showed that people with heart disease who ate a Mediterranean diet were 50 to 70 percent less likely to suffer a repeat heart attack than those on an "American" diet.[4]

The patients in the Mediterranean-diet group also had an improved rate of survival over patients on the standard low-fat diet. The Lyon study was meant to continue for five years, but the difference was so marked that researchers released the data after the first few years. They did track the patients for the full five years, and by the end 95 percent of the patients were still following the diet. In other words, not only would the Mediterranean diet help extend their lifespan, they could live with it. On the Mediterranean-style diet, you can still eat plenty of good-tasting foods. You *can* eat well when you are eating right to improve your health.

What does all this mean for you? Oftentimes in my practice, patients ask me if there is one certain food they can eat or one nutritional supplement they can take to fight heart disease. They bring in newspaper or magazine clippings with the "diet of the month" that purportedly will help them lose weight and prevent heart attack. I wish it were that simple! Preventing heart disease takes time and energy, but the bottom line remains the same: *you must eat less and exercise more.*

Research on diet's effects on the cardiovascular system has confirmed some important principles for boosting heart health:

- Balance the calories or energy you eat by expending energy with regular physical activity.
- Eat less by reducing portion size.
- Keep your intake of saturated fats low.

The Mediterranean-Style Diet

A Mediterranean-style diet is rich in whole grains, vegetables, and fish as well as omega-3 fatty acids and alpha-linolenic acid—all of which are better for your heart than the typical American fare of processed foods, meats, and saturated fats. The Mediterranean-style diet ensures that you take in optimal vitamins and antioxidants, those special nutrients that neutralize the free radicals associated with many diseases, including heart disease and cancer. In fact, this heart-healthy diet will also reduce your risk of cancer. It's the best diet for your overall well-being. Your Healthy Heart Eating Plan incorporates this diet.

DIETARY RECOMMENDATIONS

Recommendation	How Much?
Eat more complex carbohydrates (fruits, vegetables, whole grains, beans, and peas).	Optimal intake 25–40 grams per day. At least 2 servings of fruits; 1serving of citrus fruit.
Eat fewer refined carbohydrates (sugar, white breads, and pastries).	As little as possible; none if you can manage.
Limit egg yolk and red meat intake (lamb, beef, and pork).	No more than 2 egg yolks per week or one three-ounce serving of red meat per week.
Eat more fish and poultry. Eat low-fat dairy products.	No more than 2 three-ounce servings of nonred meat or fish per day or 2–3 servings of dairy per day.
Instead of butter and cream, use olive oil, canola oil, nuts, and seeds.	No more than 6 teaspoons of oils per day or 5 servings of nuts per week.
Drink alcohol in moderation (optional).	No more than one drink per day.

These recommendations were adapted from dietary guidelines prepared by Cynthia Lynch, M.A., R.D., for the Lenox Hill Hospital Women's Heart Program and from the American Heart Association, American Dietetic Association, and DASH Diet National Heart, Lung, and Blood Institute.

Depending on your risk factors for heart disease, you may need to make only a few minor adjustments to what you normally eat. Maybe you're not overweight and just need to add more fresh fruits and vegetables, replace vegetable oil with olive oil, or eat more fish high in omega-3 fatty acids. Maybe you just need to eat a little less. But if your diet is loaded with fat, calories, and highly processed foods, you may need to overhaul your nutrition completely in order to eat right for your heart. No matter how healthy or unhealthy your current diet may be, I will show you some creative, easy ways to make changes that will give you variety and help you get the right balance of protein, carbohydrates, vitamins, and minerals.

"But there's so much information out there," sighed Julianne, age thirty-nine. "I frequently check out the health sites on the Internet, and if I did all that was recommended, I'd be eating all day and weigh four hundred pounds!" She's right—a tremendous amount of information (and much misinformation!) is available on diet, nutrition, and especially supplements. But this chapter will help you decipher what's true and substantiated by science—and what may be hype or someone's opinion—so that you know for certain what's good for you *and* your heart.

One word of caution about the Mediterranean-style diet: as with any food plan or diet, you must still:

- Count your daily calories.
- Measure your portions.

If you do not count calories, you will probably gain weight, because the Mediterranean-style diet has a higher fat content than traditional low-fat diets.

Following the Mediterranean-style diet, your Healthy Heart Eating Plan gives you permission to eat plenty of fresh fruits and vegetables, beans and peas, whole grains, healthy oils in moderation, lean chicken and fish, and low-fat dairy. All of these foods have been scientifically proven to keep your heart healthy. If you stick to the following nine guidelines, and stay aware of both calories and food portions, you will maintain a normal weight. You can also make adjustments to lose weight, if you need to.

1. Lose weight and stay at your desired weight.
2. Choose foods high in antioxidants.
3. Choose foods with heart smart B vitamins.
4. Choose foods with flavonoids.
5. Choose foods with phytochemicals.
6. Choose whole grains.

7. Choose healthy fats.
8. Watch your intake of sodium.
9. Limit your alcohol intake.

Lose Weight and Stay
at Your Desired Weight

Being 20 percent or more over normal body weight—obese—is epidemic in the United States, affecting one-third of the population. Another third are constantly dieting to avoid becoming obese. According to statistics from the American Heart Association survey, Americans today are more overweight than ever before: nearly 70 percent twenty-five or older are now considered overweight.[5] When you weigh more, even as little as ten or fifteen pounds over your desired weight, it's harder to be physically active. Even ten pounds overweight can exacerbate a heart condition by elevating blood pressure and cholesterol. The good news is that while gaining weight increases your risk of heart disease, *losing weight reduces the risk.*

How Much Should You Weigh?

We used to rely on the Metropolitan Life Insurance Height/Weight Chart to give an accurate weight range, but newer studies show that your body mass index (see page 20) and waist-to-hip ratio (see page 64) give a more accurate picture of health.

Your body mass index (BMI) is your body weight (in kilograms) divided by the square of your height (in meters). The resulting BMI number or value correlates to your risk of adverse effects on your health; higher numbers show an increased risk. Women with a higher percentage of body fat tend to have a higher BMI than those who have a greater percentage of muscle. It is the extra body fat that puts you at greater risk for health problems.

CHECK THE BMI CHART

Using the BMI chart (on page 20), locate the weight closest to your weight in the left-hand column. Then, along the top, locate the height closest to your height. Where these two numbers meet on the chart is your BMI. For example, if you weigh 150 pounds and are five foot four, your BMI is 26. Looking at the BMI index, a BMI of 26 means that you are "overweight," which could increase your risk of health problems.

Once you've assessed your personal risk with the BMI and calculated your waist-to-hip ratio (page 64), you'll have a good idea of what your weight should be. If you need to lose weight, you may wish to go back to Chapter 9 and review your exercise program.

Calories Do Count

"I've tried them all—liquid, low-carb, low-fat, and high-protein diets—and none works long term to help me lose weight," says fifty-year-old Josephine, a "fad diet expert" from years of following trendy diets with no results. If you are like her, don't throw in the towel just yet. I'm going to give you a new rule for maintaining your optimal weight that will result in permanent weight loss: *Count your calories.*

Health professionals have wavered for years on the importance of calories in weight loss, but they now concur that to lose weight and keep it off, you must take in fewer calories than you expend in energy each day.

BALANCE CALORIES AND ACTIVITY

It's important to understand that each woman is different. Your best friend may be as tall as you and weigh ten pounds less, yet depending on certain variables, you both may be at your optimal weight. These variables include height, age, bone structure, amount of lean body mass, and genetics.

The best way to reach or maintain an ideal weight is to burn more calories, through exercise and activity, than you take in. Many overweight women underestimate how much they actually eat, and they may need to exercise more in order to burn enough calories for weight loss. Even after an obese person gets closer to a normal weight, this problem with eating too much may continue.

More than 95 percent of the women who succeed in keeping off weight are exercisers—and most of them are walkers. Make sure you are keeping active and working to increase your level of each activity gradually, to the point that it helps you shed the pounds you want to lose.

PLAN YOUR WEIGHT LOSS

Before you start trying to lose weight, I want you to talk with your doctor about what your ideal weight is. (Choose a reasonable weight for your height.) You can start eating Mediterranean-style *today*, but before you start trying to take off pounds, do talk with your own doctor.

Here's a formula for determining how many calories you need to eat every day to lose weight. Suppose you weigh 140 pounds and you would like to lose ten pounds to attain your ideal body weight of 130. Subtract 10 from 140, then multiply the resulting 130 by ten, to get 1,300. Try to stay around 1,300 calories each day until you reach your goal. If you are moderately to vigorously physically active, this number may need to be adjusted upward, so that you have enough calories each day.

Present body weight: 140 pounds
Weight loss goal: 10 pounds
Ideal body weight: 130 pounds

To meet your ideal body weight of 130, don't eat more than 1,300 calories each day.

There is no magic food that will help you burn calories. Instead, you need to manage your lifestyle: you need to exercise more, and stay within your body's calorie requirement. If you normally fill up on low-fat cookies or chips in unlimited amounts, thinking this will help you to lose weight, I suggest you toss out whatever's left in your pantry! The fact is that fat-free is *not* calorie-free. Unlimited calories, including those found in fat-free or low-fat snacks, will still add inches to that waistline. You're trying to whittle down that apple shape to decrease your risk for heart attack.

Eat Small to Moderate Portions

One of the biggest ways that additional calories may show up on your plate is in portion size. I'm always amazed when I ask for a simple bagel at my favorite deli in Manhattan and get this huge, doughy Life Saver. It seems that over the past decade, the simple bagel has doubled in size.

To get an idea of this increase, check out the various brands of frozen bagels in your local supermarket's frozen food section. Read the label on the side of the package. I find it curious that the calorie count can vary from 100 calories for a minibagel (about the size of the palm of your hand) to 300 calories for a bagel as big as your entire hand. Ironically, both sizes are listed on the package as a "portion." Yet as you can see from the "How Much Is One Serving?" chart on pages 266–267, one item does not equate to one portion or serving!

RELEARN PORTION SIZE TO STAY SLIM

Try this experiment. Go to your favorite restaurant, and order your favorite pasta dish. Now compare this "serving" of pasta with a normal serving you would have at home. It's probably three to four times larger—or even more! I find it amazing that in some restaurants one order of pasta can fill a serving platter. (I did not say plate!) Perhaps even more amazing is that some women eat all of it, simply because it's low fat. Low-fat food is one case when "more" is not "better": large portions of low-fat foods will add up to increase your weight.

How Much Is One Serving?

BREAD, CEREAL, RICE, AND PASTA

1 slice of bread (whole grain and pumpernickel are better choices)

½ hamburger bun (1 whole bun = 2 portions)

½ bagel (1 whole bagel = 2 portions)

½ English muffin

½ large pita or flat bread

¾ ounce pretzels

½ cup cooked cereal, pasta, or rice

¾ cup unsweetened dry cereal

FRUIT

1 medium-size piece of fruit

¾ cup berries

1 cup melon chunks

½ cup grapes

½ cup chopped, cooked, or canned fruit

½ cup fruit juice

¼ cup nectar

VEGETABLES

½ cup cooked greens

1 cup raw greens (spinach, romaine, Bibb lettuce, and more)

1 cup raw cut-up vegetables (broccoli, cauliflower, and more)

½ cup cooked cut-up vegetables (broccoli, cauliflower, and more)

1 carrot

2 stalks celery

MILK

1 cup nonfat milk

1 cup nonfat, sugar-free yogurt

1 ounce cheese
¼ cup fat-free or reduced-fat cottage cheese
1 cup reduced-fat soymilk

MEAT AND MEAT SUBSTITUTES
1 ounce cooked low-fat beef, pork, poultry, or fish
½ chicken breast
2 slices of roast beef (3 by 3 by ¼ inch)
½ to 1 cup cooked beans
¾ cup flaked fish
2 eggs or ½ cup low-cholesterol egg alternative

LEGUMES AND SOY PRODUCTS
½ cup soy nuts
½ cup cooked beans or lentils (black beans, red beans, and
   more)
3 ounces tofu
3 ounces tempeh

FATS
1 teaspoon vegetable oil or margarine
1 tablespoon salad dressing
3 teaspoons seeds or nuts
⅛ medium avocado
10 small or 5 large olives

YOUR BUILT-IN SERVING GUIDE

Starting today, I want you to push away the huge platter of pasta and reduce your portions. But don't worry, you don't have to lug around your measuring cups and spoons when you eat at your favorite restaurants! You always have with you a built-in guide to how much to eat to keep your weight at a normal level: the palm of your hand. The palm of your hand is roughly the size of a three-ounce portion of meat or fish, and three ounces make one serving. For raw vegetables, you can generally hold in your hand one cup, which equals one portion or serving. A portion of protein (one serving), together with a cup of vegetables (one serving), plus the same size serving of a grain, make a meal. You can follow the meal with a single serving—a handful—of fresh fruit. This is an easy and convenient way to figure out how much to eat—and much less stressful than measuring.

Yo-yo Dieting May Increase Your Risk

Weight cycling or *yo-yo dieting* (repeated weight loss and weight gain) is a common pattern among women who are trying to control obesity. Yet recent studies reported in the *Journal of the American College of Cardiology* conclude that weight cycling may actually increase your risk of cardiovascular disease.[6] In a November 2000 study, researchers defined weight cycling as a voluntary weight loss of at least ten pounds, followed by a weight regain, at least three times in life (except that which occurs with pregnancy and childbirth). These studies found that weight cycling is associated with a significant decrease (7 percent) in HDL ("good") cholesterol and a significant increase (8 percent) in the mean ratio of total cholesterol to HDL cholesterol.

Having low HDL cholesterol is a significant risk factor for cardiovascular disease. This journal report should give you even more impetus to lose weight and keep it off for good.

Avoid Low-Fat, High-Carbohydrate Diets

A surprising number of the overweight women I see eat low-fat or fat-free diets and yet cannot lose weight—in fact, many of them gain weight. I have several patients who eat low-fat, whole-grain muffins for breakfast and lunch. They eat only vegetables and pasta at dinnertime, with some low-fat cookies and crackers for a snack. Yet they still are obese. Can you imagine their frustration as the pounds continue to increase when they step on the scale? I believe that these women are insulin-resistant and need to give up their carbohydrate foods.

If you are insulin resistant, your insulin does not work as effectively as it should. As a result, your body does not metabolize carbohydrates properly. A high-carbohydrate diet may increase your blood's insulin level. For a woman who has insulin resistance syndrome, then, a high carbohydrate diet results in increased triglycerides.

IF YOU HAVE INSULIN RESISTANCE SYNDROME

If you are insulin resistant, you need to eat foods that are low on the glycemic index, a numerical system that shows how fast a carbohydrate triggers a rise in circulating blood sugar: the higher the number, the faster the blood sugar response, and the greater the rise in potential calories absorbed. A food that is low on the glycemic index will cause a small rise, while a food high on the glycemic index will trigger a more dramatic rise. Researchers have concluded that women who are insulin resistant are hungrier and consume more calories when they eat foods high on the glycemic index. This, of course, leads to more weight gain.[7]

GLYCEMIC LOAD OF COMMON FOODS

Food	Amount of Carbohydrates (GM)	Glycemic Index	Glycemic Load
Potato (1 baked)	37	1.21	45
White rice (½ cup)	35	0.81	28
White bread (2 slices)	24	1.00	22
Whole wheat bread (2 slices)	24	0.64	15
Pasta, cooked (1 cup)	40	0.71	28
Popcorn, air popped (1 cup)	5	0.79	4
Lentils, cooked (½ cup)	20	0.60	16
Corn Flakes (1 cup)	22	1.19	31
100% Bran (1 cup)	24	0.60	14
Carrots, cooked (½ cup)	20	1.31	10

The glycemic load of a food is the amount of carbohydrate it contains multiplied by the glycemic index. The "Glycemic Load of

Common Foods" chart will help you choose better carbohydrates for your diet without the need for a calculator. You want to choose foods that have a lower glycemic load.

From a brief glance at the chart, you can see that lentils are a better choice than white rice, potatoes, or white bread.

MAXIMIZE FOODS LOW ON THE GLYCEMIC INDEX

- Fruits
- Vegetables low in starch
- Low-fat diary (in moderate amounts)
- Low-fat protein, tofu, nuts, and legumes (in moderate amounts)
- Unrefined grains

MINIMIZE FOODS HIGH ON THE GLYCEMIC INDEX

- Pasta
- Potatoes
- Refined grains
- Sweets
- Vegetables high in starch (potatoes, corn)

VERY-LOW-CALORIE DIETS WORK— UNTIL YOU START EATING

"No matter how much I eat, if I stay on a low-fat diet, I'm famished all the time." If I could only count the number of patients who say this to me! Some new comprehensive studies shed light on the reason why your stomach may growl for hours after a low-fat meal. Scientists suggest that the amount of fat in the diet is responsible for regulating total food intake and that following a lower-fat diet alters one of the body's natural cues for telling us when we have had enough food, leading us to eat more.

"What about very-low-calorie diets? I used to lose weight easily when I cut my calories to eight hundred a day." Monica, age forty, had a history of dieting deprivation and yet currently weighed more than she ever had. A very-low-calorie diet *can* help you lose weight, but for most women who eat less, one third of what they lose is muscle. Muscle mass is metabolically active tissue, meaning that it burns calories. The more muscle mass your body has, the more calories you will burn all day, even while you are sitting still.

A host of studies also confirm that approximately 95 percent of people who go on weight-loss diets will gain all or some of it back within one year. In fact, some studies have found that after a period of five years, not one "advertised" diet program was successful in keeping the weight off.

Heart-Boosting Weight-Loss Tips for Women

TIP 1: EAT COMPLEX CARBOHYDRATES INSTEAD OF SIMPLE SUGARS, TO FILL UP—NOT OUT.

Replace simple carbohydrates with complex carbohydrates (starch and fiber) by eating plenty of fruits and vegetables each day. But do not overeat complex carbs! They can put weight on you. Eat moderate amounts, and balance them with other foods.

TIP 2: PREPARE VEGETABLES SIMPLY.

When choosing vegetables, turn down those with cheesy sauces and turn to raw or sauteed vegetables. (Use olive oil or olive oil spray.) Choose vegetables low on the glycemic index. To add taste to green salads, opt for a flavored vinegar and herbs, then lightly sprinkle with olive oil.

Try roasting vegetables with fresh herbs for a delicious way to increase your intake of fresh vegetables without heavy sauces. Choose any favorite vegetable, such as broccoli, peppers, summer squash, zucchini, onion, new potato, or sweet potato, to name a few. Slice these vegetables, then place them on a large baking pan. Coat them with a spray of olive oil, then sprinkle with fresh herbs and spices. Bake at 350 degrees for about one hour.

TIP 3: BASE YOUR PROTEIN ON LENTILS, FISH, AND SKINLESS POULTRY. USE LEAN MEAT SPARINGLY, AS A CONDIMENT TO COMPLEMENT YOUR VEGETABLES AND GRAINS.

Be sure to trim all visible fat from poultry and meat before cooking. When you are selecting cuts of meat, choose the "skinniest" cuts, such as top round, tip round, sirloin, and chuck. Buy ground beef that is at least 90 percent lean, or choose ground round or ground sirloin. For spaghetti, chili, meat loaf, or burgers, substitute ground turkey or chicken for half or even all the beef. Instead of frying chicken or fish, broil, bake, grill, steam, or sauté it in defatted broth. Use olive oil to sauté poultry or pan-fry fish.

TIP 4: USE MEAT SUBSTITUTES.

Learn how to use tofu and legumes as meat substitutes, and plan several "meatless" high-protein meals each week by combining lentils (or black beans, red beans, navy beans, or great northern beans) with pasta or rice. This low-fat meal will fill you up and keep your blood sugar stable.

Use vegetarian refried beans in your tacos instead of meat filling. Make sure you check the label for the no-fat or low-fat variety. Make vegetable dips out of puréed beans. Add herbs and a dash of olive oil for more flavor. Try hummus, which is made from garbanzo beans, with whole-wheat pita bread and fresh vegetables.

TIP 5: KEEP A FOOD DIARY.

Keeping a food diary can help you track your daily eating patterns and weight loss. Studies have shown that when obese people who say they maintain a low-fat, low-calorie diet actually record their daily food intake, the results are surprising. The same people who said they ate no more than 1,100 calories and 20 percent fat calories per day, topped off at an average of over 2,000 calories, with 60 percent fat calories per day. This tremendous difference resulted in weight gain instead of loss!

Keeping a food diary helps you know exactly where you stand nutritionally. You may think you are eating a diet high in grains and fresh fruits and vegetables, but after calculating your food intake at the end of the day, you may find that you have eaten only three vegetables—and filled up on periodic snacking.

Until you get in the "healthy heart habit," keeping a food diary will help you stay organized and honest. My patients use it as they would a checkbook, writing down each food they eat, along with the calories. There are food diaries published that you can use, but you can also use a small notebook and carry it in your purse. To have an accurate indicator of what you really eat, add up everything at the end of the day.

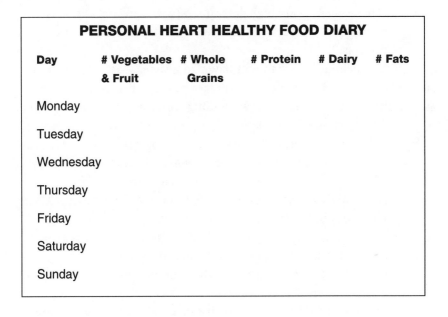

PERSONAL HEART HEALTHY FOOD DIARY

Day	# Vegetables & Fruit	# Whole Grains	# Protein	# Dairy	# Fats
Monday					
Tuesday					
Wednesday					
Thursday					
Friday					
Saturday					
Sunday					

TIP 6: WATCH FOR "EXTRAS" THAT INCREASE CALORIES—AND POUNDS.

Check out the following suggestions to make sure "extra" ingredients and foods don't add extra pounds to your body:

- Watch for the hidden fats and calories in fast foods. That juicy hamburger contains over 50 percent of its calories in saturated fat.
- Make low-fat choices with condiments and dairy products. Choose low-fat or no-fat cheeses, including cottage cheese,

sour cream, cream cheese, yogurt, skim milk, ice milk, and frozen yogurt.

- Skim the broth for soups using defatted liquids. Using canned undiluted skim milk for cream soups is an excellent low-fat choice.
- Instead of using a whole egg in a recipe, use two egg whites or egg substitute. (A quarter cup equals one egg.)
- Snack on air-popped popcorn or rice cakes.
- Pretzels usually have only one gram of fat per ounce. (Check the label.) This low-fat snack food has ten times less fat than other snack foods high in trans fats. If you are salt sensitive, watch out for the sodium content, or try unsalted varieties of pretzels.
- Use peanut butter to add flavor to a snack—as a dip for celery or a spread for a piece of whole-wheat toast. Just stay on top of how many calories you are adding with this heart-healthy food.
- Use applesauce, prune purée, or other fruit substitute instead of butter or oil in loaf cakes or drop cookies.
- Avoid anything that is *creamed, sautéed, au gratin,* or *smothered.* This means it is high in fat, usually saturated fat.
- Avoid added sauces on foods. Ask for any dressings or sauces "on the side," then use them sparingly.
- When eating out, request baked or broiled chicken or beef, and remember: extra crispy means extra calories.
- Opt for the vegetarian meal when dining out—but request no added butter to the plate.
- Instead of fries, choose brown rice or couscous. Use toppings that are low in fat and high in complex carbohydrates, such as tomatoes, mushrooms, broccoli, carrots, and cauliflower.
- Avoid high-fat meaty pizza toppings, and replace them with onions, mushrooms, bell pepper, broccoli, and other vegetable toppings.
- Do not cook with animal fat.
- Eat raw vegetables for snacks. Two carrots will give you a day's supply of vitamin A.
- Read your cereal box. If the cereal has no fiber or less than three grams, it probably has little nutritional value.

- Add fresh or dried fruits to your cereal to boost your intake of complex carbohydrates.
- Keep your vegetables crisp when you cook them instead of soft.

Choose Foods High in Antioxidants

Antioxidants, such as beta-carotene and vitamins C and E, are essential nutrients that help protect your body against life's stressors, and hence against wear and tear and slow aging. They also boost immunity. Antioxidants perform these feats by neutralizing highly reactive, unstable metabolic products called free radicals. Free radicals tear apart vital cell structures like cell membranes, making cells vulnerable to decay and pathogens. Antioxidants appear to tie up these free radicals and take away their destructive power—reducing the risk of chronic diseases such as heart disease.

Antioxidants also reduce the oxidation of LDL ("bad") cholesterol. Oxidation is the chemical process that causes iron to rust and turns a peeled banana or apple brown. It also turns LDL cholesterol from an inert substance into its most active form: free radicals. Oxidized LDL is highly vulnerable to breaking off from artery walls, stimulating the process of a heart attack. Studies show that antioxidants, particularly vitamin E, may also keep platelets from clumping together. By eating less saturated fat and more antioxidants, you'll help keep LDL in its quieter form. This is why your Healthy Heart Eating Plan requires a diet rich in antioxidants.

Beta-carotene

The antioxidant beta-carotene is converted to vitamin A in the body. Many other carotenoid compounds also have antioxidant properties, including:

- Alpha-carotene (found in carrots, cantaloupe, and pumpkin)
- Gamma-carotene (found in apricots and tomatoes)

- Beta-cryptoxanthin (found in mangoes, nectarines, peaches, and tangerines)
- Lycopene (found in guava, pink grapefruit, tomatoes, and watermelon)
- Lutein and zeaxanthin (found in beets, corn, and collard and mustard greens)

FOOD SOURCES OF BETA-CAROTENE

Apricots	Peach
Broccoli	Papaya
Cantaloupe	Pumpkin
Carrots	Spinach
Collard Greens	Sweet potato
Kale	Tomatoes
Mango	Winter Squash

BETA-CAROTENE SUPPLEMENTS

I do not recommend that you take beta-carotene supplements because they have not been proven to prevent heart disease.

Vitamin C

Like other antioxidants, vitamin C improves heart health by cleaning up free radicals, thereby preventing them from damaging tissues. While it's known that vitamin C is vital for warding off infection and aiding wound healing, some new studies suggest that it also helps people with high levels of cholesterol by improving blood flow and widening the blood vessels.

Vitamin C also plays a vital role in boosting levels of the energizing brain chemical norepinephrine. Norepinephrine produces a feeling of alertness and increases concentration, so deficiency of vitamin C can negatively influence your mood. It is essential to include plenty of vitamin C sources in your Healthy Heart Eating Plan.

FOOD SOURCES OF VITAMIN C

Blueberries	Kiwi
Broccoli	Oranges
Cantaloupe	Peppers—red, green, yellow, orange
Currants	Potatoes
Gooseberries	Strawberries
Grapefruit	Tomatoes

VITAMIN C SUPPLEMENTS

As for supplements, I am less than impressed with the studies on vitamin C supplements and heart disease. The rationale is that given its antioxidant properties, the supplements should produce preventative benefits, but studies have failed to prove that supplemental vitamin C prevents heart disease better than dietary vitamin C. Whole foods are the best way to get most vitamins and minerals. Not only do you get a specific vitamin, such as C, but you also get many essential nutrients that are necessary for energy and good health. For example, an orange not only has vitamin C but is also high in carotenoids (of which beta-carotene is the best known) and calcium—and it tastes good! To boost your intake of vitamin C through foods, eat broccoli, citrus fruits, guava, papaya, red and green peppers, and foods fortified with vitamin C.

Vitamin E

Vitamin E is important for the maintenance of cell membranes, and its antioxidant effect may slow age-related changes in the body. There is now evidence that vitamin E plays a role in lowering the risk of coronary artery disease and heart attack. In one study of postmenopausal women, those who had a higher intake of vitamin E from food reduced their risk of heart disease. Interestingly, this heart benefit occurred only in women who got their vitamin E from food, not from supplements.

It is difficult to get enough vitamin E through the foods we eat. High levels are best found in whole grains, nuts, and seed oils, which makes it hard to ingest large amounts, especially while following a low-fat diet.

Food Sources of Vitamin E

Whole grains
Dark green vegetables
Nuts and seeds
Avocadoes
Vegetable oils (olive, peanut, canola)
Sweet potatoes
Wheat germ

VITAMIN E SUPPLEMENTS

A report published in the *New England Journal of Medicine* found that when men and women over fifty-five with cardiovascular disease took 400 international units of vitamin E supplements for four years, their risk of death from cardiovascular disease and heart attack was not reduced. In another study done in China, participants took 30 mg of vitamin E for 5.2 years, along with supplements of selenium and beta-carotene. This study showed a 9 percent reduction in deaths. In yet another study done in Italy, heart attack patients taking 300 international units of vitamin E for 3.5 years had a slight reduction in risk of death by heart disease. In the same study, the chance of nonfatal heart attacks slightly increased, but neither heart benefit was statistically significant.

The jury is still out on the preventive benefits of vitamin E supplements for women without heart disease. Part of the problem with the research is that people were given different vitamin E doses and for different periods of time. The Cambridge Antioxidant Study did find a reduction in recurrent heart attack in men and women who received vitamin E supplements.[8] This was one of the few studies with positive results for vitamin E supplementation. Until we have stronger evidence that vitamin E supplementation may help prevent heart disease, you should get ample amounts of this antioxidant by eating it in whole foods.

A word of caution: It's been shown that high doses of vitamin E may increase bleeding. If you are on a blood thinner, you must talk to your doctor before taking these supplements, and even if he or she agrees that you can take it, use it with caution.

RECOMMENDED DAILY ALLOWANCE OF VITAMINS

Vitamin	Daily RDA	Special Considerations
Vitamin C	75 mg	
Folic Acid	400 mcg	pregnancy: 600mcg
		lactation: 500mcg
		heart disease: 100mcg
Niacin	14 mg	pregnancy: 18 mg
		lactation: 17 mg
Vitamin B6	1.3 mg	pregnancy: 1.4 mg
		lactation: 1.6 mg
Vitamin B12	2.4 pg*	pregnancy: 2.6 mcg
		lactation: 2.6 mcg
Vitamin E	15 mg	
Vitamin D	5 mcg	women age 19–50
	10 mcg	women age 50–70
	15 mcg	women older than 70

* pg = picograms
Source: Food and Nutrition Board, Institute of Medicine, National Academy of Sciences, 2000.

Choose Foods with Heart Smart B Vitamins

Three of the B vitamins—folic acid and vitamins B6 and B12—are key nutrients that are good for your heart. The B vitamins help boost your body's energy stores, fuel your metabolism, and normalize other bodily functions. New research indicates that many women are deficient in these micronutrients. Especially if you do not eat healthy amounts of fruits, vegetables, legumes, and whole grains, or if your diet is heavy in sugar, refined flour, coffee, and alcohol, you may have reduced folic acid and B vitamin stores in your body. If you take oral contraceptives or smoke cigarettes, you're also likely to be low in folic acid. If you are a vegetarian, you may be deficient in vitamin B12, as it is found mainly in animal products.

In scientific studies, folic acid and vitamins B6 and B12 were given to people who had suffered a stroke. Researchers concluded that as a result of taking these vitamins, homocysteine levels were lower, and biochemical "markers" in the blood that indicate injury to artery walls were improved. High levels of homocysteine may be linked to heart disease and stroke risk,[9] as a result of too little vitamin B6 or folic acid intake. Folic acid and vitamins B3, B6, and B12 contribute to the breakdown of homocysteine in the body. (For more on homocysteine, see page 71.)

Folic Acid

Folic acid is important for reducing levels of homocysteine, which is an emerging risk factor for cardiovascular disease. Low blood levels of folic acid are associated with an increased risk of fatal coronary artery disease, but a diet high in folic acid improves arterial function (the ability of the arteries to dilate). This B vitamin can also significantly lower the risk of neural tube defects, such as spina bifida, when taken by pregnant women.

Eating foods rich in folic acid is a must for a healthy heart. Most of the current research shows the benefit of folic acid in people who have received it from food sources. You can get adequate amounts through a diet rich in green leafy vegetables, beans, peas, peanuts and other legumes, and citrus fruits.

If you know you have a folic acid deficiency and want to use a supplement, you can take the Recommended Daily Allowance, which is 400 mcg for women who do not have heart disease. For women who do have heart disease or elevated homocysteine levels, doctors usually prescribe supplementation of 800 to 1200 mcg, but you should never take this much on your own, without your doctor's knowledge and approval.

FOOD SOURCES OF FOLIC ACID

Food	Serving Size	Amount (mcg)
Breakfast cereal	½ cup–1 cup	100–400
Lentils (cooked)	½ cup	180
Chickpeas	½ cup	140
Spinach (cooked)	½ cup	130
Black beans	½ cup	130
Kidney beans	½ cup	115
Orange	1 medium	40
Broccoli (raw)	½ cup	60

FOLIC ACID SUPPLEMENTS

The jury is still out on the optimal dose of folic acid needed to prevent heart disease. I usually prescribe folic acid supplements and other B vitamins, such as vitamin B6, for patients with coronary artery disease or elevated levels of homocysteine. While most multivitamins contain 400 mcg of folic acid, doctors use higher dosages to reduce homocysteine; check with your doctor for the best dosage for you. Be cautious: take a dosage larger than 400 mcg *only if* your doctor says that is advisable, because taking too much folic acid may obscure the diagnosis of pernicious anemia due to B12 deficiency. If pernicious anemia is suspected, B12 levels can be measured before giving folic acid therapy.

Niacin (B3)

The one vitamin that may lower your LDL ("bad") cholesterol, increase your HDL ("good") cholesterol, reduce your triglycerides, and reduce Lp(a) is niacin, or vitamin B3. But it does all this with some annoying and possibly serious side effects, including flushing, nausea, diarrhea, headaches, and fatigue.

Talk to your doctor before taking niacin. Because it increases blood sugar, it should not be used by diabetics. It may also increase uric acid, a concern for those with gout. Just as with statin drugs, if you take niacin, your liver function should be checked periodically.

Vitamin B6

Vitamin B6 is necessary for the metabolism of proteins, carbohydrates, and lipids. A vitamin B6 deficiency raises homocysteine levels and may make the blood more likely to form clots that obstruct blood vessels or change cholesterol levels. Many women in the United States consume less vitamin B6 in their diets than the Recommended Daily Allowance. Vitamin B6 is one of the few water-soluble vitamins that can be toxic if taken in large doses. Brown rice, peanuts, walnuts, soybeans, chicken, and fish are all sources of B6.

Vitamin B12

Vitamin B12 has been found to lower levels of homocysteine. Studies have found that people taking vitamin B12 have less thrombomodulin and less damage to the cells lining the blood vessels.

If you are a meat eater, getting adequate vitamin B12 is probably not a problem—it is found in fish, eggs, meat, and milk. Vegetarians are at risk for deficiency and may benefit from a daily vitamin B12 supplement. Vitamin B12 levels can be measured by a blood test. Your doctor can advise you if a blood test or supplementation is necessary.

EASY WAYS TO GET MORE
ANTIOXIDANTS AND NUTRIENTS

- Use a tomato or spinach sauce over pasta.
- Add "no salt added" tomato sauce to soups and stews.
- Add sliced tomatoes to sandwiches and salads.
- Add spinach, carrots, peppers, broccoli, squash, and other vegetables with antioxidants to casseroles and stews.
- Throw some greens and carrots into your vegetable soup.
- Try a veggie pizza, with broccoli, squash, peppers, and onion on top.

- Add fresh pineapple, mandarin oranges, and strawberries to your spinach salad.
- Toss grated zucchini into your next batch of muffins or loaf of bread.
- Snack on dried fruit and nuts, like apricots and cashews.
- Top off your yogurt with chopped nuts or wheat germ.
- Toss fresh blueberries onto cereal or into yogurt.

HEART-BOOSTING SMOOTHIE

This drink is high in protein as well as the essential heart-boosting nutrients discussed in this chapter, making it an excellent start to your day, or a quick afternoon power boost.

You need:

½ cup soft tofu or silken tofu (thickened with calcium sulfate), or ½ cup soy milk

½ cup plain fat-free yogurt

½ cup fat-free or low-fat calcium-enriched milk

1 cup fresh berries (blueberries, strawberries, raspberries)

½ banana

2 teaspoons flax oil (or freshly ground flaxseed)

1 teaspoon vanilla extract (or other flavored extract—optional)

Sugar or honey (sweeten to taste—optional)

2 ice cubes (optional)

To make:

Put all ingredients into a blender, and process until creamy. Makes 1 serving.

Variations:

- Instead of berries, use seasonal fruit such as peaches, pineapple, melon, or dates.
- For a thicker shake, use frozen fruit.

- Instead of two ice cubes, use two frozen milk cubes, to add more calcium.
- If you cannot tolerate soy, use ½ cup of calcium-fortified orange juice or rice milk instead of soy milk.

Choose Foods with Flavonoids

Flavonoids, the four thousand compounds responsible for the colors of fruits and flowers, have a disease-fighting, antioxidant effect in the body. A few studies show that intake of flavonoids is inversely linked with coronary artery disease; in other words, people with a low intake of flavonoids have a higher death rate from coronary artery disease than do those who consume more flavonoids. Flavonoids have been shown to inhibit the clumping of platelets (blood-clotting cells), which may help reduce the risk of heart disease.

Some recent studies indicate that the antioxidants found in green and black tea are more potent than those found in many fruits and vegetables. In a study of seventy-seven men and women with heart disease,[10] researchers found that those participants who drank two cups of regular tea (not herbal tea) each day had improvement in blood vessel flexibility. Experts do not know exactly how much tea is necessary for health benefits but remember that a diet of tea alone will not reduce your risk of heart disease!

Recent studies also conclude that certain specific flavonoids, such as those found in onions, soy, and red wine (all antioxidants), have heart-healing properties. For instance, trans-resveratrol (a natural compound found in red wine,[11] grape juice, and blueberries) may be more potent than vitamin E in fighting heart disease. Powerful flavonoids in red wine have been found to inhibit LDL ("bad") cholesterol oxidation. A superantioxidant called activin is found inside the seeds of red grapes, so by-products of red grapes—such as red wine, juice, and seeds—may offer protection against heart disease and other chronic diseases.[12] As an antioxidant, activin is up to seven times more powerful than vitamins C, E, and beta-carotene. This finding does not mean that you should begin to drink red wine if you don't, or that you should drink more than one glass a day. (More than one glass has been implicated in exacerbating fibrocystic breast disease.)

Soybean flavonoids also have strong antioxidant properties, inhibiting LDL oxidation and platelets and resulting in decreased clotting. Some citrus flavonoids, such as hesperidin, raise blood levels of HDL ("good") cholesterol and lower LDL cholesterol and triglycerides.

BLUEBERRIES: GOLD MEDAL HEART BOOSTER

Blueberries take the prize for being a superantioxidant, and the secret lies in their color. The blue pigment anthrocyanin, also found in strawberries, may help slow the ravages of aging and reduce the risk of heart disease. Blueberries are also high in fiber, iron, and vitamin C and contain no fat, sodium, or cholesterol.

HEART-BOOSTING SUPERSTARS

U.S. Department of Agriculture researchers have ranked the most common fruits and vegetables according to their ability to act as antioxidants. From highest to lowest, they are:

1. Blueberries
2. Kale
3. Strawberries
4. Spinach
5. Brussels sprouts
6. Plums
7. Broccoli
8. Beets
9. Oranges
10. Red grapes

In most cases, you can get the necessary amount of flavonoids through a diet high in fruits, vegetables, and soy products. Grape juice and fresh grapes are both high in flavonoids, as is tea, hot or cold. Even though these foods contain flavonoids, eating large amounts of them will not give you more protection—and tanking up on tea is not an excuse to stop exercising or to eat foods high in saturated fats! Tea is also a diuretic, so you have to be sure to drink as much water as you drink tea so that you do not get dehydrated. (Sometimes taking too many flavonoids can result in an allergic reaction or gastrointestinal upset. If this happens to you, reduce your intake to a comfortable level.)

Choose Foods with Phytochemicals

Phytochemicals, such as flavonoids, are biologically active substances that give plants their color, flavor, odor, and protection against disease. Some of the foods high in phytochemicals are also high in antioxidants. If you vary the ingredients and methods of preparation, a Mediterranean-style diet that includes a variety of grains, fruits, and vegetables should provide enough of both substances. Phytochemical supplements and pills do exist, but most of the research on the benefits of phytochemicals was done on whole foods, so I believe it's better to get your phytochemicals from a varied diet. Foods contain a wide array of nutrients, including many that have not yet been identified, that are essential for wellness, and that work *with* the known nutrients. If you rely on supplements for nutrition, you miss out on the compounds we don't yet know about.

Should You Use Soy?

Some new studies claim that soy foods may help to lower lipid levels and give other beneficial cardiovascular effects. Soybeans contain isoflavones, a plant sterol that mimics the hormone estrogen but appears to have no harmful side effects. Some believe that it is the isoflavone content in soy that is heart healthy. Other scientists believe that soy benefits the heart through the lowering of total and LDL ("bad") cholesterol. While these studies look promising, keep in mind that you'll have to eat more than 25 gm of soy each day to reduce your LDL cholesterol. This is the equivalent of four cups of soy milk each day.

If you think you do not like the taste of soy foods, I encourage you to keep an open mind. Today's soy products are nothing like the white, mushy foods of the past. They come in many different forms and are generally very mild tasting. Soy can be marinated and will take on the flavor of the dish it is used in, such as sauces, chili, dips, stir-fries, fruit shakes, and pasta.

Please don't think that soy sauce and soy oil contain consequential amounts of isoflavones—eating them does *not* count toward boosting your heart's health! In fact, if you have high blood pressure, you may want to avoid soy sauce altogether because of its high sodium content.

SOY SUPPLEMENTS
While soy foods may help you stay healthy, numerous studies show that supplements may pose risks. The reason is that components like phytoestrogens found in soy products have a pharmacological effect in the body. As a whole food, soy is a healthy, low-fat, low-cholesterol way to add protein to your diet. Yet scientists are not prepared to give the okay signal to taking isoflavones as a supplement.

Some people who realize that soy may boost heart health try to get as much as they can by taking lots of little tiny pills of isoflavones. The Food and Drug Administration has approved the practice of reducing cholesterol by using soy protein—but not by using supplements of isoflavones.

THE BOTTOM LINE
If you want the benefit of soy, eat whole foods—soybeans and soy products. Also, if there is early heart disease in your family medical history, then you may benefit from eating soy regularly in your diet.

Your Heart Healthy Eating Plan should contain the foods in the chart—they are loaded with phytochemicals.

FOOD SOURCES OF PHYTOCHEMICALS

Phytochemical	Food Sources	Wellness Factor
Carotenoids	carrots, apricots, sweet potatoes	prevent cancer and heart disease
Indoles	cruciferous vegetables like cabbage, broccoli, and cauliflower	prevent breast and uterine cancer
Isoflavones	legumes, soybeans	reduce cholesterol
Lycopene	tomatoes, red peppers, carrots	prevent cancer
Sulfides (allyl)	cabbage, onions, broccoli, garlic, Brussels sprouts	prevent cancer

A HEART-BOOSTING CONFETTI SALAD

In a large salad bowl, put bite-size pieces of your favorite salad greens (arugula, dandelion greens, mesclun, mustard greens, romaine lettuce, spinach, or watercress). For texture and color, use more than one variety.

To boost phytochemicals, add several of the following vegetables:
- Shredded red or green cabbage
- Sliced carrots
- Bite-size pieces of broccoli and cauliflower
- Slices of red, orange, and yellow peppers
- Chunks of green bell pepper
- Chopped chives
- Sliced beets
- Cooked soybeans or garbanzo beans (chickpeas)
- Sliced red tomatoes or sun-dried tomatoes packed in olive oil
  Top with minced garlic, basil, and parsley, then lightly drizzle with heart-boosting olive oil and your favorite flavored vinegar.

Choose Whole Grains

Ongoing studies have some researchers convinced that eating one or more servings of whole-grain foods each day may reduce the risk of heart disease. Keep in mind that whole grains do not include white bread and white rice! There are a host of natural grains that are healthy for your heart, including:

barley
bran
brown rice
bulgur
couscous
millet
oats
polenta
quinoa
whole wheat

FIBER

Fruits, vegetables, and whole grains are all high in fiber. Insoluble fiber is necessary to keep your bowels regular, and soluble fiber can help to lower cholesterol, especially when your diet is low in saturated fat and cholesterol. Foods high in soluble fiber include oatmeal, beans, peas, rice bran, oat bran, barley, citrus fruits, strawberries, and apple pulp.

Choose Healthy Fats

"Fats are now *good* for my heart and a weapon against cancer? I thought low-fat or even fat-free was better." Forty-three-year-old Sandy was conscientious in trying to lose weight, but she lived on fat-free potato chips, pretzels, cookies, cream cheese, and other cheeses. In the past two years, this mother of three had gained eighteen pounds, most of it in her waistline. As Sandy's weight gain proves, calories do count: even without fat, these foods contain a lot of calories.

The idea that some fat is actually good for the heart is fairly new. In the past two decades, scientists have gone from "All fat is bad" to "Some fat is bad" to "Certain fats may actually be healthy for your heart." What should you believe?

The reality is that not all fat is equal—and yes, some types of fat are actually healthy for you. These good fats are monounsaturated fats (found in olive oil, canola oil, peanut oils, and avocados) and polyunsaturated fats (found in fatty fish and in flaxseed, safflower, sesame, sunflower, corn, and soybean oils as well as in nuts). These fats are all *heart boosters*. Scientific guidelines from the American Dietetic Association and the American Heart Association focus on replacing other fats in the diet with these heart boosters—to keep cholesterol at healthy protective levels.

On the other hand, trans fatty acids, which are found in many baked and highly processed foods (such as pastries and snack foods) and are formed when vegetable oils solidify, are *heart busters*. A diet high in trans fatty acids may increase your risk of heart disease by lowering your HDL ("good") cholesterol and raising your LDL ("bad") cholesterol. According to studies in the *New England Journal of Medicine*,[13] the net effect of trans fatty acids may even be worse than that of saturated fat and can lead to many types of cancer, obesity, and heart disease. Researchers estimate that replacing 5 percent of total daily calories from saturated fat with unsaturated fat could reduce a woman's risk of heart disease by 42 percent. And replacing 2 percent of daily calories from trans fatty acids with unsaturated fat may reduce a woman's risk of heart disease by an estimated 53 percent.

The average Mediterranean diet consists of a high amount of fat—as much as 40 percent. But the fat in this diet is polyunsaturated, specifically omega-3 fatty acid—quite different from the typical American meal of fried chicken or a quarter-pound cheeseburger with greasy french fries, all filled with saturated fat.

Saturated fat increases LDL cholesterol, but monounsaturated fat appears to be neutral with respect to cholesterol levels. This gives a protective benefit to the heart. (Polyunsaturated fats lower LDL cholesterol.)[14]

Nuts also contain heart-healthy fats. Ever since the early 1990s "walnut diet," many people have successfully lowered their cholesterol levels by adding nuts to their diets. Walnuts, almonds, peanuts, and a host of other nuts have been touted for their LDL cholesterol–lowering qualities. Peanuts contain resveratrol, the same antioxidant found in grapes and wine (see page 284); it is associated with anticlotting effects similar to aspirin. Nut spreads, such as peanut butter, have no trans fatty acids and can help to keep your cholesterol levels healthy. They are an excellent source of omega-3 fatty acids and body-building protein.

But if you are going to eat nuts for their heart-healthy nutrients, you have to be aware that they are high in calories. For instance, only two teaspoons of walnuts or almonds contain a hundred calories. If you are on a weight-reduction program, eat nuts in moderation and stay within your calorie quota for the day. Add the other good fats, but always remember to *count your calories.*

NUT NUTRITION

Nut	Calories per Ounce	Saturated Fat (%)	Monounsaturated Fat (%)	Polyunsaturated Fat (%)
Almonds	166.41	9.9	67.6	22.5
Macadamia nuts	199.02	15.3	82.4	2.3
Peanuts	165.5	14.9	52.2	32.9
Soy nuts	128.4	15.8	23.7	60.5
Walnuts	172.1	6.8	23.3	69.9

Eat Fish High in Omega-3 Fatty Acids

My favorite sandwich is grilled tuna on a whole-grain bun, and I try to eat this heart-healthy meal a couple of times each week. Tuna is a fresh water fish rich in omega-3 fatty acids (n-3 PUFA), eicosapen-tanoic acid (EPA), and docosahexanoic acid (DHA). Although the studies are not all conclusive, these heart-healthy fatty acids are known to reduce triglycerides, reduce clotting, and lower blood pressure. Fish oil may also prevent artery reclosure (restenosis) after angioplasty, improve the flexibility of the arterial walls, and reduce the chance of sudden death.

For vegetarians, another omega-3 fatty acid, alpha-linolenic acid, is found in soybeans, canola oil, flaxseed, and nuts.

Fish High in Omega-3

Anchovy	Capelin	Shad
Atlantic herring	Dogfish	Sturgeon
Atlantic salmon	Mackerel	Tuna
Bluefish	Sardines	Whitefish

When Donna, age fifty-five, was diagnosed with atrial fibrillation, I immediately started her on warfarin (Coumadin) to prevent a stroke. She came in weekly for a laboratory test to check her level of blood thinning. A normal range for blood thinning in this situation is 2 to 2.5 international normalized ratio (INR), and for two weeks Donna had an INR of 2.3. The third week her INR was 1.5, showing practically no blood thinning effect. I was extremely concerned and asked if she had changed her medications or diet; Donna said no.

I increased her warfarin to 10 mg, then repeated the test the following week. It was unchanged. When I called her home to talk to Donna, her mother-in-law answered and said, "Dr. Goldberg, did Donna tell you she's been eating a lot of sushi lately, and a lot of seaweed?"

Donna was quite rightly trying to eat a lot of fish in her diet, but the seaweed, which has an extremely high vitamin K content, was inhibiting the action of the warfarin. I helped Donna adjust her diet, and we finally got her medication adjusted.

FISH OIL SUPPLEMENTS

Some of my patients who do not like the taste of fatty fish ask if fish oil supplements can be used instead. The studies on fish oil supplements are inconclusive. In some studies, participants who took supplements had a reduction in LDL ("bad") cholesterol levels when other saturated fats were reduced in their diet.

Still, no matter how promising the future looks, most researchers feel that omega-3 fatty acids are best obtained by eating fish. At this time I prescribe fish oil capsules only to my patients who have markedly elevated triglycerides that have not responded to improvements in diet and exercise or to medication.

THE BOTTOM LINE

For your Healthy Heart Eating Plan, try to eat fatty fish. If you have elevated triglycerides, ask your doctor about supplementation with fish oil capsules. When you consider that fish oil capsules are malodorous and fattening, not to mention upsetting to the gastrointestinal tract, it makes baked salmon or tuna burgers seem even tastier. When fish oil supplements are taken along with blood thinners such as ASA or other supplements that decrease clotting, it can produce nosebleeds and other bleeding problems.

A WORD OF CAUTION:

Because of the mercury content in some fish, including mackerel, swordfish, and tuna, the Food and Drug Administration recommends that pregnant or nursing women avoid these fish.

THE FACTS ABOUT FATS:
HEART-BUSTING FATS

- **Cholesterol**—found in organ meats and egg yolks. Food cholesterol increases the blood cholesterol, adding to your risk of heart disease.

- **Saturated fat**—found in foods that are firm at room temperature, including red meat, butter, cheese, luncheon meats, cocoa butter, coconut oil, palm oil, and cream.
- **Hydrogenated fat**—found in commercial baked products and snack foods. Hydrogenated fat is made during a chemical process called hydrogenation that changes a naturally unsaturated liquid oil into a solid and more saturated form. The greater the hydrogenation, the more saturated the fat has become. Saturated fat may raise your blood cholesterol levels.
- **Trans fats**—found in margarine, snack and fast-food products, crackers, pastries, and many processed foods. Trans fats are formed during the process of hydrogenation.

HEART-BOOSTING FATS

- **Monounsaturated fat**—found in foods that are liquid at room temperature, including canola, peanut, and olive oils, as well as avocados. These fats may actually reduce your risk of cardiovascular disease.
- **Polyunsaturated fat**—found in foods that are liquid or soft at room temperature, including sunflower, corn, soybean, safflower, and sesame oils, as well as nuts, seeds, and some seafood. Polyunsaturated fats can help to get rid of newly formed cholesterol and reduce cholesterol deposits in artery walls. Polyunsaturated fat lowers LDL cholesterol.
- **Omega-3 fatty acids**—found in fatty fish (tuna, mackerel, and salmon), flaxseed, flaxseed oil, nuts, canola oil, and soybean oil. They lower triglycerides and reduce the tendency to form blood clots. Studies show that these highly polyunsaturated fats not only reduce cholesterol but may also reduce the risk of arrhythmia.

REACH FOR HEART BOOSTERS

- Shop for margarine that has no more than 2 gm saturated fat per tablespoon and that has liquid vegetable oil as the first ingredient. Replace butter with olive oil, and if you do not care for the flavor, choose the extra-light variety.

- Always read the label to know what you are eating. If the ingredient list does not show the amount of trans fatty acids, look for "hydrogenated" or "partially hydrogenated" oils. While they may not give the amount, they signal the presence of trans fats.

HOW TO READ A LABEL

To see what type of fat is in the food you buy, it is important to read the label. Package labels list the ingredients, the calories, the fat content, nutrients, the sodium and fiber content, and much more, for the consumer's information.

SAMPLE LABEL

Commercially Available Shredded Parmesan Cheese

Ingredients: Part-skim milk, cheese culture, salt, enzymes, aged over 10 months.

Nutrition Facts

Serving size 2 teaspoons (5 gm)

Servings per container 17

Amount Per Serving

Calories 20

Calories from Fat 10

	% Daily Value*
Total Fat 1.5 gm	2%
Saturated Fat 1 gm	5%
Cholesterol less than 5 mg	1%
Sodium 75 mg	3%
Total Carbohydrate 0 gm	0%
Dietary Fiber 0 gm	0%
Sugars 0 gm	
Protein 2 gm	

Vitamin A 0%   *   Vitamin C 0%

Calcium 4%   *   Iron 0%

*Percent Daily Values are based on a 2,000 calorie diet. Your daily values may be higher or lower depending on your calorie needs.

LABELS CAN BE CONFUSING

- *Low-fat* means the product has no more than 3 gm of fat per serving.
- *Low saturated fat* means it has no more than 1 gm of saturated fat per serving.
- *Reduced fat* means it has at least 25 percent less fat per serving than the traditional item.
- *Light* means the product has 2 gm of fat or one-third the calories of the traditional item.
- *Fat-free* means it has 2 gm of fat or less per serving.

Watch Your Intake of Sodium

Sodium, potassium, and calcium are vital to normal cell functioning. But too much sodium in your diet may lead to high blood pressure. Too little potassium, calcium, and magnesium can also lead to high blood pressure, but you should not take supplements for the problem or attempt to self-medicate. Your doctor needs to monitor your electrolyte levels. There is much conflicting advice about sodium (salt) and hypertension, but the fact remains that people with high sodium chloride intake have higher blood pressure. This is especially true in industrialized nations, where people consume a lot of processed foods. The good news is that an estimated 30 to 50 percent of those who have hypertension can lower their blood pressure by restricting the amount of salt they eat.

My recommendations include:

- If you have normal blood pressure, do not take more than 6 gm of sodium chloride per day.

- Do not take oral potassium supplements unless your doctor has prescribed them.
- If you have high blood pressure, eat foods high in electrolytes (including foods high in potassium, calcium, and possibly magnesium). I commonly recommend the DASH diet (see page 299) to my patients with high blood pressure. It works to reduce blood pressure and cholesterol and is high in calcium-rich foods, helping to prevent osteoporosis.
- Watch the sodium content of processed foods.
- If you have kidney disease, you may need to watch your intake of potassium-rich foods (see page 298).

SALTY FOODS
(HIGH IN SODIUM)

FOOD	SERVING SIZE	AMOUNT OF SODIUM (mg)
Beef broth	1 cube	1150
Cheeseburger, fast food	¼ pound	1200
Chicken noodle soup	1 cup	1100
Cottage cheese	4 ounces	450
Frankfurter	1½ ounces	500
Garlic salt	1 teaspoon	1850
Ham	3 ounces	1000
Luncheon meat	1 slice	575
Meat tenderizer	1 teaspoon	1750
Olives, green	3	720
Onion salt	1 teaspoon	1620
Peas, green canned	1 cup	493
Potato, instant	1 cup	475
Salt	¼ teaspoon	500
Sauerkraut	⅔ cup	740
Soy sauce	1 tablespoon	1030

CALCIUM-RICH FOODS
(HIGH IN ELECTROLYTES)

FOOD	SERVING SIZE	AMOUNT OF CALCIUM (mg)
Broccoli	½ cup	50
Mustard greens	½ cup (cooked)	97
Orange	1 medium	54
Sardines	3 ounces	372 (omega-3's)
Tofu	1 cake	154
Yogurt (plain)	1 cup	415

POTASSIUM-RICH FOODS

FOOD	SERVING SIZE (5000 mg)
Apricots	6 fresh
Banana	1 medium
Cantaloupe	½ melon
Orange juice	1¼ cup
Prunes	7 large
Sweet potato	1 large

MAGNESIUM-RICH FOODS
(HIGH IN ELECTROLYTES)

Bran
Nuts
Peas
Soybeans
Wheat germ

A Healthy Diet Can Reduce Blood Pressure

In landmark studies published in the *New England Journal of Medicine*,[16] the clinical effects of three different diets on blood pressure were detailed:

- *Diet 1:* A "control" diet that allowed dietary potassium, calcium, and magnesium levels close to the 25th percentile of the U.S. population intake
- *Diet 2:* A diet rich in fruits and vegetables (excellent sources of vitamin K and magnesium)
- *Diet 3:* The Dietary Approaches to Stop Hypertension (DASH) diet, a diet rich in fruits and vegetables and low-fat dairy products (excellent sources of vitamin K, magnesium, and calcium)

In the study, all three diets had the same sodium content and were adjusted so that the participants would not lose weight, as researchers wanted to study only the effects of the electrolytes.

The results were quite revealing. Blood pressure reductions were seen in the groups using Diets 2 and 3, with the greatest reductions in Diet 3 (the DASH diet). The DASH diet is high in calcium, potassium, and magnesium from the fresh produce and naturally low in sodium. (Diet 3 also helps to lower LDL cholesterol.)

The study results affirmed that blood pressure is related to multiple dietary electrolytes. Participants who followed Diet 3 had an average drop of eleven points in their systolic blood pressure reading (the top number), while their diastolic pressure (the bottom number) dropped more than five points.

Talk to your doctor before making any drastic changes in your eating habits. Don't stop or alter your medication without talking with your doctor.

THE DASH DIET GUIDELINES

- Limit fat calories to 30 percent of daily amount.
- Eat eight to ten servings of fruits and vegetables.
- Eat seven or eight servings of grains.
- Eat only low-fat or fat-free dairy products.
- Eat no more than four to five servings of nuts and seeds per week.

Limit Your Alcohol Intake

The latest guidelines from the American Heart Association suggest no more than one drink per day for women. If you do not normally drink alcohol, do not start. Recent studies point to red wine as being beneficial because of the superantioxidant activin, which reduces your risk of atherosclerosis. Instead of drinking wine each day, you can easily get the same heart benefit by eating red or purple grapes or by drinking purple grape juice.

Heart Healthy Eating Plan Recap

For your Healthy Heart Eating Plan, be sure to consider the following guidelines:

- Lose weight and stay at your desired weight.
- Choose foods high in antioxidants.
- Choose foods with heart smart B vitamins.
- Choose foods with flavonoids.
- Choose foods with phytochemicals.
- Choose whole grains.
- Choose healthy fats.
- Watch your intake of sodium.
- Limit your alcohol intake.

As you start making heart-healthy food choices, try not to keep yourself from eating the foods you enjoy—this diet is for a lifetime, not something you lose interest in because it becomes boring. Even if you're counting calories, don't get too hung up on what you eat at any one meal. What is most important is how many calories you eat per day or every two days.

If you are more than 20 percent over your desirable body weight, talk with your physician. Make plans to begin a reasonable and safe weight-loss program. If other medical problems are present, they may affect the rate and success of your weight loss. A reasonable diet combined with a regular exercise program is usually successful and fairly painless.

Starting and maintaining a new way of eating—a heart-healthy diet—may not be easy at first. Becoming more active, and starting the exercise program outlined in Chapter 9, will be a difficult lifestyle change for some people. But studies show that those who stay on low-fat diets over six months or longer find that their tastes go toward foods that are naturally low in fat. And people who begin exercising start to look forward to it after a few weeks.

Now that you have a solid foundation for maintaining or losing weight, I challenge you to take your Healthy Heart Eating Plan to heart—literally! Use these ideas and implement them in your daily routine today. As you plan your weekly menu, follow the 2000 Dietary Guidelines from the American Heart Association,[17] along with the Mediterranean-style diet (page 261). Most importantly, don't keep foods around your kitchen that will cause you to fail.

It's up to you. Preventing heart attack may involve some drastic lifestyle changes—changes only you can make. But the rewards of being able to lead an active, normal life without the worry of heart problems are well worth any sacrifices you make.

11

Nonvitamin Supplements and Heart Disease

I f you're like millions of other people, you may be thinking, when it comes to supplements, "If a supplement is natural, it must be good for me." Think again! Natural dietary supplements may include vitamins, minerals, herbs, and amino acids as well as natural enzymes, organ tissues, metabolites, extracts, and concentrates. Because these natural substances can have a medicinal effect on your body, they are not safe and healthy for everyone. If not used properly, they can make some people ill or even kill them. Take my patient, Barbara, who thought she was taking charge of her health by taking a variety of natural vitamins and supplements.

An anthropology professor at a major university, Barbara had been forty-four years old when she'd had a heart attack. Four and a half years later, she began to have recurrent symptoms of unstable angina, and she underwent heart bypass surgery. She came to see me after one of her friends, who was prodding her to change her life, said, "I guess the heart attack and open heart surgery were not enough to change your unhealthy habits. What's next?"

Barbara knew she had to do something. This highly respected professor was driven and stressed, constantly researching, teaching, or counseling her students. When she wasn't at the university, she was on her computer until the wee hours of the morning, reading the latest research and data. Because of her intense schedule, her diet was simple and consisted of two words—*fast food.* To worsen this already bad situation, Barbara exercised "very rarely."

Although she was well educated and her life had been saved by medicine and surgery, Barbara was skeptical of commonly prescribed medications and wanted to get back in control of her health the "natural way." So she went to a local health food store, and after talking with the clerk at the cash register—a "nutritional consultant"—she bought a variety of vitamins and supplements.

Barbara gave me the list of supplements she was taking. Most of them actually were appropriate—B vitamins, vitamin E, calcium. It wasn't until halfway into the physical examination that she added, "Oh, Dr. Goldberg, I almost forgot to tell you that I also take potassium supplements."

In general, high potassium levels are extremely dangerous to the heart, causing arrhythmias and even sudden death. Potassium is a very important electrolyte, and so people with measurably low potassium do need to take it in supplement form. For example, people who take diuretic medications to reduce blood pressure may need potassium supplements. But if you are at risk for heart disease or have heart disease, you should take potassium *only* if recommended by your doctor.

I reassured Barbara that she was at less risk for a buildup of potassium levels than many patients because her kidneys were normal. But I told her to throw away her potassium supplements or return them and get her money back. Then I showed her how to get a safe, adequate potassium intake by eating low-fat milk, yogurt, vegetables, fruits, and beans.

Like Barbara, many of my patients (before they get to me) think they are getting great benefit from natural supplements, when in reality they may be hurting their health. So I want to go through some of the supplements with you that I hear are most commonly recommended—sometimes with medical proof—for heart disease.

Separating Fact from Fiction

Non-Western cultures have long traditions in using herbs and other supplements to treat and cure medical problems. The Chinese, for instance, have used herbs for centuries, and some of their methods have been studied recently and proved to be effective for certain illnesses. Likewise, the healing tradition of Ayurvedic medicine, which focuses on balancing the body using a combination of techniques, meditation, herbs, minerals, and dietary advice, goes back four thousand years in India's rich history. Acupuncture and acupressure have also been shown to have healing effects in Western studies.

From Aristotle's time to the present, the medical literature anecdotally documents the use of unconventional treatments. But in the mid-1960s, interest in health food and alternative medicine boomed in the United States. We Americans were exposed to Asian traditions and medical practices, and this influx of new views and methods, along with the increasing costs and our growing mistrust of our own health care system, spurred interest in alternative treatments, including the use of natural supplements. More recently, alternative medical techniques such as acupuncture have begun to be recognized by the medical community, leading to research into many of these practices.

Dissatisfaction with conventional medical care has continued to grow, and as a result many conscientious people now want to take charge of their health—to be involved in making decisions about the treatments they receive. I do commend this in my patients, but sometimes the methods they favor are not scientifically substantiated, proven, or congruent with Food and Drug Administration (FDA) guidelines. Most alternative treatments and natural supplements have not passed clinical trials. One patient, forty-one-year-old Felicia, asked me, "Why would the supermarket sell them if they were harmful? Their supplements are right next to the produce aisle, filled with organically grown vegetables." The supermarket sells them because people want them and because they are a profitable item to carry. Don't get me wrong! Many times individual supplements are quite safe. In normal situations, a multivitamin and mineral supplement can usually be taken with confidence. But dietary supplements have few regulations, and companies that manufacture them can basically make any claim they want. Laws state that the claims must be truthful, but a given claim still may represent only a single study or several poor scientific studies.

No matter what the natural food store advertising flyer claims, even the most popular medicinal herbs with pharmaceutical compounds contain ingredients that have not been tested and that are not regulated by the FDA. And they are not likely to be thoroughly tested or their quality overseen anytime soon, since in 1994 Congress exempted these products from FDA regulation. So it's important that you get your physician's approval before adding any unproven alternative therapy to your proven medical plan.

I want you to be careful about what you take. Even natural supplements can cause serious, even life-threatening symptoms or dangerous interactions with prescribed medications. When multiple supplements are taken together or along with prescribed drugs, potentially dangerous interactions may ensue. When supplements contain ingredients that are contraindicated for heart patients, serious—even deadly—problems can arise. For example, one fifty-six-year-old patient, Pat, took a "natural" supplement to help lose weight after her neighbor had used it. While the product was "natural," and Pat bought it at her local pharmacy, it contained ephedra (ma huang), an herb that stimulates the adrenal glands, increases metabolism, and causes a sudden increase in blood pressure and heart rate in some people. Pat lost ten pounds, but she also got more than she bargained for—a trip to the emergency room because of extremely high blood pressure and a rapid heart rate.

Some natural healing substances have led to very important, life-saving treatments. For example, digoxin, a medicine for congestive heart failure, comes from the usually poisonous digitalis or foxglove plant; it was initially described in 1785. Morphine comes from the opium poppy, and penicillin from mold. While all have made a dramatic contribution to medicine, their manufacture and production are carefully managed and they are prescribed according to set guidelines.

Knowing the popularity of herbs and supplements, I always make it a point to ask my patients which ones they are taking. This is very important information to have in your medical history. Your supplements act in ways similar to medications, so if your doctor doesn't ask you for this information, make sure you provide it and that it gets into your file.

In the 1970s, laetrile, the extract of apricot pits, was touted as the miracle cancer treatment. It had no scientific substantiation, and ultimately it was proven useless. No matter what advertisers claim, do not think that eating four cloves of garlic will stop a life-threatening arrhythmia or that green algae pills will reduce your blood pressure. There is no one pill or supplement that can prevent or reverse heart disease.

I've had several patients who have taken an herbal remedy along with their regular blood pressure or cholesterol medication, only to cancel out the desired effect from the herb and the medication. I warn all my patients that herbal drugs can interact dangerously with medications and the interactions can be fatal in some situations.

Become an Expert

Just as you must become an expert in preventing heart disease, you must also become an expert in natural supplements. It is my experience that once patients have been diagnosed with heart disease, they do become "experts" on it; those who tell of feeling more energetic and have fewer problems have learned how to make lifestyle changes and use alternative or natural treatments in a complementary manner—in a way that enhances both health and well-being.

Commonly Used Supplements for Heart Disease

Let's review some of the more popular natural supplements women take to protect their heart. I will share with you the latest research, the pros and cons, and the recommended daily amount to prevent heart disease, if there is one; if it is potentially harmful, I will tell you to stay away from it.

Coenzyme Q10

Coenzyme Q10 (or CoQ10), also known as ubiquinone, is present in all cells of the body. This popular vitaminlike substance is synthesized and sold as a supplement that improves heart and immune function. As an antioxidant, CoQ10 is also found in some whole foods, particularly those that are good for the heart, such as salmon, sardines, and mackerel.

Low CoQ10 levels are indeed seen in heart failure, but studies have not conclusively shown that raising them with a supplement is beneficial.

THE BOTTOM LINE

Although I do not discourage my patients from using CoQ10, I do avoid giving false hope to those with severe congestive heart failure. CoQ10 is not a cure.

Aspirin

As early as the fifth century B.C., Hippocrates prescribed a bitter powder from the bark of the willow tree to treat aches and pains. In the eighteenth century, Edmund Stone, an Anglican clergyman, discovered the healing effects of willow bark—a substance called salicylic acid. Aspirin as we know it today was developed in 1897 by chemist Felix Hoffmann, who compounded a pill of acetylsalicylic acid to treat his father's rheumatism pain.

Using aspirin to prevent a first heart attack, stroke, or other vascular event in a healthy person is referred to as *primary prevention*. But if you do not have heart disease, don't grab a bottle of aspirin out of your medicine cabinet and think it will prevent all cardiovascular problems. Researchers are just not sure about aspirin's benefit in healthy women without heart disease. For example, while the Physicians Health Study (a study of male physicians) showed that aspirin caused a 44 percent reduction in first heart attacks in men, similar findings have not yet been made for women. Until such data are available, your decision to use aspirin as primary prevention should be based on your particular risk for coronary artery disease and stroke.

If you take aspirin, you should also be changing any risk factors for heart disease that you may have and that you can control. You should not take aspirin if you are allergic to it or have bleeding problems. Do not take herbal supplements of garlic or dong quai with aspirin therapy, as they may cause hemorrhage. Talk to your doctor about any and all other medications you are presently taking, so that he or she can determine whether aspirin is advisable for you or whether you should discontinue any of the supplements.

THE BOTTOM LINE

While aspirin's role in preventing a second heart attack has been proven with women, I do not advocate the widespread use of aspirin in primary prevention. Aspirin is prescribed for women with heart disease or multiple risk factors for heart disease.

Garlic

Garlic, a pungent herb, is a member of the Allium plant family. Garlic has antioxidant properties, reduces blood clotting, and may lower blood pressure. Studies show that it may lower and inhibit the production of cholesterol. One analysis suggested that half a clove of garlic has cardioprotective benefits.[1]

THE BOTTOM LINE

Eat whole garlic on your Italian bread, in your favorite pasta sauce, or in some favorite Mediterranean recipes, and enjoy it. But large quantities are associated with allergic reactions, anemia, and bleeding, and they can interact badly with blood thinners. These problems with garlic supplements outweigh any benefit.

Cholesterol-Lowering Margarines

Fifty-year-old Jodie came to see me and brought me a container of one of the new cholesterol-lowering margarines. After being on a low-fat diet and using this margarine for several months, she wanted to show me why she thought her cholesterol had dropped 12 points.

Recently the FDA approved Benecol and Take Control as cholesterol-lowering spreads. These spreads are made of sterol esters similar in structure to cholesterol, only they are derived from plants. They work to inhibit cholesterol absorption in the intestine and have been shown to reduce LDL cholesterol approximately 7 percent with servings of 1 gm per day. If you were to stay on a low-fat diet, your LDL ("bad") cholesterol would be lowered by almost 10 percent. These new margarines, used with a low-fat diet, have a proven additive lowering effect.

THE BOTTOM LINE

While these margarines are part of a heart-healthy and cholesterol-lowering diet, keep in mind that sometimes *more is not better*— especially as calories add up with each serving. Jodie got benefits from using this margarine because she followed a low-fat diet and exercised regularly. Using the margarine alone, without a low-fat diet, will probably not lower your LDL cholesterol to healthy levels.

Herbs to Avoid

Alternative medicine proponents argue that many herbs prevent illness and promote healing, but no current laws regulate them to ensure their quality. The strength and components of an herbal medicine can vary between batches and manufacturers. Some herbal preparations, when tested, are found to have no active ingredients at all, in spite of the claims on the label. Unscrupulous manufacturers can even substitute one herb or substance for another, and they do not have to indicate this on the label. They can easily (and legally) say the substitution was an accident.

Ephedra

Herbal Ecstasy and other products containing ephedra, as Pat found out, should not be taken if you have high blood pressure. The FDA has proposed cracking down on the marketing of these supplements, citing about eight hundred injuries and at least seventeen deaths linked to them. The proposals include limiting concentrations of ephedra in any dietary supplement, requiring a warning label that its use can cause death, and banning claims that it can help people lose weight or build muscle. Ephedra is also marketed as ma huang, Chinese ephedra, and epitonin. If you are at risk for heart disease or have high blood pressure, do not take these supplements.

Phenylpropanolamine

Phenylpropanolamine (PPA), a common supplement used in appetite suppressants and some cough and cold remedies, has also been found to have a dangerous heart link. Studies in the *New England Journal of Medicine* (December 2000)[2] reported that PPA may cause hemorrhagic stroke (a stroke due to a burst blood vessel in the brain), and that women between the ages of eighteen and forty-nine are at highest risk. In one study investigators reviewed 140 cases that were reported to the FDA as possible serious side effects of PPA. Nearly one-third could directly link a serious complication to the heart or brain, and nearly half of those were heart-related, including cases of hypertension, palpitations, and tachycardia. Eighteen percent involved the brain, with strokes or seizure. Ten people died, and thirteen people were permanently disabled.

Ginkgo Biloba

Some studies indicate that ginkgo biloba protects cell membranes from damage from free radicals, but this popular herb reduces clotting time, increasing bleeding. Anyone taking warfarin (Coumadin) or other blood thinners should *never* take this herb.

Ginseng

Some of my patients ask about ginseng, since it is said to increase alertness and to stimulate the immune response. I cannot give the go-ahead on this herb, because *ginseng may cause heart palpitations and increased blood pressure.*

Cholestin

Cholestin, a Chinese red yeast rice, is a dietary supplement that contains the same cholesterol-lowering compounds found in prescribed statin drugs. The supplement is inexpensive, easily available without a prescription, and highly effective. But also like statin drugs, it may cause liver and muscle damage. The difference is that statins are regulated by the FDA. Before a doctor prescribes a statin drug, he or she assesses your total health, and once you are taking the drug, follow-up laboratory tests are necessary to ensure your continued good health. None of these precautions happens when you self-administer cholestin.

Grapefruit Juice

New studies conclude that grapefruit juice (not the fruit) may increase the potency of certain medications. They show that when grapefruit juice is ingested, the absorption of some cardiac drugs may be altered. For example, the potency of some antihypertensive medications and statins is increased when they are taken with grapefruit juice. Just be aware of this seemingly safe combination, and let your doctor know if you drink grapefruit juice. In some situations, you may have to avoid grapefruit juice when taking your medications.

Grapefruit juice increases the potency of the following medications:

Amlodipine	Lovastatin
Atorvastatin	Sertraline
Carvedilol	Simvastatin
Losartan	

POTENTIAL TOXICITY
FROM HERBAL REMEDIES

Common Name	Usage	Potential Toxicity
Black cohosh	menopause	angina, rapid heart rate
Chaparral	sedative	liver inflammation
Garlic	lower cholesterol	reduced blood clotting (bleeding), hives
Ginseng	fatigue	anxiety, depression, vaginal bleeding
Hyssop	regulate blood pressure, promote circulation	diarrhea, upset stomach
Kava kava	sedative	dermatitis, hallucinations
Licorice	immune system	edema, high blood pressure, low potassium
Ma huang	weight loss	rapid heart beat, atrial fibrillation, stroke, heart attack
St. John's wort	anti-depressant	sensitive skin in sunlight

POTENTIAL HERB-MEDICATION INTERACTIONS

Herb	Potential Interaction	Medication
Fenugreek	insulin is enhanced; hypoglycemia	oral drugs that lower blood sugar, insulin
Dong quai	aspirin is enhanced; hemorrhage	aspirin, warfarin, heparin, or other blood thinners
Feverfew	bleeding	nonsteroidal anti-inflammatory drugs (NSAIDS), aspirin, warfarin, increases effects of cholesterol medication
Garlic	bleeding	warfarin/heparin, ASA, blood thinners, increases effects of cholesterol medication
Gingko	bleeding	blood thinners
Alfalfa	warfarin's effects are negated; increased blood clotting	warfarin (Coumadin)
Ginseng	medications' effects are negated; elevates blood pressure	blood pressure medications
Ma huang	Elevates blood pressure, blood pressure medications' effects are negated, tachychardia	
Gugulipid	medications' effects are negated	propranolol, diltiazem
Foxglove	cardiac arrhythmia	digoxin
Aloe	diuretics' effects are enhanced; dehydration, hypotension	diuretics

| Buckthorn | resulting in dehydration, hypotension, arrhythmias | low potassium |

The Bottom Line on Supplements

There is no "quick cure" for obesity, high cholesterol, or hypertension. If you are taking *any* natural supplements, I want you to share this information with your doctor, to see if they are safe considering the state of your health and any other medications you may be taking. If you are considering trying natural supplements, it is important that you *first* consult with your health care professional, especially if you are already taking *any* medication.

To show you how important this is, I want to tell you about my patient Betsy. About five months ago Betsy came in to see me for a consultation on her cholesterol. At age fifty, this woman had a strong family history of heart disease. Her father had died of a heart attack at forty-eight, and her younger brother, forty-two, had recently had an angioplasty. Betsy brought me a copy of a recent cholesterol test that had been done by her primary care physician. While her total cholesterol was 340 mg/dL, her HDL ("good") cholesterol was 32 mg/dL and her LDL ("bad") cholesterol was 200 mg/dL. On the bottom of the laboratory test report was an underlined note from her physician that said, "Start atorvastatin (10 mg)."

When I asked Betsy how she was doing with the medication, she said she had not started it and wanted a second opinion. After taking a complete history and a physical, I told Betsy that I agreed with her primary care physician that the medication was necessary. I explained to her that she probably overproduces cholesterol and would benefit from an anticholesterol medication, as lifestyle changes might not be adequate. Betsy's low HDL cholesterol was an additional risk factor for heart disease.

Betsy appeared to agree with me about the medication, and she said she'd also start a treadmill exercise program. I gave her a prescription for a cholesterol test and liver function tests in one month, to make sure the medication was effective and had no side effects. I also scheduled a follow-up visit with her for six weeks later.

Well, Betsy canceled that appointment and did not return for the blood tests. Five months later she did come back and sheepishly admitted that she had not filled the prescription because she said she didn't want to depend on medication for the rest of her life. But she assured me that she'd changed her diet and was exercising regularly. Indeed, she had lost fifteen pounds in the five months since I'd last seen her. But she had also been taking a variety of supplements on the recommendation of a relative who owned a health food store. Betsy opened a large shopping bag to show me all the supplements she was now taking.

I was a bit alarmed and asked her why she hadn't shared this information earlier. Betsy admitted she wasn't sure whether I would have supported her taking all the pills. Then, surprisingly, she asked to have her cholesterol rechecked. She promised that if her "lifestyle changes" had not worked to lower her cholesterol, she would start on the medication that I had prescribed. Her brother was having a second angioplasty that week, and the reality of her family history of heart disease was really worrying her.

The following are some of the changes that Betsy had made on her own:

- She ate in line with the Mediterranean-style diet (described in Chapter 10).
- She worked out on treadmill for thirty-five to forty-five minutes each evening.
- She switched from butter to plant-based margarine.
- She used cholestin to reduce cholesterol, in accordance with the label.
- She used garlic and niacin supplements, in accordance with the labels.

At this point, I was no longer upset that Betsy had ignored my recommendations and put herself at risk for a heart attack. I could tell that she had agonized over whether to come in and be honest with me, even as her risk for heart disease absolutely frightened her.

I was curious to see if the changes in her lifestyle had helped her. I told her that I respected her honesty and was impressed by her weight loss.

I repeated the cholesterol and liver tests, as well as tests for blood sugar and other electrolytes—and was stunned to learn that Betsy had reduced her total cholesterol by 100 points and increased her HDL cholesterol from 32 to 45. This was a tremendous step in her prevention of heart disease. Her LDL cholesterol had dropped from 200 to 160, which was a big improvement, but it was still not enough to keep her safe from heart problems. Together we formulated a plan to lose ten more pounds in accordance with the guidelines in Chapter 10. She would continue to take the cholestin, garlic, and niacin, but if her LDL cholesterol was not at 130 mg/dL at the next visit, she agreed that she would consider medication.

It's always important for physicians to be open-minded as their patients consider natural supplements for boosting their hearts' health. But I also don't want patients to take unnecessary risks. When patients come to me with a new natural supplement, I ask them to consider the following:

- Does it have any known side effects?
- What is the expertise of the person administering the remedy?
- What has happened to people who have taken it over the years?
- What medications are you taking, and how will it interact with them?

Keep in mind that some alternative or complementary therapies may work for you, while others may not. Remember, continuing the Healthy Heart Eating Plan, exercising, and stopping cigarettes are vital for the prevention and treatment of heart disease. There is no one single miracle medicine, and even Betsy, with all her natural supplements, acknowledged the importance of exercise and calorie counting in her weight loss and cholesterol reduction. Please be sure to get your doctor's approval before complementing your lifestyle and medication plan with any unproven natural supplement.

12

Your Stress Reduction Program

In Chapter 5, we talked about how stress is a little-known risk factor for heart disease, especially for women who put other responsibilities before their own health. Now I want to build on that discussion to help you put yourself first and implement your own de-stressing program. While you cannot change the past stressors you've had, you can begin today to relax and take the extra burden off your heart, using the Stress Reduction Program.

"Can what I think really affect my heart's health?" my patients ask. Absolutely! A school of medicine called psychoneuroimmunology studies how the mind and body interact and how mental or emotional processes (the mind) affect physiological function (the body). Some health professionals even hold that between 90 and 95 percent of all health problems can be traced to the influence of emotions. I don't go quite that far, but I do know that de-stressing and having a calm, optimistic outlook on life can complement other positive lifestyle habits and conventional medical care.

The belief in the efficacy of mind/body therapies is not new. Aristotle gave credence to them, advising with other physicians, "Just as you ought not to attempt to cure eyes without head or head without body, so you should not treat body without soul." The two-thousand-year-old Hippocratic writings observe that "there is a measure of conscious thought throughout the body." Hippocrates taught his students to carefully assess their clients' living environment for an understanding of their diseases, since their emotional reactions to life's challenges affected their health and recovery.

Taking time for yourself should become your new priority as you start on your heart-healthy way of life. This time-out is not selfish, it's necessary. By keeping yourself healthy, you are also doing something great for those you love. After all, when women become ill with heart disease, it has a trickle-down effect, influencing spouses and children, parents and other family members, friends and co-workers.

After you've read this chapter, select mind/body exercises you enjoy, and use them for ten to twenty minutes each day. With practice, you can learn how to switch automatically from a pumped-up response to stress into a calmer, more peaceful attitude.

Relaxation Response

Harvard cardiologist Herbert Benson, M.D., founder of the Mind-Body Medical Institute, was the first physician to document scientifically the physiological benefits of meditation. In patient trials with experienced transcendental meditators in the 1970s, Benson found that once the mind reaches a state of deep relaxation, the body is also able to relax. In this state, the body's immunity is heightened and its cell-repair functions enhanced. Cardiovascular patients who practice relaxation are more compliant in taking medication and have less need of medical services.

Particularly if you are anxious or have hypertension, learning how to relax can reduce physical strain and negative, emotional thoughts—and increase your ability to manage stress. If you practice relaxation regularly, your body will soon learn to elicit the relaxation response during a stressful situation—and keep your heart rate and blood pressure from rising.

To begin your own heart-healthy Stress Reduction Program, set aside a period of fifteen to twenty minutes each day that you can devote to relaxation practice. If you cannot give up fifteen minutes to relax, then try ten—just do something to let your tensions go. Make sure no distractions will disrupt your concentration: turn off the radio, the television, and even the ringer on the telephone if possible.

RELAXATION EXERCISE

During this daily "practice," it's important to recline comfortably rather than sit, so that your whole body is supported and you are relieving as much tension or tightness in your muscles as you can. Once you are comfortable, remain as still as possible. Focus your thoughts on the immediate moment or on your breathing, and eliminate any outside thoughts that may compete for your attention. Concentrate on making your breathing slow and even and rhythmic. Notice which parts of your body feel relaxed and loose and which parts feel tense and uptight. As you exhale, picture your muscles becoming relaxed, as if with each breath you breathe away the tension.

Starting with your toes and moving gradually up your body, imagine that every muscle in your body is now becoming loose, relaxed, and free of any tension. Picture all of the muscles in your body unwinding; imagine them completely loose and limp.

At the end of your relaxation time, take a few moments to study and focus on the feelings and sensations you have been able to achieve. Notice which areas now feel more relaxed, and whether any areas of tension or tightness remain. You may want to focus on relaxing the tense parts of your body tomorrow in your next session.

Many women tell me that after several weeks of daily, consistent practice, they are able to maintain the relaxed feeling the exercise gives them beyond the practice session itself. It's worth the effort. If you have trouble with this exercise, you might want to see a clinical psychologist who specializes in relaxation for professional instruction.

Deep Abdominal Breathing

Your breathing can alter your psychological state. It can improve or exacerbate a stressful moment. As you learn how to do deep abdominal breathing, you will decrease the release of stress hormones and slow down your heart rate during stressful moments. I do deep abdominal breathing before I make a presentation before a big group, and it helps me relax and actually enjoy the moment. You can use this exercise anytime you feel anxious or stressed, and after practicing it for a few weeks, you won't have to leave a stressful scene to lie down. The slow deep breathing can interrupt a cycle of rapid, shallow breathing and get more oxygen than carbon dioxide into your blood, which will give you a more comfortable state of mind.

DEEP ABDOMINAL BREATHING EXERCISE

Lie on your back in a quiet room. Plan to have no distractions for five minutes—if necessary, unplug the phone. Place your hands on your abdomen, then slowly and deliberately breathe in through your nostrils. If your hands are rising and your abdomen is expanding, then you are breathing correctly. If your hands do not rise but your chest is rising, you are breathing incorrectly.

Inhale to a count of five, pause for three seconds, and then exhale to a count of five. Start doing ten repetitions of this exercise and then increase to twenty-five, twice daily. If your muscles are tight from tension and anxiety, you might find this exercise extremely helpful to induce relaxation as well.

Progressive Muscle Relaxation

Progressive muscle relaxation involves contracting, then relaxing all the different muscle groups in the body.

PROGRESSIVE MUSCLE RELAXATION EXERCISE

Lie in a reclining position. Focusing on your head and neck muscles, tense these muscles to a count of ten, then release to a count of ten. Next, tense and release your shoulders to a count of ten. Now tense and release your arms and hands, counting to ten. Next, tense your chest, stomach, and back for a count of ten, and release, counting to ten. Tense and release your pelvis and buttocks to the count of ten. Move your attention to your thighs, and tense and release them. Finally, tense and release your calves, feet, and toes to the count of ten.

Go slowly as you progress throughout your entire body, taking as long as you can. Get in touch with each part, and feel the tension you are experiencing there. Then as you release the muscle, notice how it feels to be tension-free.

Many patients say their progressive muscle relaxation exercise is enhanced with soothing music. You can also do it with deep abdominal breathing: breathe in while tensing the muscles; exhale while relaxing them.

Visualization

We teach visualization in the Women's Heart Program at Lenox Hill to help women control their emotional distress or anxiety and to promote relaxation at the end of the exercise class. No matter how many times I see it, I still am thrilled and amazed when I see a woman's heart rate drop on the monitor, after she's learned to use visualization. It's a simple technique that is profoundly effective in helping you heal and keeping you healthy.

If you can daydream, then you can master this simple, inexpensive technique. Granted, some of us are naturally better at imagining than others, but with practice we all can learn to visualize effectively. Much like learning any skill, from playing bridge to playing tennis, becoming skilled at visualization involves some time, patience, and practice. Once you learn the technique, it will come in handy in countless situations—including when you're stuck in a long line or in a traffic jam during rush hour.

To begin, you need to be alone in a quiet environment without distractions. During this time-out, I want you to visualize a peaceful, relaxing scene, perhaps a vacation spot you have enjoyed in the mountains or at the seashore. Whatever the scene is, focus on that place. Try to recapture the moment as you imagine the sounds, smells, textures, and feelings of being there. Become aware of your breathing as you continue your focus, and push away any outside stimuli that try to come into your special place. You are completely safe and calm in this place. Feel this calm in your body and mind.

Feel your whole self at peace, and know that you can take this peace with you into the world.

Once you have practiced visualization for three weeks, you can usually use it to reduce your anxiety during stressful times and even to lower your heart rate and blood pressure. For example, if you have an upcoming meeting with your boss and you feel nervous, switch into visualization and imagine yourself in your favorite relaxing scene. Let your body feel at peace as you briefly detach from your fears. Remember, your body knows only what your mind tells it! If you tell it that it's at peace and safe, it will feel that way. In this way, visualization significantly contributes to your own well-being and heart's health.

Some good, enjoyable books on visualization include *Healing Visualizations* by Gerald Epstein, M.D., and *Rituals of Healing* by Jeanne Achterberg.

Meditation

Meditation is another way to move beyond the negative thoughts and agitations of your busy mind, becoming "unstuck" from any fears or other disturbing emotions. Scientific studies have shown it helps to lower blood pressure, alleviate insomnia, and reduce chronic pain.

Some meditations focus on the breath, while others focus on the silent repetition of a word, such as *love* or *ohm*. As stressful thoughts intrude, you continue to concentrate on the breath or word and notice and release the other thoughts or feelings. *Mindfulness* is a traditional Buddhist approach to meditation. Intense focus is the key to mindfulness, which allows your mind to be full of whatever you are doing at that moment, whether dancing, gardening, writing, or listening to music. Many wonderful books and tapes can help you find a meditation practice that you enjoy; some classics are *Focusing* by Eugene Gendlin; *How to Meditate* by Lawrence LeShan; and *A Path with Heart* by Jack Kornfield.

Yoga

Yoga can be very helpful in de-stressing because it focuses on exercise, breathing, and meditation. Not only does it provide the benefit of relaxing your body, the various positions increase your flexibility and muscle strength. With yoga, there is no high impact or bouncing. Yoga exercise produces alpha waves in the brain that are tied to the feeling of serenity and are prominent during relaxation.

The specific yoga exercises put pressure on the body's glandular systems, thus releasing healing chemicals that promote your overall health. Using the postures and your breath, you learn to quiet the body and mind and heal from chronic stress.

You can take a yoga class at the local Y or fitness center. Or you can rent or purchase a video and do the yoga postures in the privacy of your own home. There are numerous tapes to choose from, so you can definitely find one that's right for you.

Aromatherapy

Aromas and scents can alter your mood and thoughts. Some studies have shown that inhaling scents, as well as the use of certain oils, can have beneficial effects. Each fragrance oil is said to have a specific healing power. For example, lavender and spiced apples are said to increase the activity in the back of the brain, which leads to relaxation; jasmine or lemon are used to increase beta activity in the front of the brain and heighten alertness.

Just as odors can change brain wave states, they also seem to be able to change moods. How this scent-mood link works remains a mystery. Researchers do know that when aromatic molecules drift into your nose, they lock onto receptors there and create electrical impulses that travel up the olfactory nerves to the brain's limbic system, where emotions and memories are processed.

While there have been no controlled studies to date, many people claim that aromatherapy aids in reducing stress and makes them feel better. Can scents change your mood and reduce your stress? The answer lies within you.

Relaxing Scents
- Lavender
- Sandalwood
- Orange blossom
- Spiced apples
- Vanilla

Music Therapy

Music therapy is another effective nonpharmacological approach for reducing anxiety and stress. While it may sound too easy to work, many of the sensations that arise from music are processed in the same areas of the brain that process pain. For de-stressing, music therapy may be helpful in combination with another mind/body therapy, such as visualization, deep abdominal breathing, or progressive muscle relaxation.

If you use music therapy as part of your de-stressing program, make sure that the pace of the music you choose is slightly slower than your heart rate, or approximately 60 beats a minute. This rhythm will encourage your heart rate to slow down, which some studies have shown may also lower blood pressure. Some of the quieter classical works of Vivaldi, Bach, Mozart, and Chopin would fit this category. Or you might try New Age music by artists such as George Winston with Windham Hill.

Prayer

Many of my patients tell of the importance of using prayer to give them an inner peace during times of great stress or crisis. One young mother said that prayer helped her get back in control when her father was injured in a car accident. Another patient prays for twenty minutes before she starts her day. This quiet time helps women focus on what they can do and frees them from worrying about situations over which they have no control, so that they are able to meet stress with a calm, normal heart rate and blood pressure.

Prayer allows your thoughts to take a break from your daily analytical routines and gives support to your spirit. When you pray or meditate, your body switches from the pumping "fight or flight" response into a calmer, more peaceful mood. Prayer nourishes your soul, satiates that "inner" spiritual hunger, and helps you to develop your ability to focus and concentrate. There are many prayer and daily meditation guides from all faiths and cultures from which you can choose.

Again, there is no "proof" that this mind/body therapy causes actual healing, but more and more studies show that people who find strength and comfort in their personal faith or in organized religion have greater survival rates from serious disease.

Finding the Right Stress Reduction Therapy

These are a few of the more popular stress reduction therapies. Not only are they free, but you can do them anywhere—in a conference room, in the subway, or in your bed in the middle of the night, if you wake up with your mind racing because of overcommitments. It's important that you find the methods with which you feel most comfortable. If you don't, it could cause you more stress than you had in the first place.

Not every therapy works for everyone. You may prefer deep abdominal breathing while listening to classical music in a room filled with scented fragrances. Your best friend may like a more active destressing exercise, such as doing yoga.

I am giving you a doctor's order to experiment with and find the best mind/body stress reliever for you, and to start practicing it every day so that you never feel overwhelmed by your life's pressures. You may need to try out a few of the ones I discussed, or you might find yours first off.

One patient, Marnie, age thirty-seven, would fall asleep during her meditation sessions. I thought that she must be pretty relaxed to fall asleep, but she actually needed a more active therapy to modify her daily stress response. Marnie now is a yoga instructor at a local gym. She finds that this ancient discipline boosts relaxation throughout her busy day.

It is not hard to fit relaxation time into your daily routine. Check out the Sample Five-day De-stressing Plan. It has helped many women learn how to fit mind/body exercises into their busy on-the-go routines.

SAMPLE FIVE-DAY DE-STRESSING PLAN

Day	Time	Activity
Monday	10 minutes	yoga stretches before work
	10 minutes	meditation instead of coffee break
	10 minutes	relaxation response while soaking in bath
Tuesday	10 minutes	deep abdominal breathing at lunch
	10 minutes	meditation waiting for carpool
	10 minutes	yoga stretches before bedtime
Wednesday	10 minutes	visualization (of mountain stream) instead of coffee break
	10 minutes	yoga stretches before fixing dinner
	10 minutes	meditation before bedtime
Thursday	10 minutes	yoga stretches before work
	10 minutes	relaxation response at lunch
	10 minutes	meditation waiting at dentist
Friday	10 minutes	deep abdominal breathing before work
	10 minutes	visualization (the sunset) during lunch
	10 minutes	yoga stretches before bedtime

When Counseling May Help

If your stress problems are overwhelming, I want you to consider professional counseling. Psychological intervention is for everyone, not just for people who have "psychological problems." Especially if you are trying to cope with feelings of depression, anxiety, or grief, a psychologist can do a thorough evaluation and possibly recommend some medication to help you feel better and more able to cope. Cognitive-behavioral therapy can teach you to develop appropriate, active coping strategies to deal with life's issues.

Some of the options include the following:

INDIVIDUAL COUNSELING. In one-on-one sessions with a therapist, you address individual problems. The sessions may include specific guidance for alleviating depression, anxiety, or stress, along with other personal problem areas.

For women who have a difficult time getting their priorities in order, counseling can help them assess their life situation, set personal goals for self-care, and focus more on their own needs while still caring for others. Your therapist can give you moral support as you prioritize your commitments, say no to commitments that would put you in overload, delegate responsibilities at home and at work, and stand strong when family members ask you to do more than you choose to do or can do without jeopardizing your health.

FAMILY COUNSELING. When you have difficulty dealing with life's stressors, it affects your entire family. Therefore it is often helpful for family members to get counseling with you, to help them understand and accept your personal concerns and their possible effects on them. Family members can have the best of intentions, but without specific guidance, they sometimes make things worse. Family meetings may help you to discuss problems openly and get help resolving issues that cause you great personal stress.

GROUP COUNSELING. No one can better understand you than another woman with similar problems. Group sessions led by a trained therapist allow for the sharing of feelings and the development of effective coping strategies. The exchange of ideas at group sessions is often a most productive way to revamp your thought processes. There are support groups for widows and other grieving people, for overeaters, for workaholics, and for people in all kinds of recovery.

While you cannot control life's stressors—and sometimes we all get more than we bargained for—you can change the way you respond to stress and treat yourself. As you focus more on taking care of yourself, you have my guarantee that all who love you—your spouse or significant other, children, parents, siblings, friends and colleagues—will appreciate the results: your renewed inner spirit, increased vitality, and overall good health.

13

Your Stop Smoking Program

To look at forty-nine-year-old Janet, you'd think she was the picture of health. This attractive mother of two appears to be very athletic, with toned muscles and a trim figure. She stays on a low-fat diet and even wears the same size eight jeans she wore in college.

Nonetheless, as a doctor, I know that looks can be deceiving. For Janet is my patient, and a year ago she almost died from a heart attack. Her only risk factor for heart disease was cigarette smoking—and Janet has smoked more than two packs a day since age fifteen.

For women, smoking is especially dangerous, as it triples your risk for having a heart attack and causes early menopause, which lowers the age at which heart disease risk increases. Of all the risk factors for heart disease, smoking cigarettes is perhaps the most harmful. It is also the most preventable cause of heart disease. Smoking, or even being exposed to high amounts of environmental tobacco smoke, causes several effects on your heart and blood vessels. Nicotine increases your blood pressure and heart rate. It increases the amount of blood pumped by your heart and the amount flowing in your arteries. It causes arteries to narrow and constrict, which diminishes the ability of the increased amount of blood to pass through. If the restricted blood flow is prolonged in the coronary arteries, it may result in a heart attack and stimulate the formation of blood clots.

If you have high cholesterol, smoking increases your risk for developing even higher cholesterol. Smokers are more likely to have lower levels of HDL ("good") cholesterol and higher levels of LDL ("bad") cholesterol.

Besides nicotine, the carbon monoxide in cigarette smoke gets into your blood and reduces the oxygen available to your heart and the rest of your body. Other chemicals in the smoke cause your platelets, or blood-clotting cells, to become stickier and cluster. This shortens their clotting time and results in blood clots. All of these factors have a cumulative negative effect on your cardiovascular system. Smoking will shorten your life.

HOW DOES SMOKING INCREASE THE RISK OF HEART DISEASE?

- It increases the risk of heart attack and heart attack symptoms.
- It adds to the risk of coronary artery disease in those who are already at high risk due to hypertension and high cholesterol.
- It increases LDL ("bad") cholesterol and lowers HDL ("good") cholesterol.
- It increases the risk of coronary artery disease and stroke in women who take oral contraceptives.
- It increases the risk of sudden death.
- It increases the risk of atherosclerosis and blockage of the arteries that supply the legs and feet.
- It increases the risk of atherosclerosis and blockage of the arteries that supply blood to the brain, leading to stroke.

But It Feels So Good!

Smoking addiction actually has two important aspects: biology and learning.

Nicotine, one of the key toxins in cigarette smoke, is highly addictive and has a number of pleasant but dangerous effects on the brain that create biological urges to smoke. The learned urges may cause you to habitually smoke in a variety of daily-life situations. For example, you may crave a cigarette upon awakening and before going to bed. Or you may be accustomed to having a cigarette with your morning coffee, after dinner, or at a cocktail party with friends.

The problem is that once nicotine is in your body, it "hits" the brain cell receptors and stimulates the release of neurotransmitters, the brain's chemical messengers. These chemical messengers—acetylcholine, dopamine, serotonin, and beta-endorphin—stimulate areas in the brain that are responsible for our ability to pay attention and concentrate, think, and feel pleasure. Perhaps that is why some women reach for a cigarette whenever they need to feel alert, be productive, or cope with daily anxiety and tension.

Quitting is not easy. When you stop smoking, you may experience nicotine withdrawal, with symptoms of insomnia, mood swings, depression, anxiety, nervousness, headaches, and increased appetite. For most of my patients, it is the increased appetite and food cravings that sometimes become stumbling blocks in their attempt to quit for good. But with the new nicotine patches, inhalers, and gum, these side effects are greatly diminished. Even without medication to help with side effects, the symptoms usually don't last more than ten days.

Common Misconceptions About Stopping Cigarettes

Forty-year-old Veronica needed to stop smoking—yesterday. This mother of four small children was forty pounds overweight, had hypertension and high cholesterol, and chain-smoked. I didn't have to tell Veronica that she was a walking time bomb—she knew already that stopping smoking would help save her life. But she was afraid she could not handle the side effects, even though they would be temporary. It took many sessions to convince Veronica that the benefits of stopping smoking far outweighed any temporary discomfort she might feel.

Let's look at some of the misconceptions that Veronica and other patients have shared with me.

MYTH: "I will gain another forty pounds. Everyone who stops smoking gains weight."

TRUTH: In reality, many people gain ten pounds or less in the first few months of stopping smoking; only 10 percent gain thirty pounds or more. While it's true that nicotine has a metabolism-boosting effect, its loss does not seem to be the reason for weight gain in ex-smokers. But, if you put food in your mouth every time you would have smoked a cigarette, the chances are great that you will gain weight. I encourage my patients who are quitting smoking to initially increase their level of activity and to substitute low-calorie foods (sugar-free hard candies, sugar-free gum, fresh vegetables chopped in pieces) when they have the urge to munch. Mind/body therapies to reduce stress are also helpful in relaxing and controlling that urge to overeat. If you do gain weight, know that you can lose this weight in a few months, using a calorie-controlled diet and increased exercise.

MYTH: "I've tried to quit five times already. If you try to quit and fail, there is no hope at all."

TRUTH: Anyone who smokes can quit. In fact, many of my patients tried to quit several times before finally quitting for good. It's important to realize that you need to deal with your addiction: biologically (with medication, a patch, or gum) and behaviorally (relearning how to live without smoking a cigarette). The biological part will be easier than the behavioral part, because learned habits are hard to break! But the biological part will not be successful without the behavioral part.

MYTH: "I don't have the willpower to quit smoking. I've gone a few hours without a cigarette, but when that urge hits, I usually give in."

TRUTH: When you try to kick the habit, relapse is easy. Still, you have to fight the urge to smoke *one hour at a time, one day at a time.* A cigarette craving may last one or two minutes, then subside. It will probably not last five or ten hours! When the craving comes on, grab a piece of sugarless chewing gum, or chew on cold crunchy carrot sticks. Whatever it takes to help the craving pass, do it.

When Smokers Quit

Within twenty minutes of smoking that last cigarette, the body begins a series of healing changes that continues for years.

20 Minutes
- Blood pressure drops to normal.
- Pulse rate drops to normal.
- Temperature of hands and feet increases to normal.

8 Hours
- Carbon monoxide level in blood drops to normal.
- Oxygen level in blood increases to normal.

48 Hours
- Nerve endings start regrowing.
- Ability to smell and taste is enhanced.

2 Weeks to 3 Months
- Circulation improves.
- Walking becomes easier.
- Lung function increases up to 30 percent.

1 to 9 Months
- Coughing, sinus congestion, fatigue, shortness of breath decrease.
- Cilia regrow in lungs, increasing ability to handle mucus, clean the lungs, and reduce infection.
- Body's overall energy increases.

1 Year
- Excess risk of coronary artery disease decreases by half.

5 Years
- Lung cancer death rate for average former smoker (one pack a day) decreases by almost half.
- Five to fifteen years after quitting, stroke risk is reduced to that of a nonsmoker.
- Risk of cancer in the mouth, throat, and esophagus decreases by half.

10 Years
- Lung cancer death rate continues to decline.
- Precancerous cells are replaced.
- Risk of cancer to mouth, throat, esophagus, bladder, kidneys, and pancreas decreases.

15 Years
- Risk of coronary artery disease is that of a nonsmoker.

Sources: The American Heart Association, the American Cancer Society, and the National Centers for Disease Control and Prevention.

Your Stop Smoking Program

Whether you smoke occasionally or two packs a day—to relax or to speed up your metabolism—I hope you are ready now to stop smoking to reduce your risk of heart disease. If you stopped smoking right now—today—your overall health would improve greatly. Within five years of stopping, your risk of heart disease would be cut in half. After ten years of no smoking, your heart disease risk would approach that of a nonsmoker. You have nothing to lose—except a destructive addiction—and everything to gain.

For many women, a step-by-step program specifically tailored to their personal needs is the most effective—and successful—way to stop smoking. This personalized plan has six steps that will help you stop and reduce the number and length of the side effects.

Step 1. Identify Your Reasons for Smoking

You've probably thought about why you smoke. These excuses give clues to your level of addiction and triggers to smoking. When I counsel patients on how to quit, their excuses give me clues. Women are more likely than men to smoke to reduce anxiety, ease depression, or keep weight off. Until you address the underlying reasons why you smoke, it is difficult to stop smoking altogether. The truth is that no matter what your excuse for smoking may be, every puff you take is literally taking away minutes, days, and years from your lifespan.

In the spaces provided, write down some personal excuses why you smoke, followed by reasons why you want (or need) to quit.

SAMPLE LIST OF REASONS

I smoke because:

1. It calms me down after work.
2. It helps me keep my weight down.
3. I like the taste.
4. My husband smokes.

I want to quit because:

1. It smells.
2. It's expensive.
3. It's bad for me.
4. My daughter has asthma.

YOUR LIST OF REASONS

I smoke because:

1.
2.
3.
4.

I want to quit because:

1.
2.
3.
4.

Step 2: Identify Your Past Successes and Failures

Now that you've put in writing the reasons why you smoke and why you need to quit, think about any past successes (and failures) you have had in giving up smoking. Now fill in the following blanks.

1. *What helped you give up cigarettes?* Did a friend stop smoking at the same time, giving you encouragement to stop? Did your boss reward you with a paid day off when you quit? Did your doctor affirm your efforts?
2. *What made it difficult?* Did you have great stress at home or at work? Was it during the holiday season? Did you find it made you too nervous? How much weight did you gain?
3. *Why will it be different this time?* This is up to you!

1. What helped you give up cigarettes?_____

_____

2. What made it difficult?_____

_____

3. Why will it be different this time?_____

_____

Step 3: Plan to Quit

In this step, think of how you will try to stop smoking differently this time. Just as you would plan a special meal for company or a party for a friend, set the date and time of when you want to quit—then itemize, list, and plan for overcoming both the biological and the learned parts of your smoking addiction.

THE BIOLOGICAL PLAN

If you smoke more than ten cigarettes per day or crave your first cigarette immediately upon arising, planning to address the biological addiction will help you be successful as you undertake your last time to quit smoking.

If you try to stop cold turkey, you may feel the discomfort of symptoms and decide to stop trying. But if you make a plan to prevent withdrawal, you can avoid those unpleasant symptoms.

First talk with your doctor, especially if you want to try a nicotine patch or chewing gum, both of which are available either over the counter or by prescription. These medications can help you quit, but if you continue to smoke while using them, know that you can get very high levels of nicotine in your body that may cause problems. If you are pregnant or have had serious heart trouble within the past month, be sure to speak to your doctor before taking any over-the-counter nicotine medication.

Your doctor can recommend any of several nicotine and nonnicotine prescription medications, including inhalers and nasal sprays. Some of my patients who have a rough time quitting smoking do well with prescribed medications, including bupropion (Zyban, Wellbutrin), an antidepressant that helps smokers in withdrawal. Some smokers use a patch with Zyban, but your doctor will advise you.

All these medications are most successful when combined with a smoking cessation program or behavioral counseling. Most Ys and community centers—or your doctor, employer's human resources department, or local hospital—can help you find a program convenient to where you live or work.

COMMONLY USED STOP SMOKING PREPARATIONS

Type of Preparation	Available Over-the-Counter	Available as Prescription
Nicotine patch	*	
Nicotine gum	*	
Nicotine nasal spray		*
Nicotine inhaler		*
Bupropion (Zyban, Wellbutrin)		*

THE LEARNED HABIT PLAN

Now I want you to identify those specific habits that stimulate your craving for nicotine, known as your *triggers*. Your triggers may include: freshly brewed coffee in the morning, an icy cocktail at a party with good friends, the end of an excellent meal, having out-of-control kids, work stress, or having more month than money.

No matter what triggers your craving for a cigarette, you can break the link between smoking and that activity. But changing habits or eliminating triggers is difficult. It takes time, and you'll find that the biological plan is easier to implement than the learned habit plan.

Step 4: Plan to Face the Triggers

I want you to write down the triggers—the people, places, things, and events—that make you want to light up. Use the blanks provided in the "Personal Trigger List." Once you have quit, go over this list daily—or even several times a day—to remind yourself of when and where you are vulnerable.

What says "smoke a cigarette" to you? Is it the ashtray next to the couch in the den? A half-empty pack on the kitchen counter? Before you launch your stop smoking campaign, get rid of all cigarette paraphernalia—from your home, your car, and your office. Get rid of matches and lighters too—after all, even if you found a cigarette, you could not light up without fire!

If driving to work in traffic makes you want to smoke, keep several flavors of sugar-free gum in the car and keep cigarettes out—and don't allow anyone else to smoke while you're driving. If eating with co-workers who smoke increases your desire, tell them you'll need to eat on the other side of the restaurant until you get past this hurdle, or that you'll meet them for a soda during break times. If one of your trigger situations is "smoking with the first cup of hot coffee in the morning," change to a flavored coffee or spiced tea, or buy a new coffee mug and sit in a different room—anything to break that daily trigger habit. Likewise, if a family member or your spouse smokes, ask him or her to do so away from you—and not in the house, where you can be tempted by the lingering smells. It's important to enlist the support of friends and family members for success in smoking cessation. Your example may even encourage your loved ones to quit with you.

Now look at your Personal Trigger List, and write down ten solutions to help control your urge to smoke, using the space beside each trigger.

Personal Trigger List	Personal Solution List
1.	1.
2.	2.
3.	3.
4.	4.
5.	5.
6.	6.
7.	7.
8.	8.
9.	9.
10.	10.

USE MIND/BODY COPING METHODS

Review the ways to de-stress presented in Chapter 12. You may find that lots of feelings—anger, anxiety, stress, boredom—crop up when you quit smoking. Some of these feelings are not easy to contend with. (That's why you smoked!) But learn the relaxation techniques that appeal to you, and make time several times each day to use them—to reduce negative feelings and to reduce cravings.

USE EXERCISE AS A DISTRACTION

Exercise helps many women stop smoking. A study presented in the *Journal of the American Medical Association* showed that exercise plays a key role in smoking cessation for women, particularly when combined with other techniques such as nicotine patches, Wellbutrin, and support groups.[1] It's difficult to smoke during exercise, and once you get moving, it's hard to think of smoking if you are working out hard. Use exercise to stay away from cigarettes and to boost your health at the same time.

Step 5: Plan to Reward Yourself!

It will take months or years to undo all the damage done by cigarettes. Regularly giving yourself a reward is important to keep you
motivated to stay away from cigarettes—forever.

What makes you smile? A new herb for your windowsill? An aromatherapy candle? A sugar-free gourmet ice pop? Before you stop
smoking, make a list of ten small but pleasurable rewards that you
can give yourself each day you successfully stay away from cigarettes.
These rewards should be reasonable and accessible things you enjoy.

Your Personal Reward List

1.

2.

3.

4.

5.

6.

7.

8.

9.

10.

Step 6: Set a Date

You're almost ready to put the cigarettes in the trash and start your
new heart-healthy life. So let's pick that date and write it down. I
want you to get a piece of paper and write a letter—a contract—to
yourself, making the written commitment to stop smoking cigarettes
on a particular date. In the dated letter, make the commitment fol-

low your plans about triggers and solutions, about de-stressing ther-apies, about exercising, and about rewarding yourself. Give yourself time to see your doctor and get any medication you've decided you want to help you through withdrawal, and allow yourself time to find a support group.

Once you've written the letter, tape it to your refrigerator or dresser mirror, anywhere you will see it many times each day as your reminder.

What If You Relapse?

You would not be human if you didn't relapse. One patient, Lydia, told me she and her husband followed the six-step plan compul-sively. They had no cigarettes in the house, they taped their trigger and solutions lists to the refrigerator, and they even wrapped indi-vidual rewards for themselves and kept them in a box in the den.

"We were doing great until my sister came over—my sister who smokes," Lydia said. "I watched her light the cigarette, and I was hypnotized by the smell, the action, how she must be feeling, even the way she tossed her head when she exhaled. All my knowledge about the dangers of smoking disappeared in her cloud of smoke. I knew I had to have one.

"Believe it or not, even though my sister knew I had to stop smoking, she gave me a cigarette. I think it made her feel better about smoking to see me with a cigarette again. I told her I wasn't going to use it, but later that day before Jim came home, I saw the cigarette on the coffee table and lit up. It was incredible—better than I ever experienced. I smoked for all of thirty seconds, when I heard Jim open the front door door. He definitely smelled smoke and was not happy with my relapse. I was so embarrassed and angry that I caved in.

"Since that 'last smoke,' I have not had one cigarette in three years. I gained a few pounds, but then I lost them over a few months. I found my activity level increased because I was breathing better and felt more energetic."

Smoking is one of the most difficult of the heart disease risk factors to control. Your first or even fifth attempt may not be easy, but quitting smoking is the most important action you can take for your heart's health.

If you need to stop smoking and you're following the six steps for quitting, please don't put extra pressure on yourself to follow every step of the exercise and diet programs at the same time. This could become overwhelming and reduce your chance for success at all of them. Instead, set your quitting date, and increase your physical activity. Once you've quit and are steady in your exercise program, then you can start to make some healthy diet changes.

You may have days when temptation outweighs your willpower. Take it one day at a time—that way you *can* succeed. You'll feel better, look better, breathe easier, and extend your life.

PART IV

Medical Treatments for Cardiovascular Disease

14

Medications That Can Save Your Life

"I'll do anything to lower my blood pressure—walk every day, cut out salt, even lose weight. But I don't want to take medication." Lorri, a forty-seven-year-old mother of three, was determined to avoid medication to help reduce her blood pressure, yet I knew that her heart's health—and her life—depended on it.

Why are we so hesitant to take medication, especially when it can improve our health and lengthen our life? I have had many patients like Lorri who refuse to take necessary medications to lower their blood pressure or keep blood lipids at a healthy level. These women dread making the long-term commitment to medication, and their excuses vary from not being able to afford it, to not wanting to put anything "unnatural" in their bodies, to not liking the annoying side effects, such as fatigue, that some medications do have. My patient Lorri finally admitted that her real reason for not wanting to take medicine regularly was: "It's just one more thing to worry about in my already busy day."

By now you know that I'm a firm believer in changing lifestyle habits as the best way to reduce the chance of heart attack. In some cases, however, lifestyle factors are *not* enough to make a difference, and in these cases medications can help prevent heart attacks and save lives. For example, clot busters are used to stop a heart attack in its tracks, reducing the chance of heart muscle damage.

During my cardiology fellowship, I was paged to see sixty-one-year-old Violet, a retired schoolteacher, at the Kings County Hospital emergency room. Her ECG indicated that she was in the middle of a serious heart attack, and that if we didn't stop it fast, she would lose the function of the anterior or front wall of her heart. That loss of function could result in heart failure, an increased risk of sudden death, and overall a poor quality of life.

Violet's symptoms—severe shortness of breath and nausea—had started three hours earlier, and she had called 911 about two hours after they started. Many years ago she may not have made it to the hospital.

I described for Violet how the new clot busters could actually dissolve the clot that was obstructing the artery, causing the heart attack. She agreed to the treatment, and the intravenous infusion was started, along with other medications. The next morning an ECG indicated she had avoided serious heart damage with this therapy, and an echocardiogram confirmed it.

At the beginning of the twentieth century, medical options were few, but they included nitroglycerin for angina (which is still used today). Digitalis was a main treatment for symptoms of heart failure. It wasn't until the 1940s that researchers connected high cholesterol to higher risk for heart attack, and the first medications to control cholesterol were developed in the 1980s. Beta-blockers came into widespread use in the 1970s to reduce symptoms of angina and reduce the risk of secondary heart attacks, and they revolutionized the treatment of coronary artery disease. The medications we now use to treat heart disease have been shown beyond question to prolong life. While these medications usually do not "cure" the problem, they can give much-needed control, helping to protect the heart from further damage and deterioration.

Combine Medications with Lifestyle Changes

Lenore's experience shows how effective cardiac medications, combined with healthy lifestyle changes, can keep blood pressure at a normal level and prevent heart disease. This thirty-two-year-old attorney came to see me after discovering at a local health fair that her blood pressure was elevated. Over the previous two years her blood pressure and weight had slowly crept up, and her trips to her gym were infrequent. Lenore had occasional headaches and wondered if they were due to elevated blood pressure.

Checking Lenore's blood pressure, I found that it indeed was moderately elevated at 160/100. She told me that that was the same reading that she'd had a month before at the health fair and two weeks later at her gynecologist's office. Although Lenore was reluctant to take medication, I pointed out to her that the elevated blood pressure was not an isolated incident, and that it had been consistently elevated now on three separate occasions. I felt medication was prudent at that time, at least until she started the Women's Healthy Heart Program and showed some beneficial changes in her blood pressure. I believed that once she started the Healthy Heart Eating Plan and the Exercise Prescription, she would be able to decrease or even eliminate the medication, under my supervision.

Two weeks after starting the medication Lenore's blood pressure was 130/80 and her headaches had disappeared. She began the exercise and diet programs outlined in Chapters 9 and 10, along with some mind/body exercises discussed in Chapter 12 to help reduce work stress. After three months Lenore had lost ten pounds and reduced her blood pressure to 120/70. Excited at her excellent results in managing her blood pressure, I reduced her medication. Three months later at a follow-up visit, Lenore had lost five more pounds, and her blood pressure was 112/70. At that time, I discontinued her blood pressure medication altogether. I checked her blood pressure again three months later, and it remained in a good range at 118/72. We still monitor it periodically, but as long as Lenore keeps managing her stress and weight through lifestyle habits, she can keep her heart healthy.

Now I cannot guarantee this degree of success for every woman, but lifestyle changes can reduce the need for medication in some. I share patient stories like these to show you potential outcomes and also to show you the benefits of medications in treating heart disease. In this chapter, I want to inform you about the latest treatments and about how they can work for you, if you need them, as part of a successful healthy heart program. While the medications explained here may not be appropriate for your specific problem, they have allowed millions to regain control of their illness—and their lives. Use this information to talk with your doctor as you seek professional advice about your particular health needs.

My Philosophy of Prescribing Medication

In my practice, when I prescribe medications for heart disease, I take into account the following factors for every patient:

- Sex and age
- Concurrent medical conditions or illnesses
- Pharmacological properties of all medications the patient takes
- Availability of treatment
- Economic considerations

As with all aspects of women's health, when it comes to medications, my belief that "women are not small men" continues to ring true: what works for your husband may not work for you. For decades, men and women have been categorized not by sex, size, or age but as "adults," receiving the same medications and the same dosages. In fact, older women have usually received the same doses of medication as younger women or men. In most medical practices, a petite woman who is five foot one and weighs 105 pounds gets the same dose of medication as a six-foot man who weighs 200 pounds. Researchers now realize that serious side effects of medications may have been greater in women simply because their doses were too high. But because most drug trials in the past have focused on men, we do not know all the best dosages for women. Today more trials include women, so in the near future we will have more accurate information on the efficacy of drug therapy for women.

When prescribing medication, I consider the potential side effects for each patient and explain them. I also find out whether the patient can take the medication regularly and not have it interfere with her quality of life. Before I write the first prescription, I always ask what type of herbs, natural supplements, or other medications she is taking, to avoid any dangerous drug-drug or herb-drug interactions (as I talked about in Chapter 11). If possible, I prescribe medications that can treat more than one condition, such as coronary artery disease and high blood pressure (both of which respond to beta-blockers), when the woman has both conditions. And with all my patients, I follow up to gauge the response to treatment and to make changes as needed.

QUESTIONS YOU NEED ANSWERED
BEFORE SWALLOWING A PILL

If you are already taking medications or if your doctor has told you you should, ask the following questions, so that you understand your role in managing your heart disease and preventing a heart attack:

- What is the medication intended for?
- Are there any potential side effects?
- Does the medication interact with any foods?
- Does it interact with other medicines I am already taking?
- Should it be taken with or without food?
- Will it interact with natural supplements?

Common Medications for Treating High Blood Pressure

Diuretics

WHAT THEY'RE PRESCRIBED FOR

Diuretics are commonly used to treat elevated blood pressure and reduce fluid accumulation in heart failure. They promote the excretion of water from the body. They are particularly beneficial for people with salt-sensitive hypertension.

POTENTIAL SIDE EFFECTS

Some diuretics cause a loss of potassium and magnesium, two beneficial electrolytes. If your diuretic causes your potassium levels to be low, you may experience arrhythmia, dehydration, muscle cramp, and dizziness. To replenish the reduced levels, your doctor will prescribe a potassium replacement. Triamterene is a diuretic that helps to retain potassium, so if you take that medication, you may not need potassium replacement. While not all diuretics result in potassium loss, if you are taking a diuretic, ask your doctor if a potassium replacement is necessary.

POSSIBLE INTERACTIONS

If you are using a diuretic with an ACE inhibitor, you may not need potassium replacement because ACE inhibitors increase potassium levels. Do not take triamterene if you take an ACE inhibitor.

COMMONLY USED DIURETICS		
Generic Name	**Brand Name**	**Frequency of Dosage**
Furosemide	Lasix	once a day
Hydrochlorthiazide	HydroDiuril	once a day
Hydrochlorothiazide plus triamterene	Dyazide	once a day

Calcium Channel Blockers

WHAT THEY'RE PRESCRIBED FOR

Calcium channel blockers lower blood pressure, slow heart rate, and are used to treat arrhythmias such as supraventricular tachycardia. These medications are also used to treat angina symptoms, prevent coronary artery vasospasm, and relax the heart muscle.

While *calcium channel blocker* is a specific class of medication, not all drugs in this class have the same properties. For example, diltiazem and verapamil slow the heart rate, lower blood pressure, treat anginal symptoms, dilate or relax blood vessels, and relax the heart muscle. This is the mechanism by which the medication lowers blood pressure and prevents coronary artery vasospasm.

Amlodipine is a calcium channel blocker that is used to treat hypertension and angina. While it dilates blood vessels, resulting in lower blood pressure, it does not slow the heart rate. Some recent studies suggest that heart attacks increase in those who take calcium channel blockers. This is not confirmed and is under further investigation.

POTENTIAL SIDE EFFECTS

Some of the most common side effects include constipation, dizziness, and mild leg or ankle swelling.

POSSIBLE INTERACTIONS

If you have reduced heart function or systolic failure, you should not use any calcium channel blocker except for amlodipine, as the medication may worsen the symptoms. When combined with a beta-blocker, a calcium channel blocker, such as diltiazem or verapamil, may produce a serious slowing of your heart rate or lower blood pressure, resulting in feelings of light-headedness.

COMMONLY USED CALCIUM CHANNEL BLOCKERS

Generic Name	Brand Name	Frequency of Dosage
Amlodipine	Norvasc	once a day
Diltiazem	Cardizem CD	once a day
Verapamil	Verelan	once or twice a day

ACE Inhibitors

WHAT THEY'RE PRESCRIBED FOR

ACE inhibitors (angiotensin-converting enzyme inhibitors) lower blood pressure and are also used to improve survival in those with heart failure. They reduce fluid accumulation in cases of heart failure. They are important as a preventive measure for patients who have had acute heart attacks. ACE inhibitors help prevent the development of kidney disease in people with diabetes.

ACE inhibitors also have a beneficial effect on the endothelium, the inner lining of the artery walls. The endothelia produce substances such as nitric oxide that are responsible for the blood vessels expanding and relaxing. They also reduce heart muscle thickening in hypertension. Recent studies suggest that ramipril may have more specific heart benefits. Studies have shown that when ramipril is used to treat hypertension, it lowers the risk of heart disease and heart muscle thickening caused by hypertension. It also helps to prevent the development of kidney disease in people with diabetes.[1]

POTENTIAL SIDE EFFECTS

The side effects of ACE inhibitors include a rash and a dry cough, both of which stop when the medication is discontinued. The cough is dose-related and more common in women. Some people who take ACE inhibitors get swelling and tingling around the lips. While this side effect is less common, it is serious, and the drug must be stopped immediately.

POSSIBLE INTERACTIONS

ACE inhibitors raise potassium levels. If you are on potassium supplementation, speak to your doctor before filling the prescription.

COMMONLY USED ACE INHIBITORS

Generic Name	Brand Name	Frequency of Dosage
Captopril	Capoten	3 to 4 times a day
Enalapril	Vasotec	1 to 2 times a day
Lisinopril	Prinivil	1 to 2 times a day
Ramipril	Altace	1 to 2 times a day

Angiotensin II Blockers

Angiotensin II blockers (A-II blockers), such as losartan, candesarten, and valsarten, are also used for lowering blood pressure and for those who've had heart failure. They also have similar benefits to ACE inhibitors for preventing kidney disease in diabetics. These drugs have a similar activity to ACE inhibitors, but they do not cause cough as a side effect. If you have a cough from an ACE inhibitor you are taking, ask your doctor if A-II blockers would be an alternative for you.

COMMONLY USED ANGIOTENSIN II BLOCKERS

Generic Name	Brand Name	Frequency of Dosage
Losartan	Cozaar	1 to 2 times daily
Candesarten	Atacand	1 to 2 times daily
Valsarten	Diovan	1 time daily

Clonidine

WHAT IT'S PRESCRIBED FOR

Clonidine (brand name Catapres) has been around for years and is also used to treat high blood pressure, among other things. This medication is taken two to three times per day. It is also available in a skin patch that is changed weekly.

POTENTIAL SIDE EFFECTS

Side effects of clonidine include dizziness while changing positions, such as getting up from a chair or getting out of bed. Clonidine also slows your pulse rate, yet if you stop it abruptly, you experience a rebound increase in high blood pressure. So do not stop taking it unless you have your doctor's approval and an alternative antihypertensive drug.

POSSIBLE INTERACTIONS

Clonidine may greatly reduce blood pressure when used with other blood pressure medications that lower the heart rate, such as beta-blockers and some calcium channel blockers. Because it slows the heart rate, use it cautiously.

Common Medications for Treating Coronary Artery Disease

Let's look at some of the most commonly used medications for treating coronary artery disease, including their effects and side effects, and how they can work to keep you well.

Aspirin

WHAT IT'S PRESCRIBED FOR

Ever since aspirin became a standard treatment for relieving pain, millions have taken this over-the-counter drug for arthritis, headache, and other pain-related ailments. Then around 1950 researchers discovered another beneficial effect of aspirin: as a blood thinner, it inhibits platelets in the blood from sticking together to form a blood clot; a clot that obstructs a vessel is one of the causes of heart attack and stroke.

In study after study, aspirin has been found to reduce the risk of a second heart attack in both men and women, and to be beneficial in preventing second strokes. Aspirin therapy is also beneficial for treating angina after a heart attack, angioplasty, bypass surgery, or transient ischemic attack (TIA or "ministroke"). Some researchers conclude that giving men and women who have suffered a heart attack aspirin as a treatment reduces the risk of death from a second heart attack by 25 percent, the chance of a nonfatal second heart attack by 49 percent, and the chance of a stroke by 46 percent. Still, despite its obvious proven benefits, I find that aspirin is underutilized in women with diagnosed coronary artery disease.

The standard dose of aspirin that is used to prevent a further heart attack or stroke is 81 to 325 mg. This dosage may vary, so be sure to check with your physician for your particular need. After bypass surgery, stents and angioplasty, or a TIA, your doctor may also recommend aspirin therapy.

POTENTIAL SIDE EFFECTS
Some of the most common side effects of aspirin include gastrointestinal upset and bleeding in people with bleeding tendencies. A slight increase in hemorrhagic stroke, possibly due to aspirin therapy, has been reported. Do not take aspirin if you are allergic to it. Do not take it with herbal supplements of garlic or dong quai, as this combination may lead to hemorrhages. Make sure your doctor knows any and all supplements and medications that you are taking.

Clopidogrel

WHAT IT'S PRESCRIBED FOR
While aspirin has the best benefit-to-risk ratio of any proven therapy for heart attack, there are other antiplatelet medications that your doctor may prescribe. Clopidogrel (brand name Plavix) helps to re-

duce platelets from clotting. Researchers have found that people who had a stroke, heart attack, or peripheral vascular disease and then began taking clopidogrel had a slightly lower death rate.[2,3] Clopidogrel is commonly prescribed after a stent for one month and is used along with aspirin therapy. It is also prescribed as an alternative to aspirin in people allergic to aspirin.

POTENTIAL SIDE EFFECTS
Clopidogrel has the same side effects as aspirin. You may have bleeding, and some patients experience a reduction in platelets, so make sure you get regular blood tests and platelet counts while you are on this medication.

POSSIBLE INTERACTIONS
While taking clopidogrel, do not take supplements and herbs that also reduce blood clotting, like fish oil capsules, garlic capsules, and vitamin E. You *can* eat fish and garlic, however.

Warfarin

WHAT IT'S PRESCRIBED FOR
Warfarin (brand name Coumadin) is a blood thinner that inhibits blood-clotting proteins. It is used to prevent stroke in atrial fibrillation, reduce the risk of the mechanical valves clotting, and treat pulmonary emboli and DVT. This medication also reduces the risk of growth of any blood clots that may have formed in the left ventricle after a heart attack. You must take warfarin for at least three weeks before it begins to work.

POTENTIAL SIDE EFFECTS
If your dose of warfarin is too great, you could get side effects of bleeding and hemorrhagic stroke. Too low a level may be associated with increased clotting and stroke.

POSSIBLE INTERACTIONS
Warfarin cannot be taken in early stages of pregnancy, or it will cause fetal abnormalities. It also interacts with many other medications, in-

cluding oral contraceptives. Make absolutely sure your cardiologist and any other doctors know any and all medications that you are taking. To make sure the warfarin is working, your doctor will carefully monitor you with blood tests, one to three times per month. The frequency may be increased in some situations.

Heparin

Heparin is another blood-thinning medication that makes your body's natural anticoagulant protein more effective. It is used in the hospital in patients with unstable angina heart attacks, pulmonary emboli, and DVT (deep vein thrombosis). The role of heparin for pulmonary emboli and DVT is to protect the patient until warfarin has reached therapeutic levels.

There is a new form of heparin, low-molecular-weight heparin or Lovenox (brand name), that is prescribed for use in both the hospital and for outpatients. This medication is administered by injection under the skin.

Ticlopidine

WHAT IT'S PRESCRIBED FOR
In clinical studies, over a three-year period, ticlopidine (brand name Ticlid) resulted in a 21 percent decrease in stroke over aspirin.

POTENTIAL SIDE EFFECTS
The downside is that ticlopidine costs more and has more side effects than aspirin, including side effects on the bone marrow, which can cause reduced white blood cell counts. This side effect is reversible when you stop taking the medication, but you will then need to try an alternative medication with your doctor's approval. While taking ticlopidine, get your blood and white blood cells checked regularly, as determined by your doctor.

Dipyridamole and Pentoxifylline

Dipyridamole and Pentoxifylline are both antiplatelet medications used for the treatment of claudication, or pain in the calves felt on exertion because of peripheral vascular disease—atherosclerosis of the blood vessels in the leg.

Beta-blockers

WHAT THEY'RE PRESCRIBED FOR

Since the early 1970s, beta-blockers have been used for heart patients with great success. These life-saving medications reduce the work of the heart, slow pulse rate, and lower blood pressure. In clinical trials, researchers conclude that beta-blockers reduce the risk of death *after* a heart attack and decrease the risk of a second heart attack. They are also used in congestive heart failure to reduce high levels of circulating adrenaline in the blood, so that all systems can calm down.

Beta-blockers have many uses in treating heart disease, including treatment of high blood pressure, angina, and certain arrhythmias, such as supraventricular tachycardia and some ventricular arrhythmias.

POTENTIAL SIDE EFFECTS

Some of the more common side effects of beta-blockers include fatigue, sleeplessness, and depression. With propanolol (brand name Inderal), some patients report a greater incidence of sleeplessness, fatigue, and depression than with metoprolol (brand name Lopressor). Also, it can cause loss of sexual desire. All beta-blockers can trigger asthmatic symptoms, so do not take this medication if you have asthma. Your doctor will find an alternative medication for you.

POSSIBLE INTERACTIONS

Beta-blockers lower heart rate and blood pressure, so they should be used cautiously with calcium channel blockers like diltiazem and verapamil. The combination of medications can produce greater reductions in heart rate and blood pressure.

COMMONLY USED BETA BLOCKERS

Generic Name	Brand Name	Frequency of Dosage
Atenolol	Tenormin	once a day
Metoprolol	Lopressor	twice a day
Metoprolol	Toprol XL	once a day
Propranolol	Inderal	three or four times a day

Nitroglycerin

WHAT IT'S PRESCRIBED FOR

Nitroglycerin dilates or widens blood vessels, including the coronary arteries. When used for angina, it has a quick effect in its short-acting forms, such as a tablet under the tongue or spray, and gives quick relief. These preparations are convenient and small enough to be tucked away in your purse. Nitroglycerin is prescribed for patients who have had coronary artery disease. Typically, it is taken when symptoms of shortness of breath, exertional fatigue, chest tightness, or arm numbness are experienced.

Once a bottle of nitroglycerin tablets is opened, it is good for three months. Be sure to store this bottle away from light, or the tablets will lose their potency. When you put a tablet under your tongue, you may feel a slight burning sensation. If you do not feel it, the medication may no longer be potent. Don't be caught with medicine that is no longer helpful.

POTENTIAL SIDE EFFECTS

Side effects of nitroglycerin include headache and lower blood pressure. If it is given to someone who is dehydrated or who already has low blood pressure, it may cause fainting.

POSSIBLE INTERACTIONS

When you combine nitroglycerin with other blood pressure medications, you may get a greater fall in blood pressure.

Longer-acting forms of nitroglycerin are used for chronic therapy and include:

- Isosorbide mononitrate—a pill taken once a day
- Isosorbide dinitrate—a pill taken three times a day
- Nitroglycerin patch—a skin patch applied to your chest that is changed daily
- Nitroglycerin paste—a paste available in a tube like toothpaste. The paste is applied to the skin on the chest and is then covered up with a paper patch. This is messy and is more likely to be used in the hospital than at home.
- Intravenous nitroglycerin—an intravenous substance used in the hospital setting

Common Medications
for Lowering Cholesterol

Statins

WHAT THEY'RE PRESCRIBED FOR

Statin drugs have revolutionized how cholesterol can be lowered medically and can do so by up to 40 percent. They also lower triglycerides somewhat and slightly increase HDL ("good") cholesterol. Studies show cholesterol-lowering drugs measurably reduce heart attack risk in women and senior citizens by nearly 34 percent (about the same amount as in younger men).[4] Yet many women with coronary artery disease are not receiving the life-saving benefits of statin therapy, because they are underprescribed.

Statins work by interfering with the body's ability to manufacture cholesterol in the liver. They also have an antioxidant property and help to improve function of the arterial walls, helping them maintain flexibility and contractibility. Recently a study showed that women who use statins also had increased bone density, a major bonus for prevention of osteoporosis and subsequent fractures.[5]

Your LDL ("bad") cholesterol should be less than or equal to 100 mg/dL. If the diet and exercise programs in Part III don't lower your cholesterol, you may need one of these medications.

POTENTIAL SIDE EFFECTS

In some people, the side effects of statins may include an abnormal liver function test. Your doctor will check your liver function four weeks after starting the statin medication, then periodically as long as you take the statin. If the liver function tests are twice normal, the medication should be discontinued. Sometimes statins cause muscle soreness, which is relieved when the medication is discontinued. You *must* stay in touch with your doctor when taking one of these drugs and call him or her to report any of these symptoms. If these symptoms go unchecked, they can cause serious side effects, so you should ask your doctor to change the medication.

In the summer of 2001, one of the newer statins, Baycol, was withdrawn from the market because of several deaths among people taking this medication. The deaths may have been caused by muscle breakdown that led to kidney failure. They appeared to be more common in those people who were taking Baycol with other cholesterol medications. This has not been found to occur with the other statin medications. However I cannot underscore enough that if you have muscle soreness while taking statins you should call your doctor immediately.

POSSIBLE INTERACTIONS

The side effects are increased when the statin is used with niacin or a fibric acid derivative (used to reduce elevated triglycerides). The combinations need to be closely monitored by your doctor. Also statin levels increase with erythromycin, so if you have an infection that requires an antibiotic, make sure your doctor knows that you are on a statin and prescribes a different antibiotic for you. Digoxin levels in the blood are increased if used with a statin, which means that if you take both drugs, you may need a lower dose of digoxin.

COMMONLY USED STATINS

Generic Name	Brand Name	Frequency of Dosage
Simvastatin	Zocor	once a day
Atorvastatin	Lipitor	once a day
Pravastatin	Pravachol	once a day

Fibric Acid Derivatives

WHAT THEY'RE PRESCRIBED FOR
Fibric acid derivatives, such as gemfibrozil (brand name Lopid) and fenofibrate (brand name Tricor) are another type of cholesterol-lowering medication. They work primarily to reduce triglycerides. But they also increase HDL ("good") cholesterol and reduce total and LDL ("bad") cholesterol.

POTENTIAL SIDE EFFECTS
Possible side effects include an abnormal liver function test and muscle soreness. If the liver function test's abnormality is twice the normal value, the medication should be discontinued. If you have muscle soreness, you should also discontinue it.

POSSIBLE INTERACTIONS
If you are taking warfarin, you may experience increased blood thinning when you also take gemfibrozil and fenofibrate. Your doctor will need to adjust the warfarin dosage to avoid problems. The side effects of fibric acid derivatives increase when they are used with niacin or a statin, so liver function should be monitored through blood tests.

Bile Acid Sequestrants

These cholesterol medications work by binding the cholesterol that is absorbed from the intestine (dietary cholesterol). They are effective in lowering cholesterol by 15 to 30 percent and may be used in addition to statin medications. Many women I take care of cannot tolerate them because of abdominal cramping and constipation. If you are on these medications, avoid taking them at the same time as your other medications, because bile acid sequestrants may interfere with their absorption.

COMMONLY USED BILE ACID SEQUESTRANTS

Generic	Brand Name	Frequency of Dosage
Colestipol	Colestid	1 to 2 times daily
Cholestyramine	Questran	3 times daily
Colesevelam	Welchol	1 to 2 times daily

Niacin

WHAT IT'S PRESCRIBED FOR

Niacin (brand name Niacor, Niaspan) has many benefits. It lowers total and LDL cholesterol, lowers triglycerides, and raises HDL cholesterol. Niacin also lowers Lp(a), a lipoprotein that has a structure similar to LDL cholesterol and is associated with an increased risk of heart attack (see page 73).

POTENTIAL SIDE EFFECTS

Niacin would be a wonder drug if it weren't for the side effects, which make it difficult to tolerate. Some of the most common include flushing and itching, although some new formulations are available that do not cause flushing. If you take it with alcohol, that too may increase flushing. Other problems include abnormal liver function tests, increase in uric acid, and glucose intolerance. If you have any of these side effects, the medication should be discontinued. If you have diabetes, this medication should only be taken under close medical supervision, because it can worsen blood sugar levels.

POSSIBLE INTERACTIONS

Using multiple cholesterol medications may increase the risk of abnormal liver function tests and muscle discomfort, but another drug (such as a statin or fibric acid derivative) is sometimes necessary. In all cases, you should be closely monitored by the doctor.

Drug Combinations

Drug combinations are used in many situations when a patient has several risk factors or several cardiac conditions. Several different kinds of medications are used to treat angina, for example. To reduce the work of the heart, a beta-blocker is given; a nitrate is also given to widen the arteries; and aspirin is prescribed to prevent blood clots. A cholesterol-lowering medication may be added if the patient's cholesterol is too high. All of these medications are commonly used together to treat one disease.

Whether you take one medication or a combination, always ask your doctor to explain the side effects of the medications and the symptoms that indicate you're having a side effect before you start on the medication. For example, with nitroglycerin you may feel light-headed or have a headache, which are symptoms of lower blood pressure. I ask my patients to call me if they have any symptoms, so that I can adjust the medication if necessary or find them an alternative. Because so many cardiac medications lower blood pressure and heart rate, combinations of medications may reduce them further. In some cases, the heart rate or blood pressure becomes too low. Let your doctor know of any problem you have with drug combinations. He or she can work with you until you find the right combination that treats the illness with the fewest side effects.

Make sure all your doctors—your internist, ob/gyn, ophthalmologist, dermatologist, everyone—know about all the medications and any supplements you are taking. Before you start taking any other drug for any condition other than your heart, ask your prescribing doctor if the new drug will interact with your heart medications. Also ask your cardiologist how often you need to come in for him or her to monitor your health and make sure your medications are working properly. For some conditions, you'll need to check in once a month; for others, every three to six months.

Arrhythmias

Anti-Arrhythmic Medication

WHAT IT'S PRESCRIBED FOR

If you have been diagnosed with an arrhythmia, such as atrial fibrillation, but treatment has restored your normal rhythm, your doctor may start you on an anti-arrhythmic medication such as amiodarone or sotalol to maintain this rhythm. Amiodarone converts atrial fibrillation to regular or normal sinus rhythm, slows the pulse rate, and lowers blood pressure. Amiodarone also slows heart rate, and inhibits ventricular arrhythmias.

Studies show that sotalol is less successful than amiodarone in maintaining sinus rhythm long term. While sotalol has fewer drug interactions, it also may increase the risk for ventricular arrhythmia. Beta-blockers do not maintain or convert sinus rhythm but are occasionally used with warfarin to slow heart rate.

POTENTIAL SIDE EFFECTS

Side effects of amiodarone include abnormal liver function tests, hypothyroidism, hyperthyroidism, and abnormal lung function, although this is more common with higher doses. Blood tests are done periodically to monitor the arrhythmia. Ask your doctor how often he or she wants you to come in for tests.

When taking amiodarone, if you are also taking warfarin, you must be carefully monitored and the doses of warfarin must be adjusted according to your levels of blood thinning. In some patients, radiofrequency ablation (see page 408) or surgery may be necessary to control the tachycardia.

POSSIBLE INTERACTIONS

When you are on amiodarone, you must be vigilant about exposure to the sun. Wear sunscreen and a hat when going outside. The sun can cause a bluish skin discoloration (which is reversible).

Atrial Fibrillation

Drug Options
Beta-blocker
Calcium channel blocker (diltiazem, verapamil)
Amiodarone
Sotolol

In atrial fibrillation, the two small upper chambers of the heart (atria) quiver instead of beating effectively. They do not completely pump out the blood during the heartbeat, which allows blood to pool and sometimes clot in the left atrium. Should a piece of the blood clot travel through the body to become lodged in an artery in the brain, a stroke results. Thus, the goal in treating atrial fibrillation is to maintain regular rhythm and protect against stroke. In women, atrial fibrillation has a higher mortality than in men. Amiodarone and sotalol convert atrial fibrillation to a regular rhythm. They are only 50 percent effective. If they don't work, then a beta-blocker is used to slow heart rate.

If the atrial fibrillation is new with no known cause, your doctor will start you on three weeks of anticoagulation medications. Warfarin reduces the risk of blood clots. In clinical trials, researchers have shown that oral anticoagulant therapy can reduce the relative risk of stroke in atrial fibrillation patients by up to 70 percent. For more on warfarin, see page 356.

MEDICAL THERAPY

A transesophageal echocardiogram (see page 186) is a diagnostic test that is usually done when atrial fibrillation has been diagnosed. If the test does not show a clot, your doctor will proceed with cardioversion, a procedure consisting of electric shock to the heart to try to restore its natural rhythm. The anticoagulant is started while you are an outpatient, but many people stay overnight at a hospital when an anti-arrhythmic is started. Beta-blockers are also used in patients with atrial fibrillation to slow heart rate.

Ventricular Tachycardia

Ventricular tachycardia is a fast heart rate that is serious and potentially life-threatening (see page 135). This arrhythmia requires immediate treatment, including medication. The type and length of treatment depends on what's causing the problem.

If the ventricular tachycardia is sustained for thirty seconds or more, cardioversion (electric shock to the heart) must be done to convert it back to a normal rhythm. In some cases, a cardiac electrophysiological study is done to determine the mechanism of the arrhythmia and to assess the risk of a potentially fatal heart rhythm and sudden death (see page 407).

Most patients who are found to have sustained ventricular tachycardia during the EPS need to have a defibrillator implanted. This is the most successful treatment of these life-threatening arrhythmias. Occasionally patients will be treated with amiodarone with the defibrillator or with amiodarone alone (as discussed on page 366). Simple ventricular arrhythmia that is asymptomatic with normal heart function usually requires no medical treatment.

Supraventricular Tachycardia

Drug Options
Beta-blocker
Calcium channel blocker (diltiazem, verapamil)

Supraventricular tachycardia is a fast heart rhythm that originates in the upper chambers of the heart (as discussed on page 134). Both calcium channel blockers and beta-blockers are used to treat this arrhythmia.

Congestive Heart Failure (CHF)

Drug Options
ACE inhibitor
Diuretic
Digoxin
Beta-blocker
Carvedilol

In treating congestive heart failure, the goal is to reduce the symptoms and improve the chance of survival. Treatment includes an ACE inhibitor and then a diuretic, which is added to help reduce fluids in the lungs and around the heart. If you have severely reduced function, digoxin is added to stimulate heart function. A beta-blocker or carvedilol is also used. Carvedilol (brand name Coreg) is both a beta- and an alpha-blocker and increases exercise endurance in those with congestive heart failure more than a beta-blocker alone.

Years ago, even though beta-blockers were available, they were not used in people who had congestive heart failure or reduced heart function. Because these medications relax the heart muscle, it was thought that they could actually worsen the heart failure. More recent research, however, shows that beta-blockers are beneficial because they help to reduce levels of circulating adrenaline, which tends to be high in those with congestive heart failure, and which may precipitate arrhythmias and cause destruction of heart muscle cells.

Digoxin

Digoxin is the *only* medication available that stimulates heart function. It is used in moderate to severe heart failure and for slowing the heart rate in atrial fibrillation. Side effects of digoxin include bradycardia and gastrointestinal upset. High doses may even predispose a patient to developing a life-threatening arrhythmia. The medication levels have to be monitored by your doctor seven to ten days after starting and then periodically or whenever a dosage is changed.

Other Medications

Antidepressants

WHAT ARE THEY PRESCRIBED FOR?

Antidepressants are used in the medical treatment of depression, especially after a trauma. Sometimes, your body and brain chemistry can't "right" itself, and as a result you may feel low or outright depressed. Some symptoms of depression are loss of appetite and sexual desire, a bleak, negative, or hopeless attitude about the future, insomnia, and exhaustion. The longer a depression goes untreated, the more entrenched it can become, so if you develop these symptoms and they don't go away after a couple of weeks, speak to your doctor about whether an antidepressant might be advisable for you. Your emotions do affect your health, and depression can impede your full and healthy recovery. Depression occurs frequently in patients with coronary artery disease and is associated with increased risk of dying.

Antidepressants improve mood by changing the metabolism of certain brain chemicals. Not all antidepressants are alike, so you'll want to work with your doctor in getting the one most appropriate for your condition. Whichever one you are prescribed, make sure you report any side effects to your doctor. When prescribing antidepressants to my patients, I explain to them that it is a balancing act. These medications have not been widely studied for their side effects on men and women with heart disease, other than the fact that they lift the depression. Yet depression has some serious consequences for people with heart disease; therefore the risks and benefits of these medications must be evaluated for each woman. The most commonly prescribed antidepressants are selective serotonin reuptake inhibitors (SSRIs). Another class of antidepressants is tricyclic antidepressants (TCAs).

SSRIs are the preferred treatment for depression if you have heart disease. One study comparing the SSRI paroxetine (brand name Paxil), to nortriptyline (brand name Aventyl), a tricyclic antidepressant, showed that both were effective in treating depression but the TCA caused higher heart rates.[6, 7, 8] Paxil had no effect on the heart rate, and another study showed that the patients treated with Paxil had less platelet clumping than those on the TCAs. SSRIs are preferred over TCAs for the treatment of depression.

POTENTIAL SIDE EFFECTS

SSRIs may cause weight gain, increase in blood pressure, muscle aches, and decreased libido.

TCAs may cause heart attack, stroke, arrhythmia, urinary difficulty, blurred vision, and dry mouth. An overdose can cause a life-threatening arrhythmia.

POSSIBLE INTERACTIONS

SSRIs increase beta-blocker levels, so heart rates and blood pressure should be checked after starting the medication.

COMMONLY PRESCRIBED SSRIs

Generic Name	Brand Name	Frequency of Dosage
Paroxetine	Paxil	once daily
Sertraline	Zoloft	once daily
Fluoxetine	Prozac	once daily
Citalopram	Celexa	once daily

Because every woman's situation with heart disease is unique, her treatment must be matched to her symptoms and needs. The commonly used medications discussed in this chapter are effective in most women, but if those medications are not effective, the doctor will turn to lesser-known drugs for treatment. Oftentimes one medication may cause uncomfortable side effects while you hardly notice any side effects from another. That's why you must talk to your doctor about any medication—its effects and side effects—until you find the best treatment for your problem.

Groundbreaking studies are published every year in cardiology, so the future is very bright for new medical treatments to halt and hopefully even reverse heart disease. In the meantime, follow your doctor's advice. Assess your personal risk factors, use the Women's Healthy Heart Program in Part III to reduce your risk of heart disease, and take the medications you're prescribed to keep your heart healthy.

15

The Heart Attack Survival Guide

"**I** thought I was assertive until the day I almost died from a heart attack."

Amy was talking about the reality of heart attacks to a group of other women. Her openness and her excellent recollection of her symptoms and feelings were enlightening to me and the rest of the group and helped broaden our understanding of why women hesitate to ask for medical care—even when a problem is life-threatening.

This fifty-one-year-old accountant knew all about the atypical symptoms women get. With hypertension, obesity, and a strong family history of heart disease, she was at high risk for a heart attack, and she had been warned by her doctor about it for several years. But on one cold winter day, Amy blocked this knowledge and denied the warning signs she was feeling.

"I remember getting out of bed, feeling weak and out of breath. Because I was having trouble breathing, I thought maybe it was the flu, so I got up to get a thermometer and aspirin. With each step I took, my heart pounded and palpitated. I had a dull pain in my upper abdomen and was dizzy and nauseated. Even though I'd never felt this way before and knew it was not normal, instead of calling my doctor, I crawled back in bed and tried to go back to sleep.

"After about two hours passed, there was pressure in my throat, making it even more difficult to breathe. My husband, who had been out playing tennis with some friends, came into my room and saw me lying on the bed covered with sweat. I told him something was seriously wrong, and I needed to go to the hospital. He started to call 911, but I didn't want to alarm the neighbors, so I made him drive me to the ER. On the way to the hospital, we were stuck in traffic for half an hour, and I began to panic, wondering if I would get to the hospital alive."

Amy did get to the hospital alive. After several tests confirmed that she was having a heart attack, clot-busting drugs were started—a measure that saved her life—and she stabilized in the coronary care unit.

Amy is no different from many women who deny that they are having a heart attack. In fact, a revealing study was published in the journal *Circulation* (July 2000),[1] in which 962 people were asked about the proper course of action when a heart attack was suspected. Eighty-nine percent of the people surveyed said that they would use emergency medical services to go to a hospital, but only 23 percent of the real-life cases actually arrived by ambulance at the emergency room. Like Amy, 60 percent of the real-life cases were driven to the hospital by someone else, and 16 percent even drove themselves. Those who took so long to get to the hospital said they thought that by taking aspirin or other medications they could treat the problem themselves. Although aspirin may help, you cannot treat heart attack by yourself!

Do not be like Amy and have your husband (or friend) drive you to the hospital. And do not drive yourself to the hospital because you do not want to bother family or friends! Especially don't try to treat heart attack warning symptoms with aspirin or antacids. When you feel the first warning sign, call 911 immediately for an ambulance, and get professional help.

Heart Attack: How to Respond

As a cardiologist, I've noticed that a heart attack happens when you least expect it. You may be raking leaves, preparing for a dinner party, or getting ready for work on a Monday morning. Perhaps the sudden and life-threatening nature of a heart attack is why people handle this potentially fatal illness so irrationally most of the time. But when years of plaque buildup reaches the stage of an actual heart attack, you must keep your head, be rational, and seek immediate help. At the moment of the first sign of a heart attack, your clock begins ticking, and you start the toughest race of all: the race to save your own life.

Quick Action Saves Lives

If you learn nothing else from this chapter—from this book—you must know that if you or someone close to you has any of the heart attack warning signs and symptoms, stop what you are doing and call 911 immediately for emergency assistance. Tell them outright, *"I'm having a heart attack."* Those very words will summon immediate treatment, usually from the cardiac van and special technicians of the local emergency crew who can save your life.

The optimal time to get to the hospital is *within an hour* of the start of the symptoms. You have *up to six hours* to get the full benefit of clot-busting medications, with their dissolving power, or of angioplasty, with its ability to open up arteries, and still have viable heart muscle. It is critical to receive emergency medical care with as little delay as possible from the onset of symptoms. Ignoring the symptoms or hoping they will dissipate on their own will only reduce your chances for survival. And as I emphasized in Chapter 2, even if your symptoms are not from a heart attack, it is better to risk being wrong than risk being dead!

Study after study confirms that early recognition and treatment saves the heart muscle and improves patient survival.

Emergency Treatment Starts in the Ambulance

Once you are in the ambulance or cardiac van, the emergency medical service (EMS) technicians will hook you up to a heart monitor to check your heart rhythm and ECG changes consistent with a heart attack. If the heart attack resulted in sudden collapse from a life-threatening arrhythmia such as ventricular tachycardia or ventricular fibrillation, these technicians can use the defibrillator to administer an electrical shock to alleviate it.

To make sure you are breathing properly, technicians will give you supplemental oxygen, which is delivered through nasal prongs. Or if you are very short of breath, they may administer the oxygen through a clear plastic mask strapped over your face. If necessary, a tube will be placed into your throat and airway to allow technicians to intervene and help you breathe.

The EMS technicians may put nitroglycerin under your tongue to alleviate cardiac symptoms. The pill may burn a little, but that means it's working. They will place an intravenous line in your arm in case they need to give you medications that way. While doing these procedures, the technicians will keep a constant watch on your blood pressure. If it falls or becomes elevated, they'll treat you immediately. They'll also hook you up to a heart monitor, which allows them to read your heart's electrical activity. In some cities, EMS technicians have the ability to communicate from the ambulance or van with a physician at the hospital and transmit an ECG. If appropriate, they can give you clot-busting medication right in the ambulance—a move that saves thousands of lives every year.

Priority Care at the Emergency Room

When you come into the emergency room with the EMS technicians, you are prioritized as a top emergency and placed on a cardiac monitor. Some hospitals have special chest pain centers, where the focus is on the acute management of heart attacks and unstable angina.

CARDIAC ENZYMES MAY INDICATE
HEART MUSCLE DAMAGE

The emergency room staff will continue you on oxygen, and an ECG will be done (or another one will be done if you had one in the ambulance). Your blood pressure and heart rate will still be carefully monitored. Blood tests will be done to confirm specific markers for heart muscle damage. The cardiac enzymes CPK, LDH, and SGOT are all markers of muscle damage. While the CPK enzymes tend to have peak elevation eight to ten hours into the heart attack, the LDH and SGOT do not elevate until the next day. This is why it's so important for you to get to the hospital. When women stay home with heart attack symptoms, then go to the ER or get admitted as patients at the hospital several days later, these enzymes may have normalized in the meantime, which needlessly complicates their treatment and recovery.

Recently, tests have been developed to measure the level of *troponins*, the cardiac muscle proteins that control interactions among the heart muscle fibers responsible for the contraction or squeezing of the heart. So the ER staff will give you a troponin test, a marker for plaque rupture. This test result may be elevated even before a heart attack occurs, as in the case of unstable angina.

Based on the results of tests, a decision will be made either to give you a clot-busting medication or to perform an emergency angioplasty. Studies show that clot-busting medications have been vastly underutilized in women, for several reasons.[2] Some women are too frightened to get to the hospital, or they delay getting there soon enough to get the medications because they don't recognize the symptoms. For women seventy-five years old or older, clot-busting medications increase the possibility of complications, such as bleeding and hemorrhagic stroke. So some doctors withhold clot-busting therapy. My colleagues and I look at each patient's condition and, rather than make a decision on age alone, weigh all the benefits and risks of clot-busting medication. If a patient has severe hypertension (blood pressure of 180/110 or higher) or a bleeding disorder, however, clot busters are not given as treatment.

ANGIOPLASTY HAS GOOD SHORT- AND
LONG-TERM OUTCOMES

The alternative to clot-busting therapy is angioplasty, as discussed on pages 396–401. The benefit of angioplasty is that it produces fewer bleeding complications than clot-busting therapy. The short-term outcome (thirty-day survival) is also slightly better with angioplasty (but over the long term the outcome is similar). Angioplasty has good benefits for patients whose blood pressure is elevated and for patients who are older women.

To perform an emergency angioplasty, your hospital must be equipped with the proper personnel and have them available on very short notice. I feel that if it takes more than ninety minutes to get the angioplasty from the time you are in the ER, or if the hospital does not perform more than two hundred procedures a year, then clot-busting medication is the better choice. In other words, if it takes too long to get the angioplasty, it may no longer be beneficial.

When angioplasty is performed for an acute heart attack, the artery that is the source of the heart attack is opened, and a stent may be inserted.

THE CORONARY CARE UNIT GIVES
TWENTY-FOUR-HOUR TREATMENT

Whether you receive a clot buster or angioplasty, after the procedure you are transported to the coronary care unit (CCU). The widespread use of CCUs in the 1960s was one of the important steps that helped reduce early death due to heart attack. In the CCU, you will be monitored and have continuous twenty-four-hour treatment, and if a life-threatening arrhythmia occurs, defibrillators will be immediately available.

In the CCU, you will have bed rest for the first twelve hours. (Once upon a time a heart attack patient stayed in bed for six weeks.) If you have no symptoms, your activity will gradually be increased.

If you are on clot-busting therapy, intravenous heparin, a blood-thinning medication that boosts your body's natural anticoagulant protein, is given for approximately two days (see page 357). If you have had an emergency angioplasty, you may receive heparin after the procedure, along with intravenous medications that inhibit platelets to keep the artery open and to prevent blood clots from forming. These are typically used after an angioplasty with stent.

Other Serious Causes of Chest Discomfort

Unstable Angina: A Serious Warning Sign

Sometimes patients who have had signs and symptoms of a heart attack are diagnosed with unstable angina at the hospital. The only difference between a heart attack and unstable angina is that with unstable angina there is no heart muscle damage. Early intervention is still important to treat this condition because unstable angina can turn into a full-blown heart attack.

In diagnosing unstable angina, your doctor may find ECG changes that indicate an abnormality, such as reduced blood supply to your heart muscle but no muscle damage. The treatment for unstable angina is similar to that of a heart attack and usually requires medications to reduce pain, blood pressure, and heart rate. Blood thinners are also used to reduce blood-clot formation. After you are discharged from the hospital, your doctor will keep you on medications. You will then need to address your risk factors for heart disease and make changes to prevent further problems and improve your health.

Angiography with angioplasty and possible stenting are useful in unstable angina. In most cases, the hospitalization is shorter (two to three days) than for a heart attack because there is no heart muscle damage.

Heart Attack Without Abnormal Electrocardiograms

A heart attack that does not have an abnormal ECG is as serious as a heart attack with one and usually has the same signs and symptoms. The physician clinches the diagnosis through blood tests that measure the cardiac enzymes that indicate muscle damage. In fact, the initial testing is the same as in a heart attack with ECG changes.

Your doctor will treat a heart attack lacking an abnormal ECG with treatment similar to that given for unstable angina, including a combination of cardiac medications (see Chapter 14). Like patients with unstable angina, you may benefit from immediate coronary angiography and angioplasty for the blocked artery.

After the Heart Attack

Commonly Used Medications

Several proven medical therapies should be used after a heart attack, but they are typically underutilized, particularly for treating women. For example, studies show that aspirin and beta-blockers reduce mortality and prevent a recurrent heart attack.[3] These drugs also reduce the need for surgery. Statin drugs lower cholesterol and have been shown to lower LDL ("bad") cholesterol effectively.

The following statistics are startling. In one study[4] less than 10 percent of the women on cholesterol-lowering medication had their cholesterol appropriately lowered, and in another study[5] only 3 percent of women were referred to cardiac rehabilitation. This situation is unacceptable and shocking. I consider it irresponsible for a doctor or hospital to release a patient without stressing the need for follow-up, life-preserving care. If you have not been prescribed treatment after a heart attack, ask your doctor about medications and intervention, including cardiac rehabilitation, to help make this heart attack the last one you will ever have.

PROVEN DRUG THERAPIES THAT CAN PROLONG YOUR LIFE

- Aspirin
- Beta-blockers
- ACE inhibitors
- Statin drugs

For a full discussion of how these drugs help you, please refer to Chapter 14.

From CCU to Step-Down Unit

If you have what we call an uncomplicated heart attack, where you have heart muscle damage but do not have heart failure or arrhythmias, you will remain in the CCU about forty-eight hours. After the CCU, you will be transferred to the step-down unit, which is another cardiac unit with well-trained staff. While you will still be on cardiac monitors, you will be in a regular hospital room. The estimated hospital stay is five to seven days for an uncomplicated heart attack.

During your stay in the regular hospital room, it's important to report any recurrence of chest discomfort, shortness of breath, weakness, unusual pain or pressure, or other new problems immediately. If you continue to have symptoms, your doctor may refer you for an angiogram to evaluate for blocked arteries. This blockage could be the one involved in your heart attack or an obstruction in other vessels. Based on the results, you may be referred for an angioplasty with stent, bypass surgery, or other medical therapy.

Cardiac Rehabilitation: A Lifelong Process

So one of the worst things that could happen to you has happened— and you're alive and getting good care. Once you've had a heart attack, I want you to know that it's easier from here on out. The worst is over. You can move forward and have a healthy recovery by taking control of your risk factors for heart disease and making healthy lifestyle choices. You want to make sure this never happens again.

Discharge and Continued Recovery

Before discharging you, your doctor may do further testing, such as an echocardiogram or stress test, to help determine your future risk for heart problems and the best exercise prescription for you. This can be done safely under proper supervision and can help you plan the most effective cardiac rehabilitation program when you go home. This information will help you know what the safest exercise is for you.

If you enroll in cardiac rehabilitation, the team will collaborate on your exercise program. Your doctor or team will calculate your target heart rate, or the heart rate you should be at during your exercise session; it is usually 65 to 85 percent of your maximal heart rate on the stress test (see pages 231–232). If you are enrolled in cardiac rehabilitation, you will wear a heart monitor, and a nurse will monitor your heart rate while you exercise just to make sure you are in a safe heart rate zone. Your doctor will prescribe exercises based on this heart rate.

Many hospitals provide discharge classes for patients, where they can discuss issues of self-care, rehabilitation, and caregiving (for family members). In addition, during your hospital stay you may be visited by a physical therapist who will work with you and your doctor on scheduling your postdischarge activities. During the days after your heart attack, you will be encouraged to start walking for five to seven minutes, two to three times per day. At discharge, you will be told what your level of activity and exercise should be and how soon you can begin driving, resume sexual activity, and return to work outside your home. You should also be referred to cardiac rehabilitation, and if you are not, you should ask to be referred.

How Soon Is Sex Safe?

Research shows that many people can return to sexual activity two weeks after an uncomplicated heart attack. Sexual activity is safe after successful bypass surgery or angioplasty with stent; you just have to get over the aches and pains of the procedure, and you need to feel comfortable. By that time, you will have had your first doctor's visit after your hospital discharge—a good time to discuss sexual activity with your doctor, if he or she has not brought it up with you. The goal of recovery after a heart attack or heart surgery is to help you recover a normal life, and sexual activity is very much part of that.

Many women do not return to sexual activity and do not talk to their doctor about it because they are embarrassed. You'll find that once you broach the subject of sex, your doctor can openly help you deal with any fears and will encourage you to return to sexual activity. Other women share with me that they are afraid of having cardiac symptoms or even having another heart attack during sex. Some women become worried when they experience the increased heart rate and sweating associated with sexual activity. They worry that these are signs of cardiac problems.

If you have had one of the following, talk with your doctor before engaging in sexual activity:

- A recent heart attack
- Treatment for heart failure
- Uncontrolled hypertension
- Severe valvular heart disease
- Life-threatening arrhythmia

To determine whether you can safely begin having sex again, your doctor will do a stress test to assess your cardiac status. If you are experiencing any sexual dysfunction or loss of desire, ask your doctor if medications could be the cause. Sometimes medications, such as beta-blockers or blood pressure medications, can contribute to sexual dysfunction in women by causing depression.

To decide when it's time *for you* to have sex again:

- Openly discuss returning to sexual activity with your doctor.
- Stay with your cardiac rehabilitation. Studies show it can help to reduce anxiety and symptoms during sexual activity.
- Practice your mind/body exercises to help you decrease anxiety, depression, and anger.

Be sure you understand the types of medications your doctor prescribes and any special diet you are advised to follow. Your doctor or the discharge nurse may review your risk factors before you leave and give you specific instructions about steps you can take to prevent heart attack from happening to you again.

See Your Doctor

In most cases, you will see your doctor in ten days to two weeks after your hospital discharge, then at one month and three months, unless there is some clinical indication—such as recurrent symptoms, heart failure, or an arrhythmia—for more frequent visits.

During your doctor's visits, your blood pressure and pulse will be closely monitored. Your doctor will listen to your heart and lungs to make sure the medications you are taking are correct and necessary. An ECG may be taken to check your heart rhythm.

Each time you visit, remember to bring your list of medications and supplements or the medication bottles themselves with you. This will help your doctor figure out what medication is best for you. If the doctor adds a medication during your visit, be sure you understand why you need it and receive the appropriate prescription and instructions on how and when to take it. Make sure you ask whether it will interact with anything else you're taking and whether you have to watch for any side effects.

Know Your Limits Ahead of Time

One of the biggest concerns my patients have told me they have is whether they will be able to return to their routine household duties. Before you leave for home, it is important to know if you will be able to make the bed, cook meals for your family, or even sweep the floor. Talk to your doctor about your responsibilities as a caregiver, and know up front if there are limits. Remember, men who have heart disease often have a supportive spouse or significant other to help them navigate their life after a heart attack. On whom can you depend for help during your recovery? Draw on your support network, or reach out to develop one. It's important for you now to focus on how you will get well before you can give care to others.

Some of my patients find that having a supportive friend stay with them awhile is beneficial to their recuperation. Alternatively, you could line up visits from a visiting nurse service. These trained nurses make house calls several times a week, checking your pulse and blood pressure. They may also review your medications and communicate with your doctor about your progress at home.

Referral to Cardiac Rehabilitation

After a heart attack, bypass surgery, angioplasty with stent, or medical treatment for angina, all women should go to cardiac rehabilitation. Your doctor should give you a referral. Cardiac rehabilitation is an organized program of exercise, smoking cessation, nutrition counseling, stress management, education, and social support that is personalized for your cardiac condition and is monitored by health care professionals. It will help you heal, manage your heart disease, and improve your overall health so that you reduce your likelihood of having another heart attack.

Although many insurance companies pay for cardiac rehabilitation, in most cases women are not referred to it. In fact, studies confirm that physicians are more likely to refer men than women to cardiac rehabilitation.[5] Other studies show that when women do come to cardiac rehabilitation, they are less physically fit and more anxious about participating than men.[6] Women are also more likely to drop out because of family commitments, lack of transportation, or fear or dislike of the type of exercise offered in the program. The lack of referral of and participation by women in cardiac rehabilitation is one of the many things that motivated me to create the Women's Heart Program at Lenox Hill Hospital.

Whereas most cardiac exercise programs offer traditional machines such as treadmills, stationary and recumbent bicycles, and rowing machines, cardiac rehabilitation programs give women more options. For example, in the Women's Heart Program at Lenox Hill Hospital, one of the exercise choices is a low-impact aerobics class, where the women wear heart monitors while they exercise.

Cecile, age fifty, became my patient around the tenth anniversary of her first heart attack, after her daughter suggested that she see me for a consultation. Cecile was diabetic, had not worked in five years, and could not recall a time when she was able to walk down the street without being short of breath. She felt hopeless and cheated out of a "normal life." She was very angry.

For our first meeting, Cecile marched into my office and dumped her shopping bag of medications on the top of my desk. Then she said sat down, crossed her arms in front of her, and asked, "So, what are you going to do now?" She never made eye contact.

After talking with Cecile, I empathized with her. She had reason to be angry—missing out on the best years of life because of health limitations. But I also knew the anger had to stop because it was negatively impacting her health. She had steadily gained fifty pounds over the last ten years and had increased in hostility toward herself and others, so much so that her children didn't want to spend the holidays with her because she was always so antagonistic.

To try to convince Cecile that she could make changes in her life, I asked her if she liked to dance. Her eyes lit up for a brief moment, then fell again when she said, "I can't. I'm too sick."

I invited her to the Woman's Heart Program and suggested that she watch one of the low-impact aerobics classes. After the class was over, she spoke to several of the women involved, then signed up to start the following week.

Since then, Cecile has lost about eight pounds, and her diabetes is now under control. What impressed me most was hearing her tell another participant that she liked our rehab program because it was such a "warm, friendly place." Cecile needed to feel good—to have friends—and the cardiac rehab program provided her with just that.

You'll want to ask the following questions about any potential rehab program you're considering:

- Is it supervised by a physician?
- Is a support team of health care professionals, with nurses, an exercise physiologist, a nutritionist, and a behavioral psychologist, on the premises or on call?
- Is there a support group or other social support for the women who participate?

- Does it provide educational lectures that help women become more informed health care consumers?

BENEFITS OF CARDIAC REHABILITATION FOR WOMEN

- Increases endurance
- Reduces anxiety
- Improves awareness of heart disease risk factors and how to change them
- Increases social support
- Improves self-esteem

Now That You're Home, Go Slow

After you get home, you will probably be able to do most light household chores, such as making the bed or dusting. Still, I want you to take care of yourself and get your doctor's approval before you try to do heavier chores or more vigorous activity. You may feel fatigued and anxious. I want you to take it easy and listen to your body. When you are tired, rest. Take frequent breaks throughout your day until your strength increases. Get family and friends to help you with meals and household duties until you feel strong.

If you have symptoms again, don't ignore them, especially if they are similar in quality and intensity to the first ones. Get to a hospital immediately. If you are unsure about a symptom, call your doctor. Remember that early diagnosis and treatment are the keys to saving your life during a heart attack. Don't waste time by trying to figure out what the symptom is on your own. Oftentimes it is not another heart attack, but it is better to be safe (and alive!) than sorry.

WHEN IS IT SAFE TO GO BACK TO WORK?

Physically, you may be able to return to work a couple of weeks after discharge. But you may have some concerns about stress at work and how to deal with it. After a heart attack is a good opportunity to assess the stressors in your life. Before you attribute your heart attack to your job, try to be specific. See which of the following job stressors affect you, and try to modify them as you ease back into working:

- Driving or commuting
- The dual demands of running a home and working
- The hours on the job
- The need for a sabbatical or extended vacation
- Having to take work home
- No time to exercise because of work hours

While you may love your job, aspects of it may need changing; talk to your employer about your personal needs. Many of the women I see are self-supporting, or their income is a significant contribution to their household, so they cannot just quit their job. Find things that you can change to improve your quality of life at work and then every day when you get home. I encourage my patients to take a short-term sabbatical or extended vacation, if that's possible. I also recommend that they work shorter hours or avoid taking work home. With beepers, cell phones, and Internet access at home, this may prove difficult, but you need to take steps to reduce stress on your mind and body. Please refer to Chapter 12 and learn the best way for you to de-stress.

Don't be afraid of getting back to work. If your doctor gives you a clean bill of health, the chances are great that you will continue to do well if you take the necessary medications and keep your risk factors low. For instance, one of my patients, Lucy, age forty-nine, is an elementary schoolteacher who was eligible for a six-month sabbatical. After her heart attack and surgery, she took the time off and is now back at work full time. She feels great and enjoys the diversion of caring for her students. Another woman, Pilar, age fifty-one, was allowed to leave her job as a secretary an hour earlier so she could attend the Women's Heart Program at Lenox Hill Hospital. She too is back to work now full time. She joined a gym across the street from her office and goes four days a week after she finishes her workday.

Other ways to "share the load" when you go back to work include:

- Get your family to help out with some of the household chores.
- Stop saying yes to every request for commitment.
- Find a carpool or take public transportation.

If you cannot identify your stressors or modify your lifestyle, consult with a behavioral psychologist. You need to cope with the stress in your life in order to get and stay well.

Depression Is a Common Feeling

Many women become depressed after a heart attack. Some have told me they feel as if a black cloud of "darkness and doom" hovers around them. These are actually normal feelings after hospitalization and treatment for coronary artery disease, but do not ignore or dismiss them. If these feelings do not fade in two weeks, call your doctor. Beta-blockers and medications for lowering blood pressure can contribute to depression, so make sure you ask your doctor if this could be the cause of your low mood.

In some cases, social support, as I discussed in Chapter 5, is not enough to lift you from anxious moments or depression, and you need professional counseling. My patient Miranda is a case in point.

Three months after a successful bypass operation, forty-eight-year-old Miranda couldn't get herself going again. She had been a successful saleswoman at a high-end retail store until her hospitalization. Since then Miranda had become consumed with the fear of dying and rarely left the house except for her follow-up visits with me. Her family tried to reassure her, but her daughter and son-in-law did not visit her for two months. At one visit, she appeared disheveled, as if she had just gotten out of bed. In fact, she told me she was spending a great deal of time in bed and hadn't eaten a meal with her husband in weeks.

Clearly, Miranda was depressed. I wanted to prescribe an antidepressant, but she refused to take it. She did agree to see a psychotherapist, after I explained that depression is an important medical condition that needs to be treated—just as her heart condition needed to be treated. She eventually came around with a combination of medication and cognitive therapy and has since returned to work. She has even scheduled a family vacation.

Your feelings, just like your heart, sometimes need medical attention. Keep your recovery on track by letting your doctor know how you are emotionally. Sometimes you just need a boost from medication to get back to feeling yourself again. Some medications for depression can be used at low dosages yet still be effective. The most common antidepressant prescriptions that I write for my patients are discussed on pages 369–371.

CONSIDER A GROUP ACTIVITY

As a woman and a doctor, I know women are different from men—in many good ways. It's in our nature to talk about our feelings, instead of keeping them bottled up inside as men often do. That's why I believe group activities, such as an exercise class, are good for women who have experienced the trauma of heart disease. You get to meet others who have been through what you've been through; you can compare notes, give each other tips on coping with recovery, and just have fun. Many such groups also discuss the latest treatments. It's fortifying to give and get assurance that "someone else knows what I am going through," as you share your struggles in living with heart disease. Please refer back to Chapter 5 for other suggestions.

But remember that these group activities and cardiac support groups are not intended to replace the authority of your health care professional. Before taking a new remedy that someone recommends at a group meeting, be sure always to check with your physician.

To find a group near you, check with your local hospital, your cardiac or physical rehabilitation program, or your physician.

INCREASE YOUR SOCIAL ACTIVITIES

It's also important for you to find a sense of purpose and meaning for your life. You've been through a lot, and getting a healthy perspective on it will help you heal. For many women, this meaning comes from their religious or spiritual practice. Others may be passionate about their work, hobbies, family, or volunteer activities.

Many of my patients volunteer with the American Heart Association and the Mended Hearts, a national organization of people who have had heart surgery and find that this keeps them accountable for taking care of their health while at the same time giving to others.

For example, my patient Lillian believes that it's important to show other women there is life after a heart attack. Sixty-eight years old, Lillian has lived alone since her husband died from a heart attack six years ago. On the day she began having symptoms of a heart attack, she was also flooded with memories of pleading with her husband to go to the hospital. Her husband had refused to call 911 and later died in the ambulance. Lillian could barely breathe and was sweating profusely, so she knew her symptoms were serious and called 911. After a few precarious hours in the ER and an emergency angioplasty, Lillian was released from the hospital with very little heart damage.

When Lillian finished her rehabilitation at the Women's Heart Program at Lenox Hill Hospital, I asked her if she wanted to volunteer at the American Heart Association in Manhattan. That was three years ago. This year Lillian organized a group of women from our program to participate in the American Heart Association's Heart Walk in New York City. Pouring herself into a worthwhile goal became an important part of her life.

Call the American Heart Association for Support and Information

The American Heart Association is another source of excellent support; call your local office or visit their website (www.american heart.org). Seek information about support groups and educational programs, then make a point to attend any seminars or group meetings. You will find other women just like you, with similar fears and anxieties, and you can learn coping skills to move beyond the fear and into positive and active living once again. Think of socialization not only as good for the mind and spirit but as your new weapon against further heart disease.

★   ★   ★

Using the information in this book, talk about heart disease with your spouse or significant other, family members, friends, and co-workers. Tell them what you know about your condition and what you must do to stay well. This will enable them to become more understanding and sensitized to your symptoms and to the diet, exercise, and other changes you need to make. It's vital too for those close to you to know what to do in case of emergency. An unexpected benefit of educating others about your heart attack is that they too will gain greater awareness of the reality of heart disease.

16

Heart Surgery
and Procedures

There are times when I must tell a patient that the heart disease prevention efforts that she's following are "on hold" until she is more stable. Francesca was one such patient.

After four hours of severe chest discomfort and breathlessness, this forty-seven-year-old CPA called 911 and was rushed to the emergency room by ambulance. Her electrocardiogram revealed a heart attack in progress, so I explained to her that we could limit the amount of heart muscle damage by performing an angioplasty to open the artery and place a stent.

Francesca's response: "No, thank you. I'll wait on the procedure for now. Maybe I'll lose some weight and stop smoking cigarettes to see if this helps."

I explained that she was past any *maybes* and that the procedure was not optional. Francesca finally agreed. A colleague successfully performed an angioplasty to the left anterior descending artery, which saved Francesca's life. It also prevented her from having serious heart muscle damage to the anterior wall of her heart, which would have increased her chance of developing congestive heart failure and arrhythmia and would have greatly compromised her quality of life. She started a secondary prevention program when she was discharged, including quitting smoking and losing weight to prevent another heart attack.

In this chapter, I'll discuss some of the procedures that are necessary for treating advanced heart disease or a condition that is unresponsive to medication.

Coronary Angiography

Coronary angiography is a test that examines the heart's blood vessels using X rays, producing an image called an *angiogram*. It is performed when your doctor suspects you have unstable angina, when you have had an abnormal ECG, or when you are actually having a heart attack. It tells your doctor the exact location and amount of obstruction in the blood vessel. An angiogram is necessary before bypass surgery or an interventional cardiac procedure like angioplasty and stenting, to open up the blockage.

Many times during an angiogram, an artery is identified as blocked and in need of opening. It may be decided at the time of the procedure to do an angioplasty to open the artery. If the angiogram is performed to identify a blocked artery in the middle of a heart attack so that an angioplasty can be done to open up blood flow, the best place to have this done is in a hospital that can do the procedure within ninety minutes of entering the emergency room and that does it two hundred times each year. Otherwise, it may be best to use a clot-busting medication to stop further heart attack damage, because when it comes to opening up arteries in the middle of a heart attack, time and experience count.

If you have valvular heart disease without any symptoms of blocked arteries and are over fifty, then an angiogram should be done to evaluate your arteries before you undergo valve surgery. The angiogram will enable the doctor to see if coronary artery disease is also present; if it is, bypass surgery can be performed at the same time as the valve is replaced or repaired.

Angiography can save lives, but women sometimes do not do as well with this procedure as men. Elsie, a sixty-eight-year-old political activist, had complained of throat tightness for about a year, so her internist performed an exercise electrocardiogram in his office. She felt the worrisome throat tightness while she was on the treadmill, and it kept her from continuing with the test, but the doctor discounted it as a significant symptom of heart disease. He told her that the results of the test were equivocal; the ECG did not meet the full criteria for a positive test or a negative one.

Elsie asked him point-blank, "Do I have heart disease?" But the internist told her not to worry, that she did need medication for her high blood pressure and should start a diet and exercise program for her cholesterol. In spite of the uninformative stress test, Elsie clearly had symptoms of heart disease.

Eight months later her internist referred her to the Women's Heart Program. I repeated the stress test as part of Elsie's initial evaluation. As she began the test, I saw that she was not going to start the program just yet. After only two minutes on the treadmill, she became short of breath and felt the throat tightness. The ECG was markedly positive. We stopped the test immediately, and the symptoms resolved.

A significant coronary artery blockage was a strong possibility. I called her doctor, and we admitted Elsie to the hospital for coronary angiography. The angiography found a 90 percent obstruction of the right coronary artery and a 75 percent obstruction of the diagonal branch of the left circumflex artery.

The interventional cardiologist placed stents in Elsie's right coronary and left circumflex arteries. After this procedure, both arteries had a less than 10 percent obstruction. Elsie stayed overnight in the coronary care unit, then was discharged to go home. Within one month of the procedure, she was able to go back to her meetings and join the Women's Heart Program.

Unlike the ECG or stress echocardiogram, which are done in a doctor's office, coronary angiography is performed in a hospital. Years ago you had to be admitted overnight before the test and remain as an inpatient afterward, but today you can arrive at the hospital the day of the test. Depending on the results, you may be discharged later the same day.

THE PROCEDURE:

A catheter (or tube) is inserted into the femoral artery (in your groin) and is advanced through your system to your heart. A dye that is visible by X ray is then injected into the coronary arteries. The arteries are visualized, and any blockages can be seen. The degree of narrowing of the arteries is reported as a percentage. Dye may also be injected into the pumping chamber (the left ventricle), in order to evaluate the heart's pumping function. After the test, the catheter is removed, and the small puncture where the catheter was introduced is closed, using pressure.

WHAT YOU MAY FEEL:

You will feel a pressing sensation against your groin when the catheter is inserted. You may feel some palpitations, and if the symptoms that led to the procedure are caused by blocked arteries, you may experience these symptoms during the test. But you will be fully monitored and under the close supervision of doctors and nurses who can treat any problems should they arise.

PRECAUTIONS:

Before the test, you will undergo a blood test and an ECG. Your doctor will put you on an aspirin regimen. During the procedure you will be given the blood thinner heparin. It is important to tell your doctor about any other blood thinners you may take, because after the procedure, there is a risk of bleeding from the puncture site.

Angiography is an invasive procedure and so carries some risks. It may trigger anginal symptoms, heart attack, stroke, bleeding, or arrhythmia. The dye may cause an allergic reaction or reduced kidney function, particularly in a diabetic patient. These risks are minimized in hospitals where interventional cardiologists perform angiography frequently. Make sure you talk to your doctor about the risks and benefits of the procedure in your situation. For instance, if you have unstable angina and are at a risk for heart attack, then the benefit of identifying the obstruction and opening the artery to prevent a heart attack may outweigh the risks.

For some reason, many women see heart disease as something they should hide, and so they are sometimes resistant to treatment.

Recently my colleague, an internist, and I had trouble convincing his patient to go for an angiogram while she was having unstable angina. Sophie, a sixty-four-year-old businesswoman, had been admitted to the hospital for pneumonia. On admission she had an abnormal ECG reading, and she was having numbness in her left arm that would come and go with little or no exertion. Asked to consult on the case, I explained to Sophie that it was safer to go to the cardiac floor for observation. She responded, "I can't do that! My clients will think I am dying."

She was not willing even to listen to me explain the angiogram, so I called my colleague. He told Sophie that if she were a sixty-four-year-old man, she'd be dying to have the procedure, because most of her friends would already have had it. And he was right! Finally, Sophie agreed to the room transfer and had an angiogram—which found a 90 percent blockage in an artery. It was subsequently opened, preventing a serious heart attack.

Coronary Angioplasty

Once a positive stress test has diagnosed a blockage in a coronary artery, and angiography has located it, the blocked artery must be opened. The fastest technique is a coronary angioplasty, or *percutaneous transluminal coronary angioplasty (PTCA)*. (This procedure is also known as *balloon angioplasty*.) Today more patients are treated with angioplasty than with coronary artery bypass surgery. Sometimes when a coronary artery is blocked, medication can relieve the symptoms. The Women's Healthy Heart Program, outlined in Part III, along with cardiac rehabilitation, should follow this drug therapy. The decision about which option to use is made on an individual basis, and it's important for you to know your options so you can be part of the decision-making process.

Emergency angioplasty in an acute heart attack is beneficial, but if the left main artery is blocked, then surgery is warranted. If multiple vessels are blocked, a decision will be made as to which procedure would give you a better benefit. If you are diabetic and have multiple blocked vessels or reduced heart function, surgery may give you greater benefit in the long run, especially if the blockages cannot be adequately opened with a catheter.

THE PROCEDURE:

You are awake and but sedated. A catheter is inserted into a numbed area on your groin. With the assistance of X-ray images on a screen, the interventional cardiologist guides the catheter through the arteries until it arrives at the blocked coronary artery in your heart. A second, thinner catheter is then inserted through the first one. This catheter has a miniature, deflated balloon on its tip that is maneuvered through the blocked artery. A wire is placed in the blocked artery, and at the point of blockage the balloon catheter is inflated to widen and expand the artery opening. Once the blood flow is improved, the balloon is deflated and removed (see Figure 16.1).

A *stent* is often used in this procedure. It is a tiny tube made out of wire mesh. The stent is inserted into the artery with the specially designed catheter, where it keeps the narrowed artery open to allow better blood flow. Stents also reduce the chance that the artery will become narrowed again (restenosis). Today 70 to 90 percent of angioplasty procedures use a stent.

After the procedure is completed, you are placed on aspirin indefinitely. Your doctor may also give you another blood thinner such as clopidogrel (brand name Plavix) for a month, in addition to the aspirin.

PRECAUTIONS:

Angioplasty is a relatively safe procedure. About 90 percent of patients have good results from angioplasty, reducing blockage of the artery to 30 percent or less. Complications are not common, but heart attack or the need to proceed with emergency coronary bypass surgery can happen. In some cases, the artery may close again within twenty-four hours. As many as 30 percent of cases close up within six months. Bleeding from the site of insertion of the catheter and other problems in the arteries of the extremities can happen in a few percent of cases.

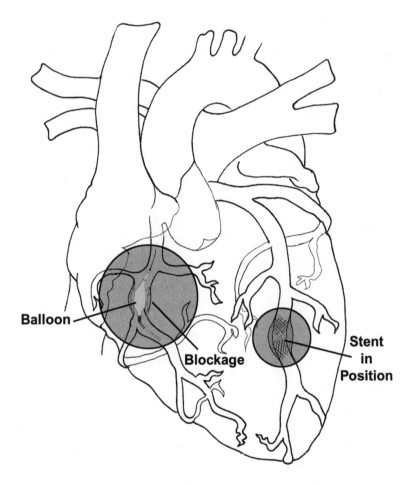

Figure 16.1
How Coronary Angioplasty Expands the Blocked Artery

Coronary Angioplasty Is Beneficial But Not Perfect

Studies show that after a positive stress test, women are less often referred for further invasive testing than are men.[1] Also, in the past women have had less successful outcomes than men with angioplasty (and surgery), perhaps because the women were older or were more likely to have diabetes, which complicates treatments, or congestive heart failure.[2] But occasionally size does matter; the catheters were once all one size, yet women have smaller arteries than men. When it comes to catheters, one size doesn't fit all. Recent studies show improved outcomes for women[3] as the technique has improved and catheters are more appropriate in size.

Still, statistics show that these procedures are less successful for women than for men and that women have more repeat procedures.[4] We don't know why; hopefully future research will explain it so that we can remedy this inequity.

A recent study from Germany published in the *Journal of the American Medical Association* revealed that in the first thirty days after a stent procedure, women had a slightly higher rate of complications than men.[4] But when men and women were compared after one year, there was no difference in outcome. (Some of the risk may be due to the higher rate of diabetes in the women subjects.)

Recurrence of Symptoms after Angioplasty

Sometime in the first few months after an angioplasty, your symptoms may recur—quite a disappointment. To see if the blockage has reoccurred, the arteries have to be reimaged with angiography. Bess, a very active seventy-two-year-old woman who was still running a catering business she had founded, had a recurrence of her shortness of breath while going up the subway stairs. She called me to ask if it was something to be concerned about. She said the symptom was not as intense as the first time, but it was very similar, and she was worried.

I told Bess to come to my office immediately. When her ECG did not indicate an abnormality, I scheduled her for a thallium stress test, which showed an abnormality in the area of heart where the artery had been stented. The diagnosis was restenosis; the stent was blocked, by a blood clot or by inflammation. An angiogram showed a narrowing in the area of the stent. In a repeat angioplasty, the artery was reopened.

Approximately 30 percent of patients experience restenosis in the first six months after a stenting, requiring a repeat coronary angiography. But in the first thirty days after angioplasty, stenting may have fewer complications. Over the long term, coronary artery bypass surgery has the edge in terms of better relief of symptoms. Yet surgery has been shown to have an increased rate of strokes in women.

If you have recurrent symptoms after an angioplasty, a repeat angiogram will be done to determine if the stent has become blocked. Sometimes the artery can be reopened, but if it cannot, depending on the artery involved and your symptoms, your other options may include surgery or medication or both. Another option is an angioplasty with stents that are coated with medication.

Studies on how we can reduce the risk of clogged stents are ongoing. One possibility is the use of localized radiation, delivered to the stent by a catheter. The theory is that the localized radiation can inhibit some of the inflammation that occurs after the stent procedure and thereby reduce restenosis.[5] There are new stents that are coated with medications that may reduce risk of restenosis.[6] The long-term success rate of this is still unknown, so make sure you are following the Women's Healthy Heart Program, and pay attention to your body's warning signs. Remember, these procedures only fix the plumbing—they do not get rid of your heart disease!

Making the Surgery Decision

In some cases, you may have a choice between coronary angioplasty and coronary artery bypass surgery. To make the decision, your doctor will assess your medical and heart history. If you have stable angina, both procedures are safe. If angioplasty is not suitable for you or if it was unsuccessful, your doctor may opt to perform off-pump coronary artery bypass surgery or minimally invasive direct coronary artery bypass surgery (see pages 405 and 404).

It's important to have an open discussion with your cardiologist, the interventional cardiologist, and the cardiothoracic surgeon, especially in situations with multiple blocked vessels or an obstructed left main coronary artery, or after multiple angioplasties with stents that have not worked.

Other factors to consider include whether you have the following:

- Blockages in one or more coronary arteries
- History of stroke
- Decreased heart function
- Lung or kidney disease
- Coronary artery bypass surgery in the past and blockages in one or two grafts

If you have any of these conditions your doctor may recommend angioplasty with stents or minimally invasive bypass surgery instead of coronary artery bypass surgery. In some cases, you have to weigh factors that are not procedure-related, such as insurance status, which may limit where and with whom you can have your surgery. With coronary artery bypass surgery, it sometimes takes six to ten weeks before you can go back to work in full force. Some of my patients return to work within a couple of weeks; most are back within a month. Some factors that affect your return to work include your work status before the procedure and your overall health.

After surgery, make sure you have help with your daily household duties, including someone to prepare meals for you upon your arrival home. You may have some soreness and will need to recover and rebuild your stamina. Follow a cardiac rehabilitation program. (We enroll our patients in the Women's Heart Program within a month after the procedure or surgery.) For more advice on managing your recovery, please refer to the sections on recovery in Chapter 15.

Choosing a Surgeon

While you may feel uncomfortable interviewing a surgeon and asking pertinent, even personal questions regarding his or her knowledge and experience, it's important to do this so that you find a professional with whom you can trust your life. If the procedure is elective, you may choose to consult with more than one surgeon. If the procedure is an emergency, an interview may not be an option.

Your cardiologist may recommend a surgeon for you to consider. Once you have been given a referral, in this age of managed care, you must check to see if this surgeon will be accepted by your insurance provider. You should also consider the surgeon's level of expertise in the procedure you are having done.

Coronary Artery Bypass Surgery

If your doctor determines that blockages in your coronary arteries are too extensive or are not suitable for angioplasty with stenting, then coronary artery bypass grafting (CABG), better known as bypass surgery, may be performed. Before the bypass surgery, you will first undergo an angiogram to give your surgeon an accurate "map" of your heart.

Bypass surgery reroutes blood flow around your clogged arteries so that your heart muscle can still get the oxygen and other nourishment it needs. First, your obstructions must be defined, so you undergo angiography. The surgeon reviews the films, then decides how many obstructions need to be bypassed. In order to bypass or go around an obstruction, veins are taken from your legs or arteries from your chest wall (internal mammary artery), wrist (radial artery), or stomach (gastroepiploic artery) and then grafted to the heart area. One end is attached to the aorta and the other end to the coronary artery, just past the obstruction. (See Figure 16.2)

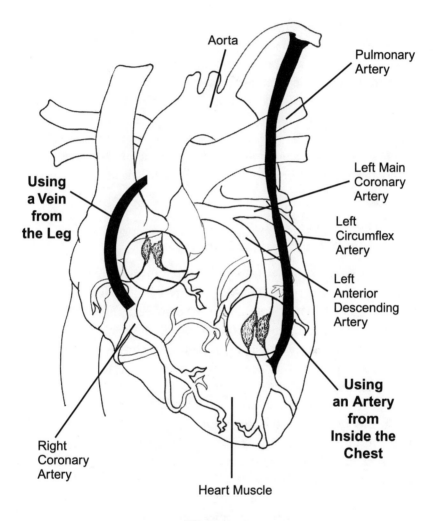

Figure 16.2
Obstructed Arteries with Bypass Grafts in Place

Open-Heart Surgery

In traditional bypass surgery, called open-heart surgery, you are put under general anesthesia, and a heart-lung machine is used to pump blood for your heart and to supply your lungs with oxygen. The surgeon then cuts through your sternum (breastbone) with a large incision and performs the surgery.

Afterward you will be on a breathing tube attached to a respirator. You'll leave the operating room still unconscious and wake up in the recovery room. After a few hours, you'll be taken to the intensive care unit for several hours, then weaned off the respirator, and the breathing tube will be removed. For patients who are severely overweight or who have a lung disease, this weaning process takes longer. Today the average stay after a bypass procedure is five to seven days.

Minimally Invasive Direct
Coronary Artery Bypass Surgery

Many hospitals are now using minimally invasive direct coronary artery bypass surgery (MIDCAB), which is less invasive than open-heart surgery. MIDCAB reroutes, or "bypasses," blood around the blocked arteries and improves the supply of blood and oxygen to the heart. If your obstruction is in the left anterior descending artery, and angioplasty is not an option, you are a candidate for MIDCAB. This less invasive surgery is also better for those who've had previous open-heart surgery and an obstructed graft.

In this procedure, the surgeon makes an incision under the left breast to obtain the artery necessary to bypass the blockages in the coronary arteries. This is usually the artery attached to the chest wall (the internal mammary artery).

Unlike traditional open-heart surgery, MIDCAB does not require a heart-lung machine. Medications are used to slow down the heartbeat, allowing the surgeon to operate on your heart while it is still beating. For someone who has had a stroke or who has lung disease or reduced heart function, MIDCAB is the preferable option.

Off-Pump Coronary Artery Bypass Surgery

If you need one or two bypass grafts but have health conditions that make surgery without the heart-lung machine preferable, your surgeon may choose to use off-pump coronary artery bypass (OPCAB) surgery. This procedure involves grafting multiple coronary arteries through an incision in your sternum (breastbone), the same incision used in CABG.

Valve Surgery

There are many instances where valve surgery is indicated. For example, if a heart valve opening becomes too narrow and tight (stenotic), the blood flow is decreased; this inhibits blood from properly flowing into the ventricle so it can be pumped out to the body. With reduced blood flow to the blood vessels to the brain and heart muscle, you may have symptoms of angina or fainting.

In other cases, a valve may not close properly, so that blood leaks back in the wrong direction (regurgitation). This causes your heart to pump inefficiently. Surgery may be warranted to replace or reconstruct the damaged valve. Your doctor may choose one of several options.

Mitral Valve Repair

This procedure reconstructs the mitral valve, to correct mitral valve regurgitation. It repairs the valve without removing the valve from its attachments in the heart. The benefits of this surgery are a reduced chance of heart failure, and if you do not have atrial fibrillation, you will not need long-term anticoagulation therapy. This surgery is particularly good for young women who are considering having children because, if heart rhythm is regular, it does not require a blood thinner. You will need antibiotics before central procedures to prevent endocarditis.

Percutaneous Balloon Valvuloplasty

Valvuloplasty, to repair mitral valve stenosis, is done by a specially trained interventional cardiologist. First an echocardiogram is done to make sure that the valve is not severely calcified and there is no clot in the left atrium. The cardiologist passes a tiny catheter with a balloon at its tip through the narrowed heart valve. Once it gets to the correct location, the tiny balloon is inflated and pulled back through the narrowed valve to widen it.

The benefit of valvuloplasty is that no anticoagulation therapy is necessary afterward, provided you are in regular rhythm (not atrial fibrillation). In fact, one of my patients opted for balloon valvuloplasty of her mitral valve because she was planning a pregnancy and did not want to be on warfarin. Antibiotic prophylaxis will be prescribed before central procedures. This procedure is most common and successful for mitral and pulmonic stenosis (usually found in children).

Valve Replacement

With a valve replacement, your valve is excised or removed from the support structures that attach it to the heart and is replaced with a new valve. Artificial replacement valves are made of Dacron or plastic, while biological valves are made of tissue taken from a pig, cow, or deceased human. Replacement with a tissue valve does not require long-term blood thinning, but if you have atrial fibrillation, you will be placed on a blood thinner to prevent stroke. If you have a mechanical valve, long-term anticoagulation therapy is indicated to prevent blood clots.

If you receive an artificial heart valve, you are at increased risk for developing an infection of the valve (endocarditis). Your doctor will give you an antibiotic to take before certain dental or surgical procedures. You will probably be placed on an anticoagulant to prevent blood clots from forming. This procedure can be done for narrowed or leaky mitral and aortic valves. One problem with this technique is that there is the risk of reduced heart function.

Surgery to Treat Arrhythmia

Electrophysiological Study

If you have a serious electrical disturbance of the heart or a difficult-to-treat arrhythmia, your doctor may use an electrophysiological study (EPS) to find the source of the arrhythmia. This invasive test is performed by a specially trained cardiologist, an electrophysiologist, and is used to evaluate ventricular or supraventricular arrhythmias.

THE PROCEDURE:

A puncture is made in your groin to access the femoral vein. A catheter that has a pacemaker at the tip is advanced through the femoral vein into the right side of the heart. Once the catheter is in the heart, the electrophysiologist records the electrical activity of your heartbeat as well as any abnormal activity. Then various areas of the conduction tissue are stimulated to see if they generate abnormal heart rhythms, or if any additional conduction tissue may be responsible for a particular arrhythmia. The EPS is done under close monitoring.

WHAT THE RESULTS MEAN:

If the test is done for the evaluation of ventricular tachycardia, the ventricle is stimulated to see if the arrhythmia is produced. If it is produced, you will probably be referred for an automatic implantable cardio defibrillator (AICD), a device that detects the arrhythmia and is programmed to deliver a shock should the arrhythmia occur, to regulate the rhythm. During the test, you will receive sedation and local anesthesia to the groin. Some of the risks of this procedure include bleeding at the groin site, a blood clot to the leg, and infection.

Radiofrequency Ablation

Once the EPS determines the mechanism of the arrhythmia, radiofrequency ablation is often used to eliminate it if it is a supraventricular tachycardia. This procedure is of particular benefit to young women, eliminating the need for long-term medication that may interfere with a safe pregnancy.

THE PROCEDURE:
The doctor will insert a catheter into the femoral vein in your groin and guide it into the heart to find the tissue that is causing the abnormal rhythm. When the tissue is located, radiofrequency-charged heat is applied, to destroy it.

WHAT YOU WILL FEEL:
Radiofrequency ablation is done under sedation and local anesthesia.

PRECAUTIONS:
While the success rate is higher than 90 percent, there are some possible complications, including soreness in the groin where the catheter is introduced, bleeding, and blood clots in the leg.

Pacemaker

If your heartbeat is too slow, your doctor may recommend a pacemaker.

THE PROCEDURE:
A pacemaker wire is inserted into the vein under your collarbone. The pacemaker is then placed under your skin. If the heart rate becomes too slow, the pacemaker automatically stimulates the heart rhythm, much as a normal heart pacemaker does.

WHAT YOU WILL FEEL:
Local anesthesia is used, and other medications are given intravenously to help you relax. In most cases, implanting the pacemaker does not require more than an overnight stay in the hospital.

Before you leave the hospital, your pacemaker will be programmed to fit your particular pacing needs. A return visit is scheduled in a month, then again at three- and six-month intervals, to make more refined adjustments to the pacemaker settings.

If your heartbeat is too fast, a medication will probably be used to slow and control it. Because a wide range of medications are available, choosing the one with the fewest side effects depends on your individual situation. This is best decided by your doctor.

Automatic Implantable Cardio Defibrillator

Sudden episodes of fainting may be caused by a rapid, irregular heart rhythm or a life-threatening arrhythmia, such as ventricular tachycardia or ventricular fibrillation (see page 135). When EPS confirms an arrhythmia of this type, a defibrillator that gives a shock to the heart may be necessary to regulate the heart rhythm.

With an automatic implantable cardiac defibrillator (AICD), a wire is inserted into the heart through the vein under the collarbone. It is attached to a small device similar to a pacemaker, except that it also has the capability to deliver an electrical shock when this abnormal heart rhythm is detected.

Other Issues Important to Women Facing Heart Surgery

Good patient-physician communication is important for receiving the highest quality of care. When I was an intern in the coronary care unit, an older woman, Joan, age sixty-three, was transferred to my hospital for coronary artery bypass surgery. Joan was on intravenous nitroglycerin and other medications and had a very serious obstruction in her left main coronary artery.

The morning of her surgery, Joan called me to her bedside and said, "Tell my doctor I'm not having the surgery. I don't want to be left with an ugly scar."

I could tell that she was frightened. I told my resident, but he just rolled his eyes. On the way back to her room, I spoke with the cardiothoracic surgeon, who had come down to see Joan before the procedure. I told him about her fears, and he went in and talked with her. After he left, I spoke with Joan. She agreed to the procedure because the surgeon said he'd try to make a different incision.

Joan's surgery took place at a time before MIDCAB. While your doctor cannot promise that you will have scarless heart surgery, you should always feel that you can express your fears and feelings and have this professional listen to what you say.

Another time during my first year of practice, I was on rounds with the residents and nurses in the coronary care unit. We were at a patient's bedside, and all of a sudden another woman in the room burst into tears. The crying woman was about sixty years old and was scheduled for bypass surgery the next day. The only problem was that no one had told her anything about it. She spoke very little English, so her husband and cardiologist had fully discussed the plan—without including her.

When the surgical resident came to pick her up for preoperative testing, a pulmonary function test, and a carotid Doppler, she refused to go because she didn't understand what was happening. I can only imagine how frightened she must have been!

The charge nurse quickly got a translator, and we found out that this woman had no idea she had triple vessel disease, much less that she was scheduled for cardiac surgery. With the help of a translator, we explained her condition so she could understand it, along with the rationale behind the preoperative testing and subsequent surgery.

The woman agreed to the preop testing but wanted to postpone the surgery until after her daughter's wedding, as she was planning a surprise bridal shower. With the help of a translator, we explained that if she had the surgery now, she would still be able to go to the wedding and even dance. If she didn't have it, however, she might not make it to the wedding at all.

Whether it's worrying about an unsightly scar on your chest or planning a bridal shower for your daughter's wedding, women are not small men! Women have specific issues that have to be addressed when surgical procedures are planned. Talk about your concerns with your health care provider.

17

The Future of Women and Heart Disease

As a national spokesperson for the American Heart Association, I'm frequently called by the media to explain a new or experimental treatment or to interpret a groundbreaking study that has been released. If you're influenced by the media and the Internet, you may have drawn the conclusion that a steady diet of wine, chocolate, tea, and garlic can prevent heart disease. In fact, one patient, Nan, told me she ate a chocolate bar every night before bedtime because she had read a "late-breaking study" on her favorite website that chocolate was important for a healthy heart. Seeing that headline was all Nan needed to confirm her need for chocolate, so she decided this was her favorite way to get healthy. In one study, researchers found that those who drank a specially formulated cocoa drink had less platelet clotting. Another study showed beneficial effects of cocoa on blood vessel function. But a chocolate manufacturing company funded both studies! These benefits were expected and proposed by the researchers—they were not proven.

Chocolate does contain heart-healthy flavonoids (see page 284), but it has other ingredients as well. The real facts about chocolate are both good and bad. The good news is that 40 percent of the fat in chocolate is unsaturated fat in the form of oleic acid, which lowers LDL ("bad") cholesterol. The bad news is that chocolate is 60 percent saturated fat—stearic acid and palmitic acid, which raises cholesterol. And as you now know, high cholesterol levels increase your risk of heart disease. While the studies on chocolate are intriguing, I probably won't be writing any prescriptions for truffles anytime soon.

The wine and chocolate theory of heart disease prevention is indeed appealing but it is unproven. We need more research on women and heart disease, not only to test the benefits of interesting foods but also to improve all heart care for women. Research is the key to changing the way doctors think about women and heart disease. Research is the driving force of clinical practice. Doctors traditionally say, "Show me the data," before they change the way they treat patients. An editorial in the March 1, 2001, issue of the *New England Journal of Medicine* addressed the differing approaches to treating heart attacks and pointed out that "the medical literature rarely enables readers to determine which patients are more likely to benefit from a procedure than to be harmed by it."[1] In other words, a lot of research is not ready for prime time: its results are interesting but cannot—and should not—be applied to treatment of patients.

So we need proven therapies for women and heart disease. Yet women still remain underrepresented in research trials[2] and will continue to be treated as small men until we have greater participation in these trials.

Many questions need to be addressed and answered through research; here are just a few.

- Why do women under fifty have twice the death rate from heart attack as men of the same age?
- Why do black women have a 60 percent higher death rate than white women?
- If we treat unique risk factors, like homocysteine, Lp(a), and C-reactive protein, will that result in fewer heart attacks and strokes for women?
- Why do women have a more complicated course of recovery after open-heart surgery and other cardiac procedures than men? Why, despite improvements in technology, do women

have more complications from cardiac surgery than men? Why are women less likely to get relief from their symptoms? How can we stop this from happening?
- Why doesn't an aspirin a day for healthy women prevent a first heart attack?
- Do vitamin supplements reduce the risk of first and second heart attacks in women?

We should have some answers to these last two questions in a few years. The Women's Health Initiative[3] is researching the effect of aspirin and hormone replacement therapy on heart disease risk in a racially and ethnically diverse population of women. The Women's Antioxidant Cardiovascular Study is looking at the role of vitamins and antioxidants in heart disease prevention and heart disease risk factors in women.[4]

This research will give doctors a new framework for preventing and treating heart disease in women. In the meantime, I want you to help yourself stay healthy and get healthier with the proven program in this book. Please, take care of yourself.

Resources

Organizations

American Heart Association

Women's Information
1-888-MY HEART
www.women.americanheart.org

MyHeart Watch
www.myheartwatch.org

To find your local American Heart Association Office, call 1-800-AHA-USA1 or visit *www.americanheart.org*.

WomenHeart

This is the National Coalition for Women with Heart Disease. Visit their website at *www.womenheart.org* or call 202-728-7199.

Exercise Videos

Skeletal Fitness®: A Workout for Your Bones

Fabulous Forever™: Easy Aerobics; Slow Down Your Aging Clock

Price: $29.95 plus $6.00 for shipping and handling

Send check or money order to NuVue, Inc., P.O. Box 866, Ridgefield, NJ 07657, or call 1-800-999-6427.

Notes

Chapter 1

1. T.D. Miller, V.L. Roger, D.O. Hodge et al., "Gender Differences and Temporal Trends in Clinical Characteristics, Stress Test Results and Use of Invasive Procedures in Patients Undergoing Evaluation for Coronary Artery Disease," *Journal of the American College of Cardiology* 38, no. 3 (2001): 690–97.
2. V. Vaccarino, L. Parsons, N.R. Every, H. Barron et al., "Sex-Based Differences in Early Mortality After Myocardial Infarction," *New England Journal of Medicine* 341, no. 4 (1999): 217–25.
3. D.K. Moser and K. Dracup, "Gender Differences in Treatment-Seeking Delay in Acute Myocardial Infarction," *Progress in Cardiovascular Nursing* 8, no. 1 (1993): 6–12.

Chapter 2

1. *Women and Heart Disease: A Study Tracking Women's Awareness of and Attitudes Toward Heart Disease and Stroke* (Dallas, TX: American Heart Association, 2001).
2. R.M. Robertson, M.D., "Women and Cardiovascular Disease. The Risks

of Misperception and the Need for Action," *Circulation* 103 (2001): 2318–20.

3. *Update 2001 Heart and Stroke Statistical* (Dallas, TX: American Heart Association, 2001).

4. D.J. Lerner and W.B. Kannel, "Patterns of Coronary Heart Disease Morbidity and Mortality in the Sexes: A 26-Year Follow-up of the Framingham Population," *American Heart Journal* 111 (1986): 383–90.

5. A.P. Burke, A. Farb et al., "Effect of Risk Factors on the Mechanisms of Acute Thrombosis and Sudden Cardiac Death in Women," *Circulation* 97 (1998): 2110–2116.

6. V. Vaccarino, L. Parsons, N.R. Every, H. Barron et al., "Sex-Based Differences in Early Mortality After Myocardial Infarction," *New England Journal of Medicine* 341, no. 4 (1999): 217–25.

7. J.S. Hochman, J.E. Tamis, T.D. Thompson et al., "Sex, Clinical Presentation, and Outcome in Patients with Acute Coronary Syndromes," *New England Journal of Medicine* 341, no. 4 (1999): 226–32.

8. S.Z. Goldhaber, D.D. Savage, P.J. Garrison et al., "Risk Factors for Pulmonary Embolism: The Framingham Study," *American Journal of Medicine* 74 (1983): 1023–28.

9. S.Z. Goldhaber, F. Grodstein, M. J. Stamfler et al., "A Prospective Study of Risk Factors for Pulmonary Embolism in Women," *Journal of the American Medical Association* 277 (1997): 642.

Chapter 3

1. H.C. McGill, A. McMahan et al., "Effects of Nonlipid Risk Factors on Atherosclerosis in Youth with a Favorable Lipoprotein Profile," *Circulation* 103 (2001): 1546–50.

2. W.B. Kannel, "The Framingham Study: Its 50-Year Legacy and Future Promise," *Journal of Atherosclerosis and Thrombosis* 6, no. 2 (2000): 60–66.

3. M.A. Austin, J.E. Hokansan, and K.L. Edwards, "Hypertriglyceridemia as a Cardiovascular Risk Factor," *American Journal of Cardiology* 81 (1998): 7B–12B.

4. J. Tuomilehto, J. Lindstrom, J.G. Eriksson et al., "Prevention of Type 2 Diabetes Mellitus by Changes in Lifestyle Among Subjects with Impaired Glucose Tolerance," *New England Journal of Medicine* 344, no. 18 (2001): 1343–50.

5. F.M. Sacks and B.W. Walsh, "The Effects of Reproductive Hormones on Serum Lipoproteins: Unresolved Issues in Biology and Clinical Practice," *Annals of the New York Academy of Science* 592 (1990): 272–85.

6. J.W. Eikelboom, E. Lonn, J. Gensest et al., "Homocysteine and Risk for Cardiovascular Disease," *Annals of Internal Medicine* 131, no. 5 (1999): 363–75.

7. K. Orth-Gomer, M.A. Mittleman, K. Schenck-Gustafsson, S.P. Wamala et al., "Lipoprotein(a) as a Determinant of Coronary Heart Disease in Young Women," *Circulation* 95 (1997): 329–34.

8. M.A. Espeland, S.M. Marcovina, V. Miller, P.D. Wood, C. Wasilauskas, R. Sherwin, H. Schrott, and T.L. Bush, "Effect of Postmenopausal Hormone Therapy on Lipoprotein(a) Concentration," *Circulation* 97 (1998): 979–86.

9. P.M. Ridker, C.H. Hennekens, J.E. Buring, and N. Rifai, "C-reactive Protein and Other Markers of Inflammation in the Prediction of Cardiovascular Disease in Women," *New England Journal of Medicine* 342, no. 12 (2000): 836–43.

10. K.J. Hanjai, "Potential New Cardiovascular Risk Factors: Left Ventricular Hypertrophy, Homocysteine, Lipoprotein(a), Triglycerides, Oxidative Stress, and Fibrinogen," *Annals of Internal Medicine* 131, no. 5 (1999): 376–86.

Chapter 4

1. L. Mosca, P. Collins, D.M. Herrington et al., "Hormone Replacement Therapy and Cardiovascular Disease: A Statement for Healthcare Professionals from the American Heart Association," *Circulation* 104 (2001): 499–503.

2. L.H. Kuller, L.R. Simkin-Silverman, R.R. Wing, E.N. Meilahn, and D.G. Ives, "Women's Healthy Lifestyle Project: A Randomized Clinical Trial: Results at 54 Months," *Circulation* 103 (2001): 32–37.

3. K.A. Matthews, L.H. Kuller et al., "Changes in Cardiovascular Risk Factors During the Perimenopause and Postmenopause and Carotid Artery Atherosclerosis in Healthy Women," *Stroke* 32 (2001): 1104–11.

4. H.C. McGill, A. McMahan et al., "Effects of Nonlipid Risk Factors on Atherosclerosis in Youth with a Favorable Lipoprotein Profile," *Circulation* 103 (2001): 1546–50.

5. C. Schaierer, J. Lubin, R. Rroisi et al., "Menopausal Estrogen and Estrogen-Progestin Replacement Therapy and Breast Cancer Risk," *Journal of the American Medical Association* 283 (2000): 485–88.

6. G.M. Darling, J.A. Johns, P.I. McCloud, and S.R. Davis, "Estrogen and Progestin Compared with Simvastatin for Hypercholesterolemia in Post-

menopausal Women," *New England Journal of Medicine* 337, no. 4 (1997): 595–601.

7. F. Grodstein, J.E. Manson, G.A. Colditz et al., "A Prospective, Observational Study of Postmenopausal Hormone Therapy and Primary Prevention of Cardiovascular Disease," *Annals of Internal Medicine* 133, no. 12 (2000): 999–1001.

8. F. Grodstein, M.J. Stampfer, J.E. Manson et al., "Postmenopausal Estrogen and Progestin Use and the Risk of Cardiovascular Disease," *New England Journal of Medicine* 335, no. 7 (1996): 453–61.

9. F. Grodstein, J.E. Manson, and M.J. Stampfer, "Postmenopausal Hormones and Recurrence of Coronary Events [Abstract]," *Circulation* 100, no. 18 (2000): supp. 1.

10. G.A. Colditz, S.E. Hankinson, D.J. Hunter et al., "The Use of Estrogens and Progestins and the Risk of Breast Cancer in Postmenopausal Women," *New England Journal of Medicine* 332, no. 24 (1995): 1589–93.

11. The Writing Group for the PEPI Trial, "Effects of Estrogen or Estrogen/Progestin Regimens on Heart Disease Risk Factors in Postmenopausal Women," *Journal of the American Medical Association* 273 (1995): 199–208.

12. Ibid.

13. S. Hulley, D. Grady, T. Bush et al., "Randomized Trial of Estrogen plus Progestin for Secondary Prevention of Coronary Heart Disease in Postmenopausal Women," *Journal of the American Medical Association* 280 (1998): 605–13.

14. P. Albertazzi et al., "The Effect of Dietary Soy Supplementation on Hot Flashes," *Obstetrics and Gynecology* 91 (1998): 6–11.

15. A. Brezinski et al., "Short Term Effects of Phytoestrogen-Rich Diet on Postmenopausal Women," *Menopause* 4, no. 2 (1997): 89–94.

16. J.W. Anderson, B.M. Johnstone, and M.E. Cook-Newell et al., "Meta-Analysis of the Effects of Soy Protein Intake on Serum Lipids," *New England Journal of Medicine* 333, no. 5 (1995): 276–82.

17. K. Reinli and G. Block, "Phytoestrogen Content of Foods—A Compendium of Literature Values," *Nutrition and Cancer* 26 (1996): 123–48.

18. J.W. Erdman and R.J. Stillman, "Provocative Relation Between Soy and Bone Maintenance," *American Journal for Clinical Nutrition* 72 (2000): 679–80.

Chapter 5

1. C. LaVecchia, A. Decardi, S. Franceschi, A. Gentile et al., "Menstrual and Reproductive Factors and the Risk of Myocardial Infarction in Women Under Fifty-five Years of Age," *American Journal of Obstetrics and Gynecology* 157 (1987): 1108–12.

2. E. Hall, "Gender, Work Control and Stress: A Theoretical Discussion and an Empirical Test," *International Journal of Health Services* 19, no. 4 (1989): 725–45.

3. K. Orth-Gomer, S.P. Wamala, M. Horsten et al., "Marital Stress Worsens Prognosis in Women with Coronary Heart Disease: The Stockholm Female Coronary Risk Study," *Journal of the American Medical Association* 284 (2000): 3008–15.

4. S.E. Taylor, L.C. Klein, B.P. Lewis, T.L. Gruenewald, R.A. Gurung, and J.A. Updegraff, "Biobehavioral Responses to Stress in Females: Tend-and-Befriend, not Fight-or-Flight," *Psychological Review* 107, no. 3 (2000): 411–29.

5. E.D. Eaker and W.P. Castelli, "Type A Behavior and Coronary Heart Disease in Women: Fourteen-Year Incidence from the Framingham Heart Study," in B.K. Houston and C. Snyder, eds., *Type A Behavior Pattern: Research, Theory, and Invention* (New York: John Wiley, 1988), 83–97.

6. A. Rozanski, J.A. Blumenthal, J. Kaplan, "Impact of Psychological Factors on the Pathogenesis of Cardiovascular Disease and Implications for Therapy," *Circulation* 99 (1999): 2192-2217.

7. E.D. Eaker and W.P. Castelli, "Type A Behavior and Coronary Heart Disease in Women: Fourteen-Year Incidence from the Framingham Heart Study," in B.K. Houston and C. Snyder, eds., *Type A Behavior Pattern: Research, Theory, and Invention* (New York: John Wiley, 1988), 83–97.

8. G. Specchia, C. Falcone, E. Traversi et al., "Mental Stress as a Provocative Test in Patients with Various Clinical Syndromes of Coronary Heart Disease," *Circulation* 83, no. 4, supplement: III 37–44.

9. C.F.M. De Leon, W.J. Kop, H.B. de Swart et al., "Psychosocial Characteristics and Recurrent Events After Percutaneous Transluminal Angioplasty," *American Journal of Cardiology* 77 (1996): 252–55.

10. R. Fleet, K. Lavoie, and B.D. Beitman, "Is Panic Disorder Associated with Coronary Artery Disease? A Critical Review of the Literature," *Journal of Psychopharmacology Research* 48, nos. 4–5 (2000): 347–56.

11. F. Lederbogen, M. Gilles, A. Maras et al., "Increased Platelet Aggrega-

bility in Major Depression?" *Psychiatry Research* 102, no. 3 (2001): 255–61.

12. S.S. Knox et al., "Hostility, Social Support, and Coronary Heart Disease in the National Heart, Lung, and Blood Institute Family Heart Study," *American Journal of Cardiology* 82 (1998): 1192–96.

13. S.E. Taylor, M.E. Kemeny, G.M. Reed, J.E. Bower, and T.L. Gruenewald, "Psychological Resources, Positive Illusions, and Health," *American Psychologist* 55 (2000): 99–109.

14. J.S. House, K.R. Landis, and D. Umberson, "Social Relationships and Health," *Science* 241 (1988): 540–45.

15. H. Bless, N. Schwarz, G.L. Clore, V. Golisano et al., "Mood and the Use of Scripts: Does a Happy Mood Really Lead to Mindlessness?" *Journal of Personality and Social Psychology* 71 (1996): 665–69.

Chapter 6

1. S. Kinlay, J.W. Leitch, A. Neil, B.L. Chapman et al., "Cardiac Event Recorders Yield More Diagnoses and Are More Cost-Effective Than 48-hour Holter Monitoring in Patients with Palpitations. A Controlled Clinical Trial," *Annals of Internal Medicine* 124, no. 1 (1996): 16–20.

2. J.M. Holroyd-Leduc, M.K. Kaprol, P.C. Austin, and J.V. Tu, "Sex Differences and Similarities in the Management and Outcome of Stroke Patients," *Stroke* 31 (2000): 1833–37.

3. L.A. Freed, D. Levy, R.A. Levine et al., "Prevalence and Clinical Outcome of Mitral-Valve Prolapse," *New England Journal of Medicine* 341, no. 1 (1999): 1–7.

4. H.M. Connolly, J.L. Crary, M.D. McGoon et al., "Valvular Heart Disease Associated with Fenfluramine-Phentermine," *New England Journal of Medicine* 337, no. 9 (1997): 581–88.

5. M.S. Sutton, "Silver Lining to the Cloud over Anorexogen-Related Cardiac Valvulopathy?" *Annals of Internal Medicine* 134, no. 4 (2001): 335–37.

6. Committee on Evaluation and Management of Heart Failure, American Heart Association Office of Science and Medicine, *Guidelines for the Evaluation and Management of Heart Failure. Report of the American College of Cardiology/American Heart Association Task Force on Practice Guidelines* (1995).

7. U. Elkayam, P.P. Tummala, K. Rao et al., "Maternal and Fetal Outcomes of Subsequent Pregnancies in Women with Peripartum Cardiomyopathy," *New England Journal of Medicine* 344, no. 1 (2001): 1567–71.

Chapter 7

1. Expert Panel on Detection, Evaluation and Treatment of High Blood Pressure in Adults, "Executive Summary of the Third Report of the National Cholesterol Education Program (NCEP) Expert Panel on Detection, Evaluation and Treatment of High Blood Cholesterol in Adults (Adult Treatment Panel III)," *Journal of the American Medical Association* 285 (2001): 2486–97.
2. "The Sixth Report of the Joint National Committee on Prevention, Detection, Evaluation, and Treatment of High Blood Pressure," *Archives of Internal Medicine* 157 (1997): 2413–46.
3. Y. Wong, A. Rodwell, S. Dawkins, S.A. Livesey, and I.A. Simpson, "Sex Differences in Investigation Results and Treatment in Subjects Referred for Investigation of Chest Pain," *Heart* 85 (2001): 149–52.
4. T.H. Marwick, T. Anderson, J. Williams et al., "Exercise Echocardiography Is an Accurate and Cost-Efficient Technique for Detection of Coronary Artery Disease in Women," *Journal of the American College of Cardiology* 26, no. 2 (1995): 335–41.
5. Y. Arad, L.A. Spadaro, K. Goodman et al., "Prediction of Coronary Events with Electron Beam Computed Tomography," *Journal of the American College of Cardiology* vol. 36, no. 4 (2000): 1253–60.
6. K.P. Alexander, L.J. Shaw, E.R. Delong et al., "Value of Exercise Treadmill Testing in Women," *Journal of the American College of Cardiology* 32, no. 6 (1998): 1657–64.
7. C.R. Cole, E.H. Blackstone, F.J. Pashkow et al., "Heart-Rate Recovery Immediately After Exercise as a Predictor of Mortality," *New England Journal of Medicine* 341, no. 18 (1999): 1351–57.
8. R.M. Steingart, M. Packer, P. Hamm et al., "Sex Differences in the Management of Coronary Artery Disease. Survival and Ventricular Enlargement Investigators," *New England Journal of Medicine* 325, no. 4 (1991): 226–30.

Chapter 8

1. L. Pilote and M.A. Hlatky, "Attitudes of Women Toward Hormone Therapy and Prevention of Heart Disease," *American Heart Journal* 129, no. 6 (June 1995): 1237–38.
2. *Women and Heart Disease: A Study Tracking Women's Awareness of and Attitudes Toward Heart Disease and Stroke* (Dallas, TX: American Heart Association, 2001).

3. J. Prochaska and W.F. Velicer, "The Transtheoretical Model of Health Behavior Change," *American Journal of Health Promotion* 12, no. 1 (1997): 38–48.

Chapter 9

1. A.M. Jette and L.G. Branch, "The Framingham Disability Study: II— Physical Disability Among the Aging," *American Journal of Public Health* 71 (1981): 1211–16.
2. C.M. Morganti, M.E. Nelson, M.A. Fiatarone, G.E. Dallal, and C.D. Economos, "Strength Improvements with One Year of Progressive Resistance Training in Older Women," *Medicine and Science in Sports and Exercise* 27 (1995): 906–12.
3. M.E. Nelson, G.E. Dilmanian et al., "A One-Year Walking Program and Increased Dietary Calcium in Postmenopausal Women: Effects on Bone," *American Journal of Clinical Nutrition* 53 (1991): 1304–11.
4. Ibid.
5. I. Thune and A.S. Furberg, "Physical Activity and Cancer Risk: Dose-Response and Cancer, All Sites and Site-Specific," *Medicine and Science in Sports and Exercise* 33 (2001): 530–50.
6. M.L. Stefanik, "Exercise and Weight Control," *Exercise and Sport Sciences Reviews* 21 (1993): 363–96.
7. I.-M. Lee, K.M. Rexrode, N.R. Cook, J.E. Manson, and J.E. Buring, "Physical Activity and Coronary Heart Disease in Women: Is 'No Pain, No Gain' Passé?" *Journal of the American Medical Association* 285 (2001): 1447–54.

Chapter 10

1. D. Steinberg, "The Cholesterol Controversy Is Over: Why Did It Take So Long?" *Circulation* 80 (1989): 1070–78.
2. F.B. Hu, M.J. Stampfer, J.E. Manson et al., "Dietary Fat Intake and the Risk of Coronary Heart Disease in Women," *New England Journal of Medicine* 337, no. 21 (1997): 1491–99.
3. T.A. Wilson, M. McIntyre, and R.J. Nicolosi, "Trans Fatty Acids and Cardiovascular Risk," *Journal of Nutrition, Health, and Aging* 5, no. 3 (2001): 184–87.
4. M. de Lorgeril, P. Salen, J.L. Martin et al., "Mediterranean Diet, Traditional Risk Factors, and the Rate of Cardiovascular Complications After

Glossary

ACE inhibitor (angiotensin-converting enzyme inhibitor)—a class of medications used to lower blood pressure and treat congestive heart failure. One of the benefits is improved survival in congestive heart failure.

Alpha linolenic acid—a type of omega-3 fatty acid.

Angina (angina pectoris)—chest discomfort due to decreased blood flow to the heart muscle. The decrease in circulation is caused by atherosclerosis, the buildup of cholesterol in the walls of the blood vessels. Women's angina symptoms may be atypical.

Angiography (coronary angiography and carotid angiography)—a diagnostic procedure that uses dye to image the coronary arteries. It evaluates the arteries for obstructions responsible for angina or a heart attack. The image produced in angiography is an angiogram.

Angioplasty (coronary angioplasty, PTCA)—a procedure that opens up a coronary artery without surgery and that usually inserts a stent to keep the artery open.

Angiotensin II blocker (A-II blocker)—medication used to lower blood pressure and treat congestive heart failure.

Aortic regurgitation—the incomplete closing of the aortic valve, which causes the blood to leak backward into the left ventricle. Also called aortic insufficiency.

Arrhythmia—a deviation from the regular heartbeat; arrhythmias range from very slow to abnormally fast or irregular.

Atherosclerosis—the narrowing of arteries due to the buildup of cholesterol.

Atrial fibrilliation—an arrhythmia that originates in the heart's upper chambers and impairs the normal emptying of blood from the atria to the ventricles.

Atypical symptoms—symptoms of heart attack other than chest discomfort, such as shortness of breath, fatigue, back pain, and lower chest discomfort. Atypical symptoms are more common in women.

Beta-blockers—a class of medication used to treat high blood pressure, symptoms of coronary artery disease, and certain arrhythmias. Beta-blockers slow heart rate and lower blood pressure.

Blood pressure—the pressure that blood exerts against the inside walls of major arteries. It is measured in millimeters of mercury (mm Hg). Systolic pressure is pressure at the time when the heart is pumping blood out to the body; it is the top number of a blood pressure reading. Diastolic pressure is pressure at the time when the heart is relaxed. It is the bottom number of the reading.

Blood thinner—a class of medications used to reduce blood clotting.

Bradycardia—a type of arrhythmia in which the pulse rate is slower than 60 beats per minute.

Calcium channel blocker—a class of medications that lower blood pressure, slow heart rate, and treat arrhythmias such as supraventricular tachycardia.

Cardiac catheterization—a dye study (angiogram) to evaluate the coronary arteries and the pumping chamber of the heart.

Cardiovascular disease—any disease of the heart, heart valves, blood vessels, and arteries, including stroke, hypertension, rheumatic fever, and heart attack.

Cardioversion—an electrical shock to the heart, used to regulate its rhythm.

Carotid endarterectomy—a surgical procedure to remove plaque from the carotid artery.

Cholesterol—a waxy, fatlike substance found in the blood that helps produce hormones and cell structures necessary for the body to function normally. Elevated cholesterol is a risk factor for heart disease and stroke.

Claudication—pain in the calves on exertion because of peripheral vascular disease, or atherosclerosis of the arteries in the legs.

Coronary angiography—*see* angiography.

Coronary angioplasty—*see* angioplasty.

Coronary artery—a blood vessel that supplies blood to the heart muscle.

Coronary artery bypass surgery grafting (CABG)—open-heart surgery that uses arteries and veins from elsewhere in the body to go around obstructions in the coronary arteries to improve blood flow to the heart muscle. This procedure uses a heart-lung machine.

Coronary artery disease (CAD)—a condition in which arteries to the heart muscle are blocked. CAD is responsible for heart attack, unstable angina, angina, and atypical symptoms of angina.

C-reactive protein—a protein that is increased in the blood in response to inflammation. It is a marker of increased heart disease risk.

Defibrillation—a high-energy electrical shock to the heart intended to normalize the heart rhythm. The machine used to deliver the shock is called a defibrillator.

Diabetes—a disease caused by elevated blood sugar. In type 1 diabetes, the cause is undersecretion of insulin; in type 2, insulin is underproduced or underutilized and the body's cells are unresponsive to it. Diabetes is a risk factor for coronary artery disease and stroke.

Diastolic heart failure—a type of heart failure where heart muscle function may be normal but the pressure within the heart is elevated, resulting in symptoms of shortness of breath, chest tightness, and wheezing. This type of heart failure is seen in coronary artery ischemia, hypertension, and diabetes.

Diastolic phase—in the heart's two-phased pumping sequence, the filling phase.

Dietary cholesterol—cholesterol that is found in foods from animals (meat, poultry, seafood, and dairy products). Egg yolks and organ meats are

especially high in dietary cholesterol. Dietary cholesterol can raise your blood cholesterol level and increase your risk of heart disease.

Digitalis—one of the first heart medications used to treat heart failure. It is still used to increase heart muscle contractility. Digoxin is one of the most commonly prescribed types of digitalis.

Diuretic—a class of medications commonly used to treat elevated blood pressure and to reduce fluid accumulation in heart failure. Also known as water pills.

Dysphagia—impairment of the ability to swallow.

ECG stress test (exercise electrocardiogram)—a diagnostic test that evaluates for coronary artery disease. You exercise on a treadmill while you are hooked up to an ECG. The doctor monitors the test for ECG changes that indicate narrowed blood vessels.

Echocardiogram—a diagnostic test that uses an ultrasound probe (with sound waves) to produce images of the heart. The images show the shape, texture, and movement of the valves and measure the size of the heart and its chambers. The test also assesses heart function, a very important determinant of survival after a heart attack.

Electrocardiogram (ECG)—a diagnostic test that records electrical currents to detect abnormal heart rhythm.

Endocarditis—infection of a heart valve.

Endothelium—the lining of an arterial wall. The endothelium helps to maintain normal function of the artery, including the ability to dilate and contract.

Fibric acid derivative—a class of cholesterol-lowering medications that work primarily to reduce triglycerides and increase HDL ("good") cholesterol.

Framingham Heart Study—a federally funded study that has tracked 5,209 adults in Framingham, Massachusetts, since 1948 to find out the epidemiology of cardiovascular disease.

Glycemic index—a numerical system of measuring how fast a carbohydrate triggers a rise in circulating blood sugar; the higher the number, the faster the blood sugar response.

HDL cholesterol—high-density lipoprotein or "good" cholesterol.

Heart attack—an incident of heart muscle damage due to the complete blockage of blood flow through a coronary artery. The blockage may be caused by a blood clot or a spasm of the artery.

Heart disease—collectively, the diseases of the heart muscle, the heart valves, and the coronary arteries.

Heart rate—the number of times a heart beats per minute.

Holter monitor—a small device worn over a twenty-four-hour period, that allows continuous ECG recording.

Homocysteine—an amino acid derived from the metabolism of methionine, an essential amino acid predominant in animal protein. At high levels, homocysteine may damage arterial walls, which can cause cholesterol to build up and block the vessels.

Hormone replacement therapy (HRT)—therapy that combines estrogen and progestin to treat menopausal symptoms and osteoporosis in postmenopausal women who have a uterus.

Hydrogenated fat—a fat that is produced during hydrogenation, a chemical process that changes a naturally unsaturated liquid oil into a solid and more saturated form. The greater the amount of hydrogenation, the more saturated a fat becomes. Saturated fat may raise your blood cholesterol levels.

Hypertension (high blood pressure)—elevated pressure in the arteries and a risk factor for heart disease and stroke.

Insulin resistance syndrome—a lack of responsiveness by the body to the actions of insulin. Despite high levels of insulin, blood sugar levels rise and eventually type 2 diabetes results.

Ischemia—a reduced supply of blood to the heart because of severely obstructed coronary arteries.

LDL cholesterol—low-density lipoprotein or "bad" cholesterol.

Lp(a)—a substance that is structurally similar to a blood-clotting protein and LDL ("bad") cholesterol. Lp(a) may worsen atherosclerosis by promoting the production of plaque and blood clots.

Minimally invasive direct coronary artery bypass surgery (MID-CAB)—surgery that uses a "keyhole" to bypass obstructed coronary arteries; distinguished from open-heart surgery.

Mitral valve regurgitation—leakage of the mitral valve, in which the blood is pumped backward into the left atrium. Also called mitral valve insufficiency.

Monounsaturated fat—a fat that comes from plant foods that are liquid at room temperature, such as canola, peanut, and olive oils, as well as avocados.

Myocardial infarction—heart attack.

Nitroglycerin—a medication that dilates or widens the blood vessels, including the coronary arteries, and that is used to treat symptoms from obstructed coronary arteries.

Off-pump coronary artery bypass surgery (OPCAB)—surgery for an obstructed coronary artery that does not use the heart-lung machine.

Omega-3 fat—a highly polyunsaturated fat found in certain fatty fish (albacore tuna, mackerel, and salmon), flaxseed, flaxseed oil, nuts, canola oil, and soybean oil. The heart benefits of these fats reduce cholesterol; they may also reduce the risk of arrhythmia, lower triglycerides, and lessen the tendency to form blood clots.

Paroxysmal atrial fibrillation—a type of atrial fibrillation that comes and goes.

Percutaneous transluminal coronary angioplasty (PTCR)—*see* angioplasty.

Pericarditis—an inflammation of the sac that surrounds the heart.

Peripartum cardiomyopathy—reduced heart function during the last trimester of pregnancy.

Plaque (atheroma)—the buildup of fatty substances, cholesterol, cellular waste products, calcium, and other inflammatory substances in the inner lining of an artery.

Polyunsaturated fat—a fat that comes from foods that are liquid or soft at room temperature, including plant foods, nuts, seeds, and some seafood. Examples include sunflower, corn, soybean, safflower, and sesame oils. Polyunsaturated fats can help to get rid of newly formed cholesterol and reduce cholesterol deposits in the arterial walls.

Pulmonary artery—the artery that carries oxygen-depleted blood from the right side of the heart to the lungs.

Pulmonary hypertension—a rare condition in which the blood vessels in the lung become constricted, resulting in an inability to oxygenate blood properly and subsequent lung damage.

Regurgitation—a backward leakage of blood that occurs when a heart valve does not close completely.

Restenosis—a recurrent blockage in an artery that has previously been opened by an angioplasty or angioplasty with stent.

Sarcopenia—the age-related loss of muscle mass, associated with reduced muscle strength and reduced aerobic power.

Saturated fat—a fat that comes from foods that are firm at room temperature, including fats from animal sources, whole milk dairy products, and some oils.

Selective estrogen receptor modulator (SERM)—a class of medications, such as raloxifene (Evista) and tamoxifin (Nolvadex), that are used to build bone in osteoporosis.

Sinus node—the heart's natural pacemaker that establishes the heart rate. It consists of cells that generate electrical currents to stimulate the heart's muscle cells.

Sphygmomanometer—a medical instrument used to measure blood pressure.

Statin—a class of cholesterol-lowering medications.

Stenosis—the narrowing of a heart valve, impeding blood flow.

Stent—a tiny wire mesh that is inserted into an artery after it has been opened by angioplasty.

Stress echocardiogram (exercise echochardiogram)—a diagnostic test that evaluates for coronary artery obstruction, using ultrasound to image the heart while you exercise. The test looks for exercise-related or wall-motion abnormalities that indicate the presence of coronary artery disease.

Stress nuclear test (nuclear stress test)—a diagnostic test that evaluates for coronary artery disease, using a radioactive isotope to image the heart while you exercise. The test looks for exercise-related abnormalities on a scan of the heart, which indicate the presence of coronary artery disease. The radioactive isotopes used are thallium or technitium sestimibi.

Stroke—brain tissue damage due to blood vessel disease. Stroke may be caused by plaque rupture in an artery to the brain that has atherosclerosis, hemorrhage of a blood vessel, or obstruction of a blood vessel by a clot.

Syndrome X—a heart condition in which chest pain and ECG changes suggest ischemic heart disease but without angiographic findings of coronary artery disease.

Systolic heart failure—reduced heart muscle function, resulting in shortness of breath and leg swelling. Systolic heart failure may result from long-standing and untreated hypertension, untreated mitral and aortic insufficiency, a viral infection to the heart muscle, hypothyroidism, incessant tachycardia, or a heart attack that causes a large amount of muscle damage.

Systolic phase—in the heart's two-phase pumping sequence, the emptying phase.

Tachycardia—a rapid heart rate that exceeds 100 heartbeats per minute.

Total cholesterol—the sum of LDL and HDL cholesterol and triglycerides in the bloodstream.

Trans fat—a fat that is produced commercially to harden vegetable oils into shortening and margarine. Trans fats are used in many prepared and processed foods and stick margarines. Trans fats appear to have an effect on blood lipid levels that is worse than that of saturated fats, increasing the LDL cholesterol while decreasing HDL cholesterol.

Transient ischemic attack (TIA)—a little stroke or "ministroke."

Triglyceride—a type of blood fat that boosts the process of atherosclerosis.

Unstable angina—angina in which the symptoms change: they happen for the first time, or they become more frequent or longer lasting, or they occur at rest.

Valvular heart disease—a condition in which a heart valve does not close completely (regurgitation), resulting in backward leakage of blood, or when it is narrowed (stenosis), impeding blood flow, or both.

Ventricular fibrillation—a rapid and disordered heart rhythm from the lower heart chambers. The heart cannot effectively pump blood, which may result in sudden collapse and death unless there is immediate defibrillation.

Ventricular tachycardia—a rapid heartbeat originating in the lower chambers, associated with fainting and sudden death.

Index

Page numbers in *italics* refer to illustrations.

About the Author

NIECA GOLDBERG, M.D., is a cardiologist and chief of the Women's Heart Program and of Cardiac Rehabilitation and Prevention at Lenox Hill Hospital. She is clinical assistant professor of medicine at New York University.

Dr. Goldberg received her undergraduate degree from Barnard College and her medical degree from SUNY Downstate Medical School. She received her postgraduate medical training with a medical residency at St. Luke's–Roosevelt Hospital in New York City and her cardiology fellowship at SUNY Downstate.

Dr. Goldberg is also medical director of the Coronary Detection Intervention Center at the 92nd Street Y and is a member of the board of directors of the American Heart Association/New York City. She is chairperson of the AHA/NYC's Women Take Wellness to Heart and Stroke Initiative. In this capacity, she lectures to physicians and organizes continuing medical education programs on the topic of women and heart disease. She gives numerous public lectures and contributes to the writing of articles and public education. She has contributed to heart disease–related research and has published articles in the *American Heart Journal, American Journal of Cardiology, Preventive Cardiology*, and *The Journal of Geriatric Cardiology*.

Dr. Goldberg lives in Manhattan with her husband, Dr. Robert Shapiro.